D1712898

Supporting Families Experiencing Homelessness

Mary E. Haskett • Staci Perlman
Beryl Ann Cowan
Editors

Supporting Families Experiencing Homelessness

Current Practices and Future Directions

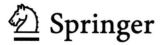 Springer

Editors
Mary E. Haskett
Department of Psychology
North Carolina State University
Raleigh, NC, USA

Beryl Ann Cowan
Boston, MA, USA

Staci Perlman
Department of Human Development
 and Family Studies/Delaware Education
 Research & Development Center
University of Delaware
Newark, DE, USA

ISBN 978-1-4614-8717-3   ISBN 978-1-4614-8718-0 (eBook)
DOI 10.1007/978-1-4614-8718-0
Springer New York Heidelberg Dordrecht London

Library of Congress Control Number: 2013950904

Springer is part of Springer Science+Business Media (www.springer.com)

To my father who believed every family deserved a home; he built affordable homes for over 50 years.

To my parents who provided my first (and continuing) lessons in positive parenting. Additional gentle lessons in parenting are provided daily by my husband Stewart and daughters Hannah and Natalie. To Sarah Sabornie and Peter Donlon of Project CATCH who led me into this field; I'm grateful for the learning opportunity. …MEH

To Matthew: For the absolute joy of being your mom. To my parents—especially my father, Earl Peckham—who taught me that anything is possible and who continues to be my role model.

To Lisa Christian, Kelly Durand, Malkia Singleton, and, especially, Joe Willard of People's Emergency Center: I continue to learn so much from, and am inspired by, each of you. I am deeply grateful for y partnership…SMP

To Gabriel and Amara: For te joys and humility of parenti

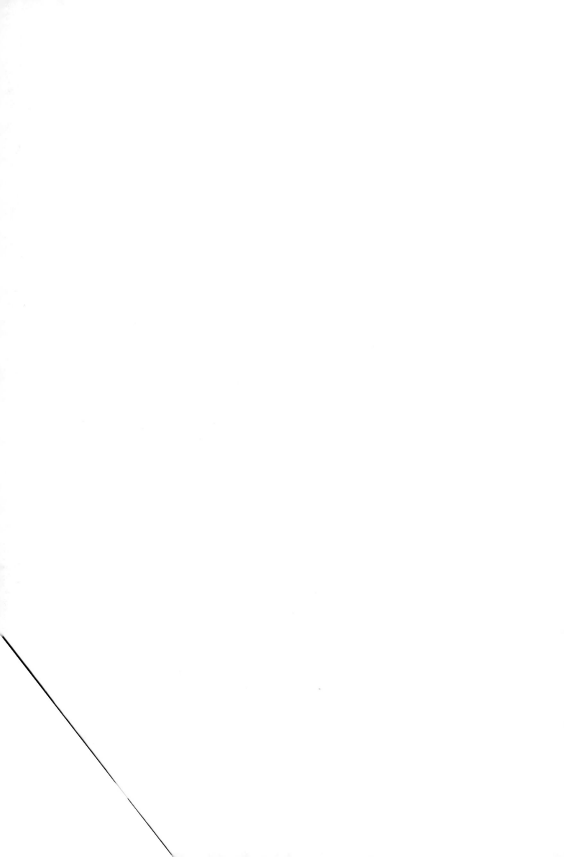

Foreword

The numbers of families and children experiencing homelessness in the United States have steadily increased over the last three decades, reaching a historic high in 2010. Few Americans fared well during the Great Recession, but the numbers of families that sank into poverty outstripped all other groups. Families now comprise more than one-third of the overall homeless population and are the fastest growing segment. Generally comprised of women parenting two children alone, these families are particularly vulnerable in this housing market and are among the poorest families—poorer even than our disabled or elderly populations. With extreme poverty, the lack of affordable housing, and our nation's shredded safety net as the primary structural drivers of homelessness, many families that lose their housing turn to the homelessness service system to seek safe haven and assistance. However, homelessness is more than the loss of housing; it represents disconnection from relationships, possessions, beloved pets, reassuring routines, neighborhoods, and community. The impact on families—and especially on children—can be devastating, frequently leaving long-lasting and profound scars. The road back is often very bumpy and protracted.

Despite this bleak picture, this may be a time of opportunity. Various policy developments suggest that we may be able to galvanize a genuine response to family homelessness that will begin to reverse its adverse effects, and ultimately prevent homelessness in the first place. After almost a decade of attention focused on the needs of chronically homeless people to the exclusion of the families, the federal Interagency Council on Homelessness published "Opening Doors: Federal Strategic Plan to Prevent and End Homelessness" in 2010 and committed the nation to ending family, child, and youth homelessness in 10 years. The plan focused on expanding affordable housing, increasing work opportunities, reducing financial vulnerability, and supporting homelessness prevention and rapid re-housing (e.g., "Housing First"). Shorty afterwards, passage of the Hearth Act aligned the HUD definition of homeless families with the longstanding definition in the McKinney-Vento Homeless Assistance Act by including doubled-up and precariously housed families—a subgroup that comprises the majority of homeless families not included in the previous HUD definition. Additionally, passage of the Affordable Care Act expanded health care coverage, holding out the promise of integrating medical and behavioral health services—a trend that already has momentum. A recent Massachusetts report indicated that almost one in four pediatric practices are now sharing space with mental health groups, "sending the message that treating children's depression and behavioral issues is as important as following their asthma and diabetes" (Boston Globe, P. Wenn, March 18, 2013).

Within this context, *Supporting Homeless Families: Current Practices and Future Directions*, coedited by Mary Haskett, Staci Perlman, and Beryl Ann Cowan, is an extremely welcome addition to the literature on homelessness, and the only one solely devoted to the needs of families and children. This timely volume is a creative compendium of articles that explores every aspect of the issue and describes the cutting edge of the field. The authors discuss the ecology of family homelessness; identify subgroups with varied and often unique needs and characteristics; highlight the pressing needs of children, especially preschoolers; describe best practices within the context of cultural and racial/ethnic issues; emphasize the importance of trauma-informed care; highlight progress, gaps, and barriers towards implementing high-quality programs; encourage collaboration among multidisciplinary service systems; highlight the importance of following families during transitions; and recommend how we can move forward to achieve these goals. Stakeholder perspectives provide differing viewpoints that further illuminate the complexity of these issues. The editor's stated goal for this volume is right on target: "to raise the standard of services" by providing strengths-based, culturally competent, trauma-informed services and to ensure their implementation by disseminating critical information to frontline providers.

Although the authors describe various promising practices and the evidence base that have started to emerge, services for homeless families and children with reliable outcomes are still in their infancy. Few services for low-income families and their children have been adapted for use by homeless programs, and the evidence base for existing programs remains strikingly limited. For example, although various programs for homeless families have shown some positive outcomes, such as those documented in the What Works Clearinghouse (2011) of the DOE Institute of Educational Sciences (2013), there are no interventions for homeless families that meet the rigorous criteria for having Positive Effects—primarily because there is as yet no robust evidence base. Similarly, although a variety of parenting prevention programs show some promising outcomes, the evidence base is only just beginning to emerge and additional research is critically needed. Once the range of best practices is more fully identified, frontline providers will need to be supported through training and career development to implement these interventions with fidelity to the models. In a resource-scarce environment such as the homeless service system, this is a challenging task. Training is often a low priority—and providers are often overworked, underpaid, and inadequately supported—leading to staff burnout and high rates of turnover. Thus, the translation of research into practice remains limited and the quality chasm is deep (IOM, 2009). Some of the authors describe strategies for providing cost-effective, supportive, and ongoing training. To improve the quality of service delivery, we must begin by transforming the workforce.

Despite the considerable challenges of "raising the standard of services" for homeless families and children, the authors in this volume remind us about our accomplishments thus far and the progress we are making. Based on an understanding that housing is essential but not sufficient to attain the outcomes necessary to ensure well-being and stability, the authors discuss the central importance of the Earned Income Tax Credit, the Homeless Prevention and Rapid Re-Housing Program, the Rental Assistance Programs, and the promise of the Affordable Care Act.

This volume also highlights the central importance of addressing the needs of children and youth experiencing homelessness. Without a place to call home, these children and youth are severely challenged by unpredictability, dislocation, and frequent exposure to violence—placing them at high risk for poor educational, socioemotional, and mental health outcomes. To date, the needs of these children and youth have been largely ignored and, with the important exception of the McKinney-Vento Homeless Assistance Act and the Education of Homeless Children and Youth Program, few services are solely devoted to supporting their growth and development. This volume describes the challenges of serving these children within a developmental framework, offering frontline staff, administrators, and policy-makers critical resource information as well as tips and tools. Chapters are also devoted to the developmental and mental health needs of infants, preschoolers, youth aged 6 through adolescence, and unaccompanied youth including those who have identified as lesbian, gay, bisexual, and transgendered and those who have aged out of foster care.

This volume should be required reading for all those interested in ending and preventing family, youth, and child homelessness. It brings together in one place state-of-the-art information that we need to ameliorate this tragic social problem. Although the research to date is limited, the authors describe the fundamental principles necessary to make the goals of "Opening Doors" a reality—and to ensure the residential stability, self-sufficiency, and well-being of families, youth, and children experiencing homelessness. Without this commitment, we stand to lose another generation of children and youth.

Ellen L. Bassuk, M.D.
Needham, MA, USA
Cambridge, MA, USA

Preface

As noted by the authors of chapters in this volume—leading researchers, practitioners, and policy-makers in the field of homelessness—the face of homelessness has changed dramatically in recent decades. Historically, individuals who struggled with homelessness were single males, often characterized by serious mental illness and/or substance abuse; currently, the fastest growing segment of the homeless population is comprised of single mothers with young children. Homelessness among families with children is rising at alarming rates due to the economic downturn in the United States in recent years combined with a deteriorating safety net of medical and mental health care; a stagnant minimum wage in spite of rising costs of living; inadequate, inaccessible substance abuse treatment; and laws that fail to protect women from domestic violence.

Pioneers in the field of family homelessness began to publish research on characteristics of parents and children experiencing homelessness in the mid-1980s and early 1990s. Those studies were valuable in terms of shedding light on the potentially devastating impact of homelessness on children and parents. Currently it is recognized that although the experience of homelessness has the potential for devastating and long-lasting consequences, many parents and children continue to function relatively well in spite of enormous risks. The increased understanding of the broader ecological context in which homelessness occurs has resulted in reduced emphasis on parental pathology and personal limitations and a greater focus on societal responsibility for supporting families at risk for homelessness and those living in shelters and "doubled-up" with family or friends. Throughout this book, authors reflect this strengths-based view of families without homes.

Homelessness and associated risks place families at jeopardy for many hardships. Episodes of homelessness build upon histories of significant stress, many of which predate housing instability. Most families that are homeless are extremely poor and are headed by single females with young children; racial and ethnic minorities are vastly overrepresented. Increasingly, two-parent families and older children are joining the ranks of those without homes. Many children and adults in this population have endured child maltreatment, physical assault, and sexual victimization.

The loss of housing can create a surge in stress for already fragile families. Once homeless, families can become disconnected from familiar neighborhoods and community supports, relatives, and child and adult peers. Living in a shelter can increase stress by creating separations between family members when regulations restrict admission to specific numbers of family members or ban adolescents and adult males. Families endure the loss of privacy and autonomy and are expected to adjust their routines to conform to shelter regulations. Given these factors, it is not surprising that children living in shelters have higher-than-average rates of medical illness, emotional and behavioral disturbance, and developmental delays when compared to more advantaged peers. Academic achievement by homeless children often is hampered by undiagnosed learning disabilities, poor school attendance, grade retention, and drop out. Adult members of families experiencing homelessness have higher rates of chronic illness, medical disorders, domestic violence, substance abuse, and emotional and behavioral disturbances than the general population.

Although the impact of homelessness on families has been outlined in the literature, a consolidated approach to translating research findings into interventions and program practices that support families has been lacking. Providers in the field often report that they lack full understanding of the behavioral and emotional needs of families and methods to successfully address those needs in ways that will empower families. Other providers associate high rates of staff burnout with the perception that they are consumed by "putting out fires" and struggle to make a positive or sustainable difference in the lives of family members. Many providers lack knowledge of "what works" because there is no centralized treatise that summarizes best practices. Furthermore, while research in the area of family homelessness has been conducted within many professional disciplines, investigators tend to operate within "silos" and are unaware of important trends in research outside their areas of expertise. Finally, policy-makers lack access on current research pertaining to family homelessness and must search for information using multiple and sometimes unreliable and outdated sources.

Our envisioned goal for this volume is to raise the standard of services provided to families without homes through practices that are strengths-based, trauma-informed, and culturally competent, and as such, are more likely to have a positive lasting impact. The specific aim is to disseminate accessible information about family homelessness to frontline service providers, researchers, policy-makers, and students across disciplines. We hope this volume will be used as a text and reference source across disciplines of education, child welfare, psychiatry and psychology, social work, public health, human development, law, and pediatrics.

The first part of this book describes a contextual overview of family homelessness and the impact on children and youth who experience homelessness. An ecological and developmental framework for understanding the implications of homelessness from infancy through adulthood is presented, with reference to existing research. Specifically, Buckner (Chap. 1) describes the complex structural components of homelessness and the psychosocial factors that underscore why some impoverished families are more vulnerable to housing instability than others. Volk (Chap. 2), Cowan (Chap. 3), and their coauthors review the empirical literature on the developmental, mental health, and academic status of children and adolescents exposed to homelessness. This part also includes Perlman and colleagues' (Chap. 4) summary of research on the characteristics of women and men who struggle to provide safe, stable, and nurturing parenting in the context of homelessness, followed by DeCandia and colleagues' (Chap. 5) description of current knowledge of parents without homes who are members of special populations with unique challenges.

In the second part of the book, frameworks and innovative designs for providing collaboration between and among diverse services that interface with families experiencing homelessness is discussed. Parents without homes must navigate multiple systems designed to support their families, including schools, child welfare, housing, and mental health care; the critical importance of collaboration among these systems is discussed by Bray and Link (Chap. 6). A trauma-informed approach to supporting these families is provided by Guarino (Chap. 7). Finally, methods to provide families with culturally competent services that support them during episodes of homelessness as well as the period of rehousing are highlighted by Garrett-Akinsaya (Chap. 8).

In the final part of the book, examples of empirically proven interventions and best practices are showcased and roadblocks that impede success and sustainability are discussed. Gewirtz and colleagues (Chap. 9) provide a review of programs designed to promote positive parenting in the context of homelessness and transitional housing, and Herbers and Cutuli (Chap. 10) summarize the literature on programs designed to address the needs of homeless children and youth. The closing chapter in the book, authored by da Costa Nunez and Adams (Chap. 11), is a discussion among primary stakeholders (parents, practitioners, service providers, researchers, policy-makers, parents) on provision of services to families without homes.

It is our shared hope that this volume will be a catalyst for providers, researchers, policy-makers, and students alike to more fully understand families without homes through the perspectives of strength, diversity, and cultural competence. Translating knowledge into practice in service of empowering vulnerable families is achievable through the consolidated commitment of us all.

Raleigh, NC, USA	Mary E. Haskett
Newark, DE, USA	Staci M. Perlman
Boston, MA, USA	Beryl Ann Cowan

Acknowledgements

The springboard for this book was the Task Force on Promoting Positive Parenting in the Context of Family Homelessness of the American Psychological Association, Society for Child and Family Policy and Practice, Section on Child Maltreatment. Mary E. Haskett and Staci Perlman served as Cochairs of the task force, and Beryl Ann Cowan was an active and valued member. The task force conducted a symposium on parenting in the context of family homelessness at the annual convention of the American Psychological Association in 2011, and the topic attracted the attention of Jennifer Hadley of Springer. Ms. Hadley convinced us to develop this book and we thank her for lending her enthusiasm and support.

Together, we extend our sincere appreciation to the many families residing in shelters, in transitional housing, doubled-up, on the streets, and in rural communities who have patiently taught us as we endeavored to learn about the challenges of parenting while living without stable housing. We are also indebted to the providers on the front line who, with limited budgets and resources, commit themselves each day to serving families without homes. We acknowledge the community groups and policy-makers who have joined forces to identify ways to end homelessness. We thank our mentors, our colleagues, and our students who have helped formulate our research, asked very hard questions, and assisted us in seeing our projects through every step of the way.

Contents

Part I
Needs of Children and Families
Experiencing Homelessness

Chapter 1
The Why and the Who of Family Homelessness

John C. Buckner

Abstract This chapter provides a structural explanation of the problem of family homelessness that draws from population-based public health and epidemiologic principles. A "simplifying model," or metaphor, is used to explain homelessness from a top-down, macro-perspective. The metaphor fosters an understanding of the root causes of homelessness and distinguishes these causal factors from the attributes of individuals and families who have become homeless. Specifically, the game of musical chairs is used as a metaphor to aid in understanding *why* homelessness exists as a social problem and *who* is most vulnerable to becoming homeless. Risk and protective factors for homelessness are discussed. Policy implications of the metaphor for lowering the incidence and prevalence of family homelessness—an extremely complex social and structural challenge—are provided. It is argued that the structural imbalance between affordable housing supply and demand must be addressed through an increase in the supply of housing. Furthermore, addressing the health, mental health, and related service needs of homeless individuals and families can be important in shortening the duration of an episode as well as lowering the reoccurrence rate of homelessness. Such service-based interventions can be important in improving the quality of life of persons, both when they are homeless and once rehoused. In addition, policy makers, researchers, and advocates must systematically consider the base population at risk of family homelessness and alleviate pressures emanating from insufficient incomes that make existing housing units unaffordable to many families.

J.C. Buckner, Ph.D. (✉)
Children's Hospital, Boston, MA, USA

M.E. Haskett et al. (eds.), *Supporting Families Experiencing Homelessness:*
Current Practices and Future Directions, DOI 10.1007/978-1-4614-8718-0_1,
© Springer Science+Business Media New York 2014

During the early to mid-twentieth century, homeless individuals in the USA were a rather homogenous population comprised mostly of alcohol-abusing men who lived in the inner cities (Caton, 1990; Hopper, 2003). In the late 1970s and continuing throughout the 1980s, the homeless population increased in size and became more diverse. A number of factors contributed to this change. Persons with severe mental illness joined the ranks of the homeless population due in part to deinstitutionalization—the release of large numbers of patients from state mental hospitals back to communities that had insufficient housing and social service supports (Caton, 1990; Jencks, 1994). The destruction of cheap housing in the inner cities and reduced federal spending for new housing construction, restoration, and rental assistance were also important contributing factors in swelling the number of individuals without a home (Jencks, 1994).

It was not until the early 1980s that families began to appear at homeless shelters for single adults and, as their numbers grew, a specialized type of shelter facility was developed across America that could address the needs of one or more parents with young children in tow (Bassuk, 1991; Weinreb & Rossi, 1995). Nowadays, the composition of the homeless population consists of three distinct subgroups: single adults, families (i.e., one or more parents accompanied by children), and adolescents who are unaccompanied by an adult.

According to the 2010 Annual Homeless Assessment Report to Congress (HUD, 2012), approximately 650,000 people (242,000 persons in families) were homeless on a single night in January 2010. This is a conservative estimate given that HUD survey emphasizes urban locations and can overlook persons living in rural and suburban areas. Just three states (California, New York, and Florida) accounted for 40 % of all homeless persons on the night of the January 2010 point-in-time count. Over the course of a year, many more individuals and families experience homelessness. The US Department of Housing and Urban Development estimates that about 567,000 persons in families became homeless and spent time in a shelter over the 12 month period between October 2009 and September 2010. This estimate excluded families living outside of the shelter system, such as in vehicles, camp grounds, or in doubled-up situations with other families who own the home or hold the rental lease. During 2007–2010, there was a 20 % rise in number of persons in homeless families. In large part, this was due to the Great Recession, which was an outgrowth of a global financial crisis the roots of which lay in an unprecedented number of home foreclosures both in the USA and in Europe. Members of families now make up a larger percentage of the homeless population than has ever previously been the case (HUD, 2012). This subgroup has also become increasingly diverse in recent years as more families who were home owners have increasingly found themselves unable to remain stably housed due to job loss and increased mortgage payment costs.

In this chapter I provide a structural explanation of the problem of family homelessness that also draws upon population-based public health and epidemiologic principles. I elaborate upon a "simplifying model," or metaphor, that has been used over the years to better explain homelessness from a top-down, macro-perspective. The metaphor fosters an understanding of the root causes of homelessness and distinguishes these causal factors from the attributes of individuals and families who have become homeless.

A simplifying model employs a metaphor to explain a concept or phenomenon. A new or poorly understood idea is linked to a much more familiar concept by way of analogy. Simplifying models are routinely used by educators as a teaching aid and have captured the attention of communication specialists who use them in crafting messages to the general public (Frameworks Institute, 2002). They are most helpful when the analogy to a more familiar concept can be utilized to develop a better understanding and draw accurate deductions about the more complex or novel idea; the metaphor becomes an inferential tool for more fully grasping the complexities of a new subject matter. However, a simplifying model can do a disservice if it produces representations of the more intricate idea or phenomenon that leads to erroneous conclusions or if the simplification process obfuscates nuances that are important to appreciate. Hence, they need to be applied with care and scrutinized for their worthiness.

A Simplifying Model for Homelessness

Sclar (1990), in a short editorial in the *American Journal of Public Health*, introduced the game of "musical chairs" as a metaphor to better grasp the then rapidly emerging problem of homelessness. Liking it, I have utilized and expanded upon it over the years to develop a simplifying model to better understand *why* homelessness exists as a social problem in the first place as well as to explain *who* it is that is most vulnerable to becoming homeless (Buckner, 1991, 2004, 2008; Buckner, Bassuk, & Zima, 1993).

Musical chairs is an useful metaphor to explain homelessness because it forces attention on two important, but separate, levels-of-analysis: the individual-level and the more structural-level that represents the balance between the supply and demand for housing. Because of its two levels of analysis quality, the metaphor is useful in distinguishing the root causes of homelessness from those factors that are qualities or characteristics of individuals and families who are homeless.

The game of musical chairs is premised on the creation of a structural problem within a small group: When the music stops there are too few chairs available for each person who is playing to grab his/her own seat. By design, one or more people will be left standing; the ratio of chairs to people needing them is not one-to-one. The question of "why are their people left standing when the music stops?" can only be answered in a meaningful fashion by pointing to the structural imbalance between the supply of chairs and the demand that had been created at the outset. If there are only five chairs for six people, one person has to be left standing. The seeds of the problem were sown from the start at a level of analysis above that of any qualities pertaining to individuals who are playing the game.

Now, the question of "who is it that is most vulnerable to being left standing when the music stops" is an entirely separate matter. In part, this predicament can be the result of bad luck and circumstances (i.e., being in the wrong place at the wrong time when the music halts), but also has much to do with certain attributes of the individuals playing the game. In comparison to fellow competitors, those who have slower reaction times, or who are less aggressive, or more polite in scurrying for the nearest available seat will be at the greatest risk of not finding a chair to sit in when the music stops.

Likewise, in adopting this metaphor to better understand the problem of homelessness (whether family homelessness or in general), we should distinguish between matters relevant to *why* homelessness occurs from *who* is most vulnerable. Families (and individuals) become homeless when the demand for affordable housing exceeds the supply in a locale. It is this structural imbalance that explains, at a fundamental level, *why* homelessness occurs in the first place. Alternatively, *who* becomes homeless under such conditions can have a great deal to do with vulnerabilities that make some families (or individuals) less able to successfully compete for a relatively scarce resource, namely housing. But the "why" and the "who" questions are entirely separate matters. The attributes of individuals and families should never, in themselves, become explanations for why the problem of homelessness has arisen. Doing so leads to very misguided, "blaming the victim," forms of judgment.

The *musical chairs* metaphor for understanding homelessness is best suited to the most ubiquitous form of homelessness that manifests within the broader context of poverty rather than through natural disaster (such as a hurricane, tornado, earthquake, forest fire, flooding); or a localized event (such as a house fire). Why homelessness occurs in the wake of a natural disaster is readily apparent; although what caused the natural disaster, itself, may be less clear-cut. In addition, who is affected by a disaster or event is usually fairly *indiscriminate* (e.g., many homes will be destroyed in a bad earthquake or flood) or *random* (e.g., the path of destruction left by a tornado). Moreover, homelessness due to a natural disaster or an event permanently destroys housing units or temporarily leaves them unfit for human habitation. The housing units of people rendered homeless due to financial reasons remain intact. Having said this, poverty contributes to the *duration* of a homeless episode for individuals and families who have been displaced through natural disaster. In the aftermath of a large natural disaster, the poorest in a geographic area will likely struggle the most to regain housing and can, over time, increasingly come to represent the population who remain homeless.

Structural Factors

Keeping in mind the musical chairs metaphor, to better understand homelessness from a macro-perspective, it is helpful to understand factors that influence the *absolute supply of housing* in a given area, circumstances that influence the *absolute number of individuals (and families)*, and alterations in the *ratio* between these two.

Absolute Supply of Housing

To a great extent, the rate of private sector financed construction of housing in the USA rises and falls with the state of the overall economy. Speculative interest by housing developers in the private sector to construct housing is influenced by projections in the need for housing in future years and by the cost of building. As housing construction requires a great deal of upfront capital expenditure, the cost of building is heavily dependent on the cost of credit (i.e., the amount of interest necessary to pay over time when issued a construction loan). The construction of new lower-cost housing is built by the private, public, and nonprofit sectors. About 1.2 million households live in public housing (housing built by a government entity). Through the federal housing voucher program (known as "Sect. 1.8"), close to 1.4 million households receive financial assistance to live in existing housing units that are privately owned. For households receiving such housing assistance, the program makes payments directly to their landlords to cover the gap between fair market rent and 30 % of the household's income. The federal government and state governments influence housing construction mostly indirectly through tax credits to developers, mortgage interest deduction to taxpayers, and the Sect. 1.8 housing voucher/certificate program as well as additional housing assistance programs (Crowley, 2004).

Adding an important level of nuance to more fully capture the complexities of homelessness, it is important to differentiate between the absolute number of housing units available in a given locale and the subset of these units that are actually "affordable." According to the US Department of Housing and Urban Development (HUD), housing is considered "affordable" if it costs no more than 30 % of one's income. The percentage of housing units that can be considered affordable will fluctuate depending upon a broader array of factors, including the supply of jobs that pay a decent wage as well as the availability of government supported housing subsidies that can be used to help pay rent. It is only the supply of *affordable* housing units that are relevant to homelessness. In any city, luxury apartments that lie vacant are of no use to homeless families in the area due to their expensive rents.

Across the 50 states in America, it requires between 63 and 175 h of work in a week for a minimum wage earner to afford a two-bedroom apartment (National Low Income Housing Coalition, 2012). In many states, this level of weekly work hours is completely unrealistic (a 7 day week has 168 total hours). As a result, if not receiving a housing subsidy, many families with a single, low-wage earner must spend well beyond 30 % of their incomes to be a primary tenant. Furthermore, in order to stay in housing, many families lack adequate income for other basic needs such as for food, clothing, child care, and health care. Using this 30 % HUD income threshold, a deficit of as many as 2 million housing units may exist in the USA between the number of households in the bottom income quintile (lowest 20 %) and the number of rental housing units these households can afford (Crowley, 2004).

Housing affordability is tied to the availability of jobs that pay a decent wage. Over the past 20 years, the USA has seen a slow, steady erosion in the manufacturing base leading to a loss of better paying jobs for working class families (Bivens, 2008).

Many American businesses have shifted their manufacturing facilities oversees where labor costs are much cheaper. According to the US Bureau of Labor Statistics, in 2011 the hourly way of an average manufacturing worker in the USA was $35.53 compared to $6.48 wage for Mexico, $2.65 in China, and $2.01 for the Philippines. Globalization of the manufacturing work force has cost millions of American jobs and placed a steady downward pressure on worker's wages. From 2001 to 2011, the Economic Policy Institute (2012) estimated that 2.1 million American jobs were displaced by China alone. Bivens (2008) reported that since 2006 the typical full-time median-wage earner in the USA loses about $1,400 per year in income due to globalization. Without a commensurate decline in housing costs, this steady decline in income reduces housing affordability.

Absolute Numbers of People

When evaluating the adequacy of the absolute supply of affordable housing in an area, it is necessary to consider the absolute demand for it. A major component of absolute demand is simply how many people there are in an area and how this population size is changing. "Demography is destiny" is an often used phrase. Forecasting demographic trends is a bit like predicting a flood after a long period of intense rain over an extended area. Weather forecasters can accurately foretell the time it will take for heavy rainfall to make its way through streams and tributaries and, days later and hundreds of miles away, swell rivers to levels where they will cause flooding. Likewise, significant changes in the birth rate of a population will show its inevitable effects both in the short and longer term as infants grow older. Patterns of migration within the USA can contribute to regional changes in population size; immigration is also a notable factor in some cities and states. But likely the biggest consideration, at least on a national scale, is demographic trends in the overall population.

Examining change in the total population of an area is important in understanding homelessness from a macro-perspective (with changes in housing supply the other critical factor). Demographic changes in the US population during the mid-twentieth century represented a very relevant structural factor in the rise of homelessness during the late 1970s and throughout the 1980s. Yet, these trends went largely unappreciated by policy makers, advocates, and researchers for the role they played. In the aftermath of World War II from 1946 to 1963, the USA experienced a rapid and long sustaining increase in the number of annual births. The 76 million children born during this period are known as the "baby boom" cohort. The increase began in 1946, peaked in the mid-1950s, and did not return to "normal" level until the mid-1960s. From a "demography is destiny" perspective, the baby boom cohort began to reach young adulthood in the mid-1960s with the number of young adults peaking in the late 1970s-early 1980s and only returning to more common historical levels of in the early 1990s.

During this time period, the baby boom cohort put well-documented pressure on schools and colleges to expand their size capacities (Cheung, 2007). Entrance to young adulthood marks a time when many individuals traditionally move out from their families of origin, enter the workforce, and begin forming separate family units. The emergence of family homelessness during the early 1980s, at a time when the USA was experiencing a sustained rise in new family formation, does not seem like a coincidence. A long and continuous rise in the absolute number of people in a population entering young adulthood each year will put pressure on the balance between housing supply and demand, especially if it is not planned for in advance, which was the case in the last quarter of the twentieth century in America. Given that not enough new family-suitable housing units had been built in communities across America ahead of their arrival into young adulthood, the baby boom cohort itself, through the absolute increase in the number of individuals reaching young adulthood, helped to set off the housing equivalent of musical chairs among individuals leaving their families of origin.

The baby boom cohort also caused strain to the mental health system. The developmental period between late adolescence and young adulthood also marks the peak age of onset for severe mental illnesses such as schizophrenia and for alcohol and other substance use disorders (Eaton, 1995). This fact, in combination with an absolute increase in the number of young adults during the late 1970s and 1980s, was partly to blame for the spike in the number of persons with severe mental illnesses and substance use disorders who became homeless during this time period. In hindsight, the outcome was predictable; yet in the moment it was difficult to discern the impact that demography was having on the mental health system (as well as other systems such as education).

Besides change in the absolute number of people, there can be alterations in the number of people (within a fixed total population size) whose incomes are not sufficient such that just 30 % of their earnings can be applied toward housing costs. An economic recession leading to extensive job loss can lower the average cost for housing (whether through mortgage payment or rent) that individuals and families can afford. In a rare study of structural causes of family homelessness, Gould and Williams (2010) found the unemployment rate associated with an increase in the number of individuals in family shelters in Missouri over an 8 year period (1992–2001).

In the context of a stable number of rental units and a worsening economy, if rent prices are not lowered, more people will find these rates unaffordable. In the Great Recession from 2007 to 2009, large numbers of home owners became unable to afford their mortgage payments due to job loss and/or sudden jumps in their monthly mortgage payments due to "teaser" loans that had been commonly made by mortgage financers to unsuspecting borrowers. These home owners added to the pool of individuals and families across the nation who were in need of affordable housing— or at least more affordable than their current homes. Given that the supply of low cost housing remained fairly constant during this time period, a sizeable source of new demand for affordable housing set off an even more competitive struggle.

Ratio of Housing Supply and Demand

As previously mentioned, within any given geographic area, a structural imbalance between housing units (whether these are single family homes, multifamily complexes, condominiums, or apartments) and the number of people within that area in need of housing sows the conditions for homelessness to occur. Said differently, too many people seeking housing in relation to the supply sets the stage for individuals and families to become homeless. As this ratio becomes increasingly less favorable, it also leads to more people "doubling up" in their living situation; a circumstance which, for some, can be a way station on the path to becoming literally homeless.

The ratio between housing supply and demand can become less favorable due to a *decrease* in the number of affordable housing units (e.g., the outright destruction of single room occupancy hotels in the inner cities of America during the 1960s); or an *increase* in the demand for affordable housing (e.g., due to demographic trends or economic conditions); or both of these factors can be in operation at the same time. More generally, *change* in the quantity of available housing in relation to *change* in the number of people in need of housing interplay in such a manner as to determine whether the supply and demand is in balance or not.

Distinguishing Incidence and Prevalence

This overall supply–demand ratio for affordable housing can fluctuate over time, thereby altering both the incidence and prevalence rates of homelessness in a geographic area. The *incidence* rate of homelessness is the number of *new* entrants into the status of homeless divided by the total number of people in a defined area over a specified period of time (e.g., 1 year). When the supply–demand ratio for affordable housing becomes less favorable, the incidence rate of homelessness should rise.

The prevalence rate of homelessness is the number of people meeting the status of being "homeless" (by whatever definition) over a specified period of time (e.g., on a given night, in a 1 year period). A prevalence rate is a function of the *incidence rate* times the *duration* of the "condition" (i.e., Prevalence = Incidence × Duration). In the case of homelessness, the average length of time that persons in an area remain homeless has substantial influence over the total number of people who are homeless in that area, within a specified period of time. For instance, keeping the incidence rate the same, doubling the average duration of homelessness from 3 to 6 months in a region should approximately double the total number of persons experiencing homelessness over a 12 month period (the annual prevalence). It should be noted that factors that alter the average duration of homelessness are not likely to influence the incidence rate of homelessness—but will change the prevalence of homelessness for better or for worse.

Risk and Protective Factors

As described earlier, the musical chairs metaphor highlights two separate levels of analysis that are each important to consider in better understanding homelessness. The previous section provided an overview of structural factors that help to account for the problem in the first place. In this section, I move to reviewing matters that help to differentiate *who* is most at risk of experiencing homelessness. As mentioned earlier, these individual or family-level variables are not germane to explaining *why* homelessness is a problem in a country, region, or locale, but are very pertinent in accounting for who is most at risk.

When observing the game of musical chairs, it is somewhat predictable who among the participants will be left standing. Similarly, in attempting to secure and retain affordable housing in locales where the supply does not meet the demand, those less competitive will find it more difficult. Those "losing out" may have to "double-up" with friends or extended family members in order to have a place to live or it could mean becoming literally homeless.

Vulnerability (Risk) Factors

In the competition for affordable housing it is income that is the primary differentiator between those who can successfully compete for housing and those who cannot. It takes financial resources (income or savings) to afford to pay the mortgage on a housing unit or to pay monthly rent, deposit and security fees, as well as utilities. (In the case of ability to pay rent, a housing subsidy could also be considered a financial resource.) In addition, the availability of instrumental support from members of one's social network is a second important factor. Some individuals or families can remain one step above literal homelessness through the instrumental support of others who own a home or hold the primary lease agreement.

Vulnerability factors that increase an individual's or family's likelihood of becoming homeless share in common a propensity to make it harder to have a well-paying job (hence income and savings) and/or strain the willingness of one's social network to provide housing supports over an extended period. Broadly speaking, when considering the major homeless subgroups in the USA, their noteworthy characteristics can present significant obstacles to being in the work force. Also, if they are not the primary lease holder or home owner, these attributes can be sources of strain for friends and family with whom they are living. Among single adults, these issues include severe mental illnesses and substance abuse disorders. Among families, a single parent with sole responsibility for the care of young children can often find it difficult to work full-time and must usually pay for childcare, thereby reducing net pay. Also, relatives and friends may be more reluctant to share their living quarters over an extended period with families, especially those with infants and toddlers. Lastly, for unaccompanied adolescents, many of who are experiencing a myriad of life challenges, it is rare to find a youth who has sufficient education or skills to be competitive in the labor market.

The remainder of this section will review research findings on these risk and protective factors for families. It should be noted that because the vast majority of homeless families in the USA are headed by single mothers, the epidemiological research that has been conducted on adults in these households pertains almost exclusively to mothers. The most comprehensive study of family homelessness was conducted in Worcester, Massachusetts during the 1990s (Bassuk et al., 1996, 1997) and will be referred to from here on out as the "Worcester study." This epidemiological investigation involved a comparison of 220 homeless mothers and 216 low-income housed, never homeless, mothers and their combined total of 620 children.

Young Children and Pregnancy

In most areas of the country, homeless families are overwhelmingly headed by single women. Typically, these mothers are in their mid-to-late 1920's and have an average of 2 younger age children with them (Shinn & Bassuk, 2004). Having children in general, especially infants and toddlers, places a single parent at a competitive disadvantage in terms of holding a job and can increase a household's cost of living for rent, childcare, food, and other expenses. In addition, pregnancy has been found to be a risk factor for homelessness (Shinn et al., 1998). In a comparison of homeless public assistance families in New York with a sample of housed families on public assistance, 35 % of the homeless women were pregnant at the time of the study and 26 % had given birth in the past year, while only 6 % of the housed group were pregnant and 11 % had recently given birth (Weitzman, 1989).

Race/Ethnicity

Being a member of a minority group heightens chances of being poor as well as being homeless (Burt et al., 1999). Racial discrimination, including and especially pertaining to housing, may help to explain this fact. The race/ethnic status of homeless families in a city typically reflects the composition of the broader population of poor housed families in that locale (Rog & Buckner, 2007).

Financial Resources

The average income of homeless mothers is significantly below the federal poverty level (Bassuk et al., 1997, 1996; Rog, McCombs-Thornton, Gilbert-Mongelli, Brito, & Holupka, 1995; Shinn & Weitzman, 1996) and their incomes are almost always too low to obtain adequate housing on their own without subsidies (Burt et al., 1999).

Education and Employment

It is common for adults in both homeless and other poor families to have low levels of educational attainment, little or no job training, and minimal work histories (Brooks & Buckner, 1996). Whereas 75 % of adults in the USA have graduated from high school or have a GED, this figure ranges from 35 to 61 % across a number of studies of homeless mothers (Bassuk et al., 1996; Burt et al., 1999; Lowin, Demirel, Estee, & Schreiner, 2001; Rog et al., 1995; Shinn & Weitzman, 1996). Not surprisingly, studies indicate that most homeless mothers (84–99 %) are not working (Bassuk et al., 1996; Lowin et al., 2001; Rog et al., 1995). The majority of homeless mothers have had some work experience, however, ranging from 67 % in the Worcester study (Brooks & Buckner, 1996) to over 90 % in the RWJF/HUD Homeless Families Program (Rog et al., 1995). Among homeless and housed low-income mothers in the Worcester study, becoming pregnant before the age of 18 significantly lowered a woman's chances of having been employed (Brooks & Buckner, 1996).

Social Networks and Supports

Over the years, studies that have examined the extent and nature of homeless mothers' social support have produced contrasting results. Several investigations have found that, compared to housed poor women, mothers in the midst of an episode of homelessness have less available instrumental and emotional support and less frequent contact with network members (Bassuk & Rosenberg, 1988; Culhane, Metraux, & Hadley, 2001; Passero, Zax, & Zozus, 1991). Having a network marked by interpersonal conflict may be a risk factor for homelessness (Bassuk et al., 1997). In contrast, one study found no differences in support between homeless and housed mothers (Goodman, 1991). Shinn and colleagues (1991) reported contrasting findings in that newly homeless mothers reported *more* recent contact with network members than poor housed mothers, and over three-quarters had stayed with network members before turning to shelter. In a follow-up 5 years later, Toohey, Shinn, and Weitzman (2004) found that the social networks of the (now) formerly homeless mothers in this sample were quite similar to those of their housed counterparts.

Differences across these study findings may have to do with the timing of when homeless mothers were interviewed in the course of their homelessness episode: In the months prior to a homelessness episode contact with network members may increase, whereas a mother may have depleted most of her social network resources by the time she and her children enter shelter.

Partner Violence

Homeless mothers, like poor women in general, have experienced high rates of both domestic and community violence (Bassuk et al., 1996; Browne & Bassuk, 1997). Many women report having been both victims and witnesses of violence over their lifetimes. In the Worcester study, almost two-thirds of the homeless mothers had been severely physically assaulted by an intimate partner and one-third had a current or recent abusive partner (Browne & Bassuk, 1997). More than one-fourth of the mothers reported having needed or received medical treatment because of these attacks (Bassuk et al., 1996). Supporting these findings, Rog and her colleagues (1995) reported that almost two-thirds of their nine-city sample of homeless women described one or more severe acts of violence by a current or former intimate partner. Not surprisingly, many of these women reportedly lost or left their last homes because of domestic violence.

While so endemic in the past and present of homeless mothers, the Worcester study failed to demonstrate that partner violence was a risk factor for homelessness (Bassuk et al., 2007) due to the equally high rates found in a comparison group of housed, never homeless, mothers. This is not to say that violence is not a serious issue in the lives of homeless mothers, but illustrates how pervasive a problem it is for poor women in general, whether currently homeless or never homeless.

In addition to adult violent victimization, many homeless mothers have experienced severe abuse and assault in childhood. The Worcester study documented that more than 40 % of homeless mothers had been sexually molested by the age of 12 (Bassuk et al., 1996). Sixty-six percent of the women in this study experienced severe physical abuse, mainly at the hand of an adult caretaker. Other studies have found similar results (e.g., Rog et al., 1995).

Mental Health

Given the high levels of stress and the pervasiveness of violence, it is not surprising that, in the Worcester study, homeless mothers had high lifetime rates of post-traumatic stress disorder (PTSD) that was three times the rate in the general female population and major depressive disorder twice the rate (Bassuk, Buckner, Perloff, & Bassuk, 1998). While mental health problems are a significant issue for women living in poverty, like violence, it is less clear that mental health poses a risk factor for family homelessness. Bassuk and colleagues (1998, 1996) found, however, few mental health differences between homeless and poor mothers. Thirty-six percent of homeless mothers and 34 % of poor housed mothers had lifetime prevalence of PTSD and 18 % of homeless mothers compared to 16 % of poor housed mothers reported current PTSD. Depression among homeless mothers is also common, as it is for poor women generally (Bassuk et al., 1998; Shinn & Bassuk, 2004). While the prevalence rates of mental disorders that Bassuk et al. (2007) reported were roughly equivalent between homeless versus housed low-income mother, homeless mothers were three times more likely to have been hospitalized at some point in their life for a mental health problem, which suggests that their issues with mental health were more severe. Between one-quarter and one-third of homeless mothers report attempting suicide at least once in their lifetime (Bassuk et al., 1996; Rog et al., 1995).

Women who have borne children and who then develop a severe psychiatric disorder, especially a psychotic disorder, are at risk for losing custody of their children. Unlike single adults, psychotic disorders are rare among homeless mothers with children (Bassuk et al., 1998). However, among single adult homeless women, some are mothers who have lost custody of their children, often due to a severe mental illness such as schizophrenia (Fischer & Breakey, 1991; Hoffman & Rosencheck, 2001; Smith & North, 1994).

Substance Abuse

In the Worcester study, lifetime prevalence rates of alcohol/drug dependence are somewhat higher for homeless mothers (41 %) than housed poor mothers (35 %), but are almost twice that found among women of equivalent age in the same population rates (Bassuk et al., 1997). Rates are much lower for current abuse as exemplified by a reported illicit drug use of 5 % in the Worcester study (Bassuk et al., 1996, 1998) and a 12 % rate of illicit drug use in the past year in the Rog et al., 1995 study. Heavy use of alcohol or heroin over the prior 2 years was found to be a risk factor for homelessness in the Worcester study (Bassuk et al., 1997). In addition, homeless mothers were four times more likely to have been hospitalized for a substance abuse problem than their housed counterparts (Bassuk et al., 1997).

Protective Factors: The Role of Subsidies

Protective factors are variables that, when present, reduce the likelihood of a negative outcome. Major federal government assistance programs such as the Earned Income Tax Credit (EITC), the Supplemental Nutrition Assessment Program (food stamps), Temporary Assistance for Needy Families (TANF or cash assistance), Sect. 1.8 housing assistance, Medicaid, and the Low Income Home Energy Assistance Program (LIHEAP) comprise the bulk of the social safety net for low-income families. As such, they are important in alleviating poverty. Moreover, they likely play an important role in reducing the incidence of homelessness for families who participate in these programs as well as shortening its duration for families who subsequently apply and begin receiving one or more of these benefits after becoming homeless. The EITC provides critical income support for parents holding minimum wage jobs (anywhere from about $3,000 to $6,000 depending upon the number of dependent children), yet one must have earned income in order to be eligible, thereby reducing the value of the program for those who do not work or have very limited earned income. The benefit derived from the EITC is much more substantial for workers who can claim one or more dependent children on their tax returns than workers who are not parents or who do not have a child living with them to claim.

Participation in the Sect. 1.8 housing program as well as receiving cash assistance have both been found to lower the risk of being homeless for poor families. In the Worcester study, Bassuk and colleagues (1997) found that, controlling for other explanatory variables, cash assistance in the form of AFDC and housing subsidies in the form of Sect. 1.8 vouchers/certificates were important protective factors. Ninety-three percent of low-income housed families had received cash assistance in the past year as compared to 72 % of homeless families in the year prior to their homeless episode. For housing subsidies, these respective figures were 27 and 10 % (Bassuk et al., 1997).

For currently homeless families, other research studies have indicated that obtaining subsidized housing helps to reduce the duration of homelessness and lessening the chances of becoming homeless again (Shinn et al., 1998; Zlotnick, Robertson, & Lahiff, 1999). In a longitudinal study of first-time homeless families and a comparison random sample of families on public assistance, residential stability 5 years after initial shelter entry was predicted only by receipt of subsidized housing (Shinn et al., 1998). Eighty percent of the formerly homeless families who received subsidized housing were stable (i.e., in their own apartment without a move for at least 12 months), compared to just 18 % who had not received subsidized housing (Shinn et al., 1998). Additional studies have found that families receiving subsidized housing upon discharge from shelter are less likely to return to shelter than families receiving some other type of placement (Stretch & Kreuger, 1992; Wong, Culhane, & Kuhn, 1997). Similarly, after a policy of placing homeless families in subsidized housing was adopted in Philadelphia, the number of families reentering shelter dropped from 50 % in 1987 to less than 10 % in 1990 (Culhane, 1992). Finally, two separate demonstration initiatives that have studied the provision of housing with supportive social services also found high residential stability rates among formerly homeless families (Rog & Gutman, 1997; Weitzman & Berry, 1994).

Implications

A simplifying model is most helpful if it can be employed to form accurate deductions about the more complex phenomenon it is being used to explain. In this regard, what are some logical outgrowths about family homelessness that can be developed from the "musical chairs" metaphor while keeping in mind the epidemiologic concepts that were introduced earlier in this chapter?

Lowering the Incidence Rate of Homelessness

Perhaps the most obvious deduction from the musical chairs metaphor is that the incidence rate of homelessness cannot be meaningfully reduced in a society (or defined geographic area) without addressing the structural imbalance between housing supply and demand that explains how the problem developed in the first place. Usually, the most straightforward solution is to construct more affordable housing; in essence, additional chairs are needed. The metaphor also suggests that solutions that only target a specific vulnerable subgroup without increasing the supply of affordable housing will likely only change the complexion of who is "left standing when the music stops." For instance, if a reduction in the number of military veterans who are homeless is sought by policy makers and, through intervention, this subgroup becomes more competitive for housing, such efforts can be effective for this subgroup. But it may come at the expense of making other subgroups relatively disadvantaged in the competitive struggle for affordable housing should the supply remain fixed. In order to truly lower the incidence and prevalence rates of homelessness, a society must increase the supply of affordable housing, not simply render specific subgroups of individuals or families more competitive within this limited supply.

The ratio between housing supply and demand is not static; rather, it can dramatically shift over time, either becoming more problematic or more favorable with changing economic circumstances, social policies, and demographic trends. When conditions conspire to make this ratio lead to increased numbers of people who are homeless, policy makers need to step back and recognize that an insufficient supply of affordable housing is the principal culprit—either more housing needs to be built, or units that sit vacant need to become more affordable (e.g., via housing subsidies or improvement in the job market), or both.

Lowering the Prevalence Rate of Homelessness

As previously mentioned, the prevalence rate of homelessness is a function of its incidence rate and average duration: $(P = I \times D)$. Interventions and policies directed at people due to the attributes they possess (e.g., mental illness, substance abuse) are unlikely to alter the incidence rate of homelessness; a focus on a higher level of analysis is needed to accomplish this objective. Nonetheless, such efforts can lower the prevalence of homelessness by reducing its average duration. For instance, shelter-based case management services that help families secure permanent housing and shorten their duration of time homeless, from say 6 to 3 months, should, if implemented on a large scale, lower the 1-year prevalence rate of homelessness, assuming a constant incidence rate.

Likewise, addressing the health, mental health, and related service needs of homeless individuals and families can be important in shortening the duration of an episode as well as lowering the reoccurrence rate of homelessness. A family (or individual) that finds an affordable housing unit and who has unmet service needs may quickly lose their housing and be back in shelter or on the streets. Moreover, such service-based interventions can be important in improving the quality of life of persons, both when they are homeless, and once rehoused.

The Challenge of Ending Homelessness

From a public health perspective, the outright prevention of a problem requires lowering the incidence rate of new "cases" to zero. Cases—individuals who have the issue or problem that is the target of prevention—emerge from a much larger "base population" of those at risk. The base population can change as a function of the problem or condition. For example, the population at risk for ovarian cancer is women, whereas those at risk for lung cancer include both genders. In terms of family homelessness, the base population at risk consists predominantly of families living in permanent housing with limited income, few monetary assets to fall back on in an emergency, and whose ties to the workforce may be more tenuous than most. Wealthier families do not have a realistic risk of becoming homeless, at least for an extended period and only through a natural disaster or local fire. They are not playing the game of musical chairs with low-income families; they are not even in the same "building" where the game is being played.

The Great Recession of 2008–2009 and its aftermath provide an important illustration of the structural forces in play that can increase the incidence and prevalence of homelessness. Changes in the economy that negatively affect a sizeable population at risk of homelessness can send these rates skyrocketing and can overwhelm a homeless shelter system that typically deals with much smaller numbers of individuals and families. Existing resources must then be diverted to sheltering the newly homeless and cannot be used for plans that were in place to limit the duration of homelessness among those who had been living in shelter.

The population of households at risk for family homelessness in a region is somewhat difficult to estimate, but is usually considerably larger than the number of families who are homeless at any moment in time. As this at-risk population is poor (below or slightly above the official poverty line), the challenge of lowering the incidence rate of homelessness is that concerted efforts must be made to address broader issues of poverty that foster homelessness. This, in turn, entails tackling the structural causes of housing—increasing the supply of affordable housing and/or making existing homes more affordable to families (either through subsidies or through work opportunities that pay a sufficient amount to afford market rents). Yet, housing is expensive to build and housing subsidies are costly as well. Making significant structural improvements in the US labor market that would lead to better paying jobs would require substantial enhancements to the educational system and America's labor force is increasingly up against global labor competition. Needless to say, addressing the problem of homelessness and poverty more broadly is a formidable task.

Unfortunately, tackling poverty in a meaningful way has not been a priority within the USA since the 1960s and was an issue barely discussed in the last presidential election. Within such a political climate, it becomes very difficult to propose solutions for preventing homelessness that could have a meaningful impact on the incidence rate. Undertaking to resolve the broader issues is seen as untenable for most policy makers as it is too expensive and politically impractical. As a result, narrower, more limited approaches are considered, which usually represent efforts that can only make a dent in the prevalence rate of homelessness by shortening its duration for those living in shelter and elsewhere.

Over the years there have been many calls by homelessness advocates and policy makers to eliminate or "end" homelessness. This objective is a noble one but requires both preventing homelessness outright among potential new entrants and addressing the housing needs of those who are currently homeless. A consideration of structural factors that explain why homelessness is occurring in a population should lead to a realistic sense of what can be accomplished for any given intervention or policy change. For family homelessness to end in the USA, two major developments will need to unfold. First, the structural imbalance between affordable housing supply and demand will have to be addressed in a profound manner through an increase in the supply of housing. Second, policy makers, researchers, and advocates will all have to systematically consider the base population at risk of family homelessness and alleviate pressures emanating from insufficient incomes that make existing housing units unaffordable to many families. Anything less than this underestimates what are the true challenges ahead if we are to end family homelessness.

References

Bassuk, E. L. (1991). Homeless families. *Scientific American, 265*, 66–74.

Bassuk, E. L., Buckner, J. C., Perloff, J., & Bassuk, S. S. (1998). Prevalence of mental health and substance use disorders among homeless and low-income housed mothers. *The American Journal of Psychiatry, 155*, 1561–1564.

Bassuk, E. L., Buckner, J. C., Weinreb, L. F., Browne, A., Bassuk, S. S., Dawson, R., et al. (1997). Homelessness in female-headed families: Childhood and adult risk and protective factors. *American Journal of Public Health, 87*, 241–248.

Bassuk, E. L., & Rosenberg, L. (1988). Why does family homelessness occur? A case–control study. *American Journal of Public Health, 78*, 783–788.

Bassuk, E. L., Rubin, L., & Lauriat, A. S. (1986). Characteristics of sheltered homeless families. *American Journal of Public Health, 76*, 1097–1101.

Bassuk, E. L., Weinreb, L. F., Buckner, J. C., Browne, A., Salomon, A., & Bassuk, S. S. (1996). The characteristics and needs of sheltered homeless and low-income housed mothers. *Journal of the American Medical Association, 276*, 640–646.

Bivens, L. J. (2008). *Everybody wins, except most of us: What economics teaches about globalization*. Washington, DC: Economics Policy Institute.

Breakey, W. R., Fischer, P. J., Kramer, M., Nestadt, G., Romanski, A., & Ross, A. (1989). Health and mental health problems of homeless men and women in Baltimore. *Journal of the American Medical Association, 262*, 1352–1357.

Brooks, M. G., & Buckner, J. C. (1996). Work and welfare: Job histories, barriers to employment, and predictors of work among low-income single mothers. *The American Journal of Orthopsychiatry, 66*, 526–537.

Browne, A., & Bassuk, S. S. (1997). Intimate violence in the lives of homeless and poor housed women: prevalence and patterns in an ethnically diverse sample. *The American Journal of Orthopsychiatry, 67*, 261–278.

Buckner, J. C. (1991). Pathways into homelessness: An epidemiologic analysis. In D. Rog (Ed.), *Evaluating programs for the homeless* (New directions in program evaluation, Vol. 52). San Francisco: Jossey-Bass.

Buckner, J. C. (2004). Epidemiology. In D. Levinson (Ed.), *Encyclopedia of homelessness* (Vol. 1, pp. 130–135). Thousand Oaks, CA: Sage.

Buckner, J. C. (2008). Understanding the impact of homelessness on children: Challenges and future research directions. *American Behavioral Scientist, 51*, 721–736.

Buckner, J. C., Bassuk, E. L., & Zima, B. (1993). Mental health issues affecting homeless women: Implications for intervention. *The American Journal of Orthopsychiatry, 63*, 385–399.

Burt, M. R., Aron, L. Y., Douglas, T., Valente, J., Lee, E., & Iwen, B., et al. (1999). *Homelessness: Programs and the people they serve. Findings of the National Survey of Homeless Assistance Providers and Clients*. Technical Report. Washington, DC: The Urban Institute.

Burt, M. R., & Pearson, C. L., & Montgomery, A. E. (2005). *Strategies for preventing homelessness*. Washington, DC: U.S. Department of Housing and Urban Development.

Caton, C. L. M. (1990). *Homeless in America*. New York: Oxford University Press.

Cheung, E. (2007). *Baby boomers, generation X and social cycles* (North American long-waves, Vol. 1). Toronto: Long wave Press.

Crowley, S. (2004). Low-income housing. In D. Levinson (Ed.), *The encyclopedia of homelessness* (pp. 365–370). Thousand Oaks, CA: Sage.

Culhane, D. P. (1992). The quandaries of shelter reform: An appraisal of efforts to "manage" homelessness. *Social Service Review, 66*, 428–440.

Culhane, D. P., Metraux, S., & Hadley, T. (2001). *The impact of supportive housing for homeless people with severe mental illness on the utilization of the public health, corrections, and emergency shelter systems: The New York–New York initiative*. Washington, DC: Fannie Mae Foundation.

Eaton, W. W. (1995). Studying the natural course of psychopathology. In M. T. Tsuang, M. Tohen, & G. E. P. Zahner (Eds.), *Textbook in psychiatric epidemiology* (pp. 157–177). New York: Wiley.

Economic Policy Institute. (2012). *The China toll: Growing U.S. trade deficit with China*. Washington, DC: Author. Briefing paper #345.

Fischer, P. J., & Breakey, W. R. (1991). The epidemiology of alcohol, drug, and mental disorders among homeless persons. *The American Psychologist, 46*(11), 1115–1128.

Frameworks Institute. (2002). *Framing public issues*. Washington, DC: Authors.

Goodman, L. (1991). The relationship between social support and family homelessness: A comparison study of homeless and housed mothers. *Journal of Community Psychology, 19*, 321–332.

Gould, T. E., & Williams, A. R. (2010). Family homelessness: An investigation of structural effects. *Journal of Human Behavior in the Social Environment, 20*, 170–192.

Hoffman, D., & Rosencheck, R. (2001). Homeless mothers with severe mental illnesses: Predictors of family reunification. *Psychiatric Rehabilitation Journal, 25*, 163–169.

Hopper, K. (2003). *Reckoning with homelessness*. Ithaca, NY: Cornell University Press.

Jencks, C. (1994). *The homeless*. Cambridge, MA: Harvard University Press.

Lowin, A., Demirel, S., Estee, S., & Schreiner, B. (2001). *Homeless families in Washington state: A study of families helped by shelters and their use of welfare and social services*. (Report No. 11.98).

National Housing Affordability Coalition. (2012). *Out of reach 2012*. Washington, DC: Authors.

North, C. S., & Smith, E. M. (1993). A comparison of homeless men and women: Different populations, different needs. *Community Mental Health Journal, 29*(5), 423–431.

Passero, J. M., Zax, M., & Zozus, R. T. (1991). Social network utilization as related to family history among the homeless. *Journal of Community Psychology, 19*, 70–78.

Rog, D. J., McCombs-Thornton, K. L., Gilbert-Mongelli, A. M., Brito, M. C., & Holupka, C. S. (1995). Implementation of the homeless families program: 2. Characteristics, strengths, and needs of participant families. *American Journal of Orthopsychiatry, 65*, 514–528.

Rog, D. J. & Buckner, J. C. (2007). Homeless families and children: Paper presented at the *2007 National Symposium on Homelessness Research*. Washington, DC.

Rog, D. J. & Gutman, M. (1997). The homeless families program: A summary of key findings. In S. Isaacs & J. Knickman (Eds.). *To improve health and health care: The Robert Wood Johnson Foundation Anthology 1997*. San Francisco: Jossey-Bass.

Rossi, P. H. (1989). *Without shelter: Homelessness in the 1980s*. New York: Priority Press Publications.

Schteingart, J. S., Molnar, J., Klein, T. P., Lowe, C. B., & Hartmann, A. H. (1995). Homelessness and child functioning in the context of risk and protective factors moderating child outcomes. *Journal of Clinical Child Psychology, 24*, 320–331.

Schwartz, D. C., Devance-Manzini, D., & Fagan, T. (1991). *Preventing homelessness: A study of state and local homelessness prevention programs.* New Brunswick, NJ: American Affordable Housing Institute.

Sclar, E. D. (1990). Homelessness and housing policy: A game of musical chairs (editorial). *American Journal of Public Health, 80*, 1039–1040.

Shinn, M. (1992). Homelessness: What is a psychologist to do? *American Journal of Community Psychology, 20*, 1–24.

Shinn, M., & Bassuk, E. (2004). Causes of family homelessness. In D. Levinson (Ed.), *Encyclopedia of homelessness* (pp. 153–156). Thousand Oaks, CA: Sage Publications, Inc.

Shinn, M., & Baumohl, J. (1999). Rethinking the prevention of homelessness. In L. Fosburg & D. Dennis (Eds.), *Practical lessons: The 1998 national symposium on homelessness research* (pp. 13-1–13-36). Washington, DC: DHHS.

Shinn, M., Knickman, J. R., & Weitzman, B. C. (1991). Social relationships and vulnerability to becoming homeless among poor families. *American Psychologist, 46*, 1180–1187.

Shinn, M., & Weitzman, B. C. (1996). Homeless families are different. In J. Baumohl (Ed.), *Homelessness in America* (p. 109122). Phoenix, AZ: Oryx.

Shinn, M., Weitzman, B. C., Stojanovic, D., Knickman, J. R., Jiminez, L., Duchon, L., et al. (1998). Predictors of homelessness from shelter request to housing stability among families in New York city. *American Journal of Public Health, 88*, 1651–1657.

Smith, E. M., & North, C. S. (1994). Not all homeless women are alike: Effects of motherhood and the presence of children. *Community Mental Health Journal, 30*, 601–610.

Smith, E. M., North, C. S., & Spitznagel, E. L. (1993). Alcohol, drugs, and psychiatric comorbidity among homeless women: An epidemiologic study. *The Journal of Clinical Psychiatry, 54*(3), 82–87.

Stojanovic, D., Weitzman, B. C., Shinn, M., Labee, L. E., & Williams, N. P. (1999). Tracing the path out of homelessness: The housing patterns of families after exiting shelter. *Journal of Community Psychology, 27*, 199–208.

Stretch, J., & Kreuger, L. W. (1992). Five-year cohort study of homeless families: A joint policy research venture. *Journal of Sociology and Social Welfare, 19*(4), 73–88.

Toohey, S. M., Shinn, M., & Weitzman, B. C. (2004). Social networks and homelessness among women heads of household. *American Journal of Community Psychology, 33*, 7–20.

U.S. Department of Housing and Urban Development. (2012). *The 2010 Annual Homeless Assessment Report to Congress.* Washington, DC

Weinreb, L., Buckner, J. C., Williams, V., & Nicholson, J. (2006). A comparison of the health and mental health status of homeless mothers in Worcester, Mass: 1993 and 2003. *American Journal of Public Health, 96*, 1444–1448.

Weinreb, L., & Rossi, P. H. (1995). The American homeless family shelter "system". *Social Service Review, 69*, 86–101.

Weitzman, B. C. (1989). Pregnancy and childbirth: Risk factors for homelessness? *Family Planning Perspectives, 21*(4), 175–178.

Weitzman, B. C. & Berry, C. (1994). *Formerly homeless families and the transition to permanent housing: High risk families and the role of intensive case management services. Final report to the Edna McConnell Clark Foundation.* New York: Wagner Graduate School.

Wong, Y. L. I., Culhane, D. P., & Kuhn, R. (1997). Predictors of exit and reentry among family shelter users in New York city. *Social Service Review, 71*(3), 441–462.

Zlotnick, C., Robertson, M. J., & Lahiff, M. (1999). Getting off the streets: Economic resources and residential exits from homelessness. *Journal of Community Psychology, 27*, 209–224.

Chapter 2
The Developmental Trajectories of Infants and Young Children Experiencing Homelessness

Katherine T. Volk

Abstract Children under age six are disproportionately more likely than their peers to experience homelessness. Recent advances in developmental science indicate that these are among the most critical years developmentally. This chapter explores the cognitive, social-emotional, and physical developmental paths of infants, toddlers, and preschoolers who have experienced homelessness. Additionally, the prenatal experiences of these children and recommendations for intervention and future research are also provided.

> "Recalling that, in the Universal Declaration of Human Rights, the United Nations has proclaimed that childhood is entitled to special care and assistance...recognizing that the child, for the full and harmonious development of his or her personality, should grow up in a family environment, in an atmosphere of happiness, love and understanding..."
>
> —Preamble, UN Convention on the Rights of the Child

Maya spends most of her day in her stroller, absorbing the chaos around her. Zachary shows little interest in playing and clings to his mother. John is thriving in his preschool program, but once back at the shelter, gets frustrated easily and often has tantrums. What should be happening developmentally for Maya, Zachary, and John? How is homelessness shaping their experience of the world around them, their relationship to their caregiver, and their long-term well-being? What can research tell us about their developmental trajectories and what are the gaps in our knowledge? In this chapter, I explore the cognitive, social–emotional, and physical developmental path of infants, toddlers, and preschoolers who have experienced homeless. I also discuss the prenatal experiences of these children and make recommendations for intervention and further research.

K.T. Volk, M.A. (✉)
Center for Social Innovation

M.E. Haskett et al. (eds.), *Supporting Families Experiencing Homelessness:*
Current Practices and Future Directions, DOI 10.1007/978-1-4614-8718-0_2,
© Springer Science+Business Media New York 2014

In *From Neurons to Neighborhoods*, the authors outline three key domains that characterize the lives of young children from birth to age 5:

1. Acquiring the capacities that undergird communication and learning, including language development, reasoning, and problem-solving (cognitive development).
2. Learning to relate well to others, including the ability to trust, form friendships, nurture, and resolve conflict constructively (social development).
3. Negotiating the development of self-regulation skills, including behavior, emotions, and attention (emotional development).

(Adapted from National Research Council and Institute of Medicine, p. 92).

Children from birth to age 5 also master significant physical tasks—gross and fine motor skills, walking, self-feeding, and potty training, just to name a few. Undergirding all of these developmental pathways is the relationship between the child and his primary caregiver. We are biologically primed to be in attachment relationships—intimate, reliable, nurturing bonds that begin at birth and form the template for all future relationships. Secure attachment relationships enable children to learn self-regulation skills and self-efficacy. They receive the nurturing and love that they need to grow and develop along healthy pathways. Strong attachments help children manage stress, handle novel or fearful situations more confidently, and understand how to trust (Gerhardt, 2004; National Research Council and the Institute of Medicine, 2000).

The well-being of young children is inextricably linked to the well-being of their primary caregivers. The experience of homelessness itself, as well as the experiences of mothers who are homeless, places children at significant risk for insecure or disrupted attachment relationships. Most families (84 %) experiencing homelessness are headed by single women; approximately half of whom have a high school diploma, GED, or less (Burt et al., 1999). Nearly all have experienced severe violent victimization and over one-third have post traumatic stress disorder (PTSD). Half are clinically depressed (Weinreb, Buckner, Williams, & Nicholson, 2006). Maternal depression, particularly when children are very young, has been linked to behavioral and cognitive problems for children in early childhood, including lack of school readiness and delayed language skills (Knitzer, Theberge, & Johnson, 2008). Many mothers who are homeless also struggle with substance use (41 %) and poor physical health (The National Center on Family Homelessness, 2009; Weinreb et al., 2006). These parents must parent their children in public, while facing the stress, shame, and fear of living without a home (Friedman, 2000; Gerson, 2006).

Children who are homeless are separated from their caregivers more often than other children. Over 30 % have been the subject of a child protection investigation and the rates of foster care placement are much higher than in the general population: 12 % compared to slightly more than 1 %. Twenty-two percent of children experiencing homelessness have been separated from their families at some point (David, 2010; The National Center on Family Homelessness, 1999). As noted by Guarino and Bassuk (2010), "An unsafe or disrupted relationship with a primary caregiver is one of the most traumatic experiences that a child can face and has a profound impact on health and well-being" (p. 12). The impact of separation on the caregiver, child, and family unit is not to be underestimated.

Much has been written about the lives of children experiencing homelessness, but rarely have children's lives at each developmental stage and across developmental domains been discussed. This is particularly important in early childhood—which represents the period of most rapid growth. The following sections will provide an overview of the influence of homelessness on early child development by developmental stage and developmental domain.

Prenatal Experiences

An infant's prenatal experience informs how the architecture of his brain develops, what his cognitive abilities and early learning experiences may be, and his physical health and well-being (National Research Council and the Institute of Medicine, 2000; Rouse & Fantuzzo, 2008). It also may inform how the mother and baby are able to bond and attach. Thus, the prenatal experiences of children who experience homelessness are critical to understanding their developmental trajectories, especially in infancy. Sadly, the "parental characteristics during pregnancy that lead to optimal development stand in stark contrast" to the situations facing mothers experiencing homelessness (David, Gelberg, & Suchman, 2012, p. 3).

Children experiencing homelessness are more likely to have been born at low birth weight, which puts them at risk for other developmental challenges, including fair or poor health, asthma, and hospitalization (Richards, Merrill, & Baksh, 2011; Richards, Merrill, Baksh, & McGarry, 2010; Weinreb, Goldberg, Bassuk, & Perloff, 1998). Furthermore, their mothers are less likely to receive adequate prenatal care (Richards et al., 2011, 2010), which is associated with additional adverse health outcomes such as preterm delivery, being small-for-gestational age, and infant mortality. "There is evidence that a broad spectrum of critical post-natal parenting tasks, including responding to the physical and emotional needs of the infant, teaching and exposing children to new cognitive experiences, and promoting children's emotional growth and autonomy are predicted by pre-birth psychosocial characteristics of the parent" (David et al., 2012, p. 2–3).

Older children with a history of biological birth risks such as those just described are more likely to experience other risks as well (Rouse & Fantuzzo, 2008), including academic and social difficulties. As Rouse and Fantuzzo (2008) describe, "basic early childhood competencies that are necessary for school success are significantly compromised by multiple risk factors in the first few years of life…including premature birth, low birth weight, and inadequate prenatal care…[these risks] compromise early cognitive ability and hinder children's capacity to capitalize on early educational opportunities" (p. 1).

Infancy (Birth: 12 Months)

Developmental scientists have documented that there are sensitive periods in a child's development. Sensitive periods are defined as limited spans of time when experiences are particularly impactful on brain development (Knudsen, 2004). Infancy is the first of these. The primary developmental tasks in infancy are the formation of attachment relationships which provide a foundation for developing an increasing capacity for future developmental achievements. These relationships are formed in the context of intense physical growth. In *Why Love Matters: How Affection Shapes the Brain*, author Sue Gerhardt describes the profound impact of early attachments: "Expectations of other people and how they will behave are inscribed in the brain outside conscious awareness, in the period of infancy, and… they underpin our behavior in relationships through life" (p. 24).

Cognitive and Social–Emotional Development

At birth, infants have approximately 100 billion neurons, most of which are not yet connected. In fact, their field of vision is only 9–12 in. As the baby is introduced to stimuli, her neural pathways are either reinforced or pruned (Shore, 1997). Secure attachment relationships, appropriate exposure to and protection from stimuli, and nurturing attention to physical needs all help to create a healthy brain that will enable the toddler, the child, and eventually the adult, to form relationships, think analytically, regulate emotions, and cope effectively with stress.

The shelter environment is often the opposite of what infants need for healthy cognitive and social–emotional development. Shelters are noisy, crowded, too hot or too cold, and may struggle with bedbugs and other pests (Fantuzzo, LeBoeuf, Brumely, & Perlman, 2013; Friedman, 2000; Gerson, 2006; Giraud, 2013; Perlman & Fantuzzo, 2010). Infants need controlled access to healthy stimuli, but instead may become "emotionally flooded and overcome by hunger, physical discomfort, and frustration" (David et al., 2012, p. 4).

For homeless infants, mothers are typically their primary (and often only) caregiver. As described above and in Chap. 5 of this volume, these women face significant challenges to their own well-being. Half struggle with depression while homeless and 85 % have had a major depressive episode in the past (Weinreb et al., 2006). In the midst of these challenges, caregiver responses to infant stress cues may be misaligned or missed altogether. These circumstances set the infant up for insecure attachment (Easterbrooks & Graham, 1997; Guarino & Bassuk, 2010) because the mother is more likely to be physically and/or emotionally unavailable or an unpredictable source of comfort and regulation.

A handful of studies have examined the long-term effects of homeless on young children. Shinn and colleagues (2008) compared formerly homeless children with their housed peers 55 months after shelter entry. Findings demonstrated that 4–6 year old children who experienced homelessness during infancy and toddlerhood were the group most impacted in terms of development. In addition, these children exhibited more internalizing and externalizing problems than housed children. Similarly, Fantuzzo et al. (2013) studied a cohort of approximately 10,600 third-graders, 9.8 % of whom had experienced homelessness. Study results showed that experiences of homelessness in infancy were uniquely related to lower rates of classroom engagement. Another related study demonstrated that children who experienced their first episode of homelessness as infants scored three and a half to four points lower than their housed peers on second grade standardized assessments of language, reading, and math (Perlman & Fantuzzo, 2010). As Shinn and colleagues concluded, very young children "may have been at a particularly vulnerable stage of development and particularly sensitive to maternal stress" (p. 804).

Physical Development

Infants' physical growth is impressive. In addition to the burst of brain development described earlier, most babies will double their weight in the first 5 months of life. They learn to suck, coo, and focus their gaze. They develop muscles, hold up their heads, roll over, reach and grab, sit up, and eventually, crawl. Shelter environments may not provide safe, clean places for infants to develop these skills. As one mother living in a shelter described, "I never put him on the floor. It's filthy." Even if floors are clean, caregivers may not have the space to put a blanket on the floor for their infants to move. They may be worried that the baby will be stepped on by other children or that the floor may be too cold or hard. Furthermore, research demonstrates that infants born to mothers who were homeless had significantly longer hospital stays, were more likely to require intensive care, and had a lower duration of breastfeeding (Richards et al., 2011, 2010).

Touch also plays a vital role in infant development. For example, when a caregiver strokes a baby's foot, it reinforces neural pathways that help the baby map the boundaries of her body. When held close, the caregiver's body temperature helps to regulate the body temperature of the baby. It provides safety and security that helps form the solid attachment relationships described earlier. Infants experiencing homelessness seem to spend much of their time in strollers or carriers, physically separated from their caregiver. Maternal depression can further inhibit physical bonds.

Toddlerhood (13–36 Months)

Toddlers can be extraordinarily frustrating, as many parents will describe. The National Network for Child Care sums it up this way: "Toddlers are long on will and short on skill" (Malley, 1991). In the context of homelessness, toddlers and their developmental needs face new challenges: lack of safe spaces to explore, crowded facilities that are overstimulating, and lack of ability for a parent to have privacy with his/her child (David, 2010; Fantuzzo et al., 2013; Friedman, 2000; Perlman & Fantuzzo, 2010). Furthermore, as children grow older, the accumulation of stressors begins to take its toll.

Cognitive Development

By age 3, the brains of children are two and half times more active than adult brains, a level of activity that remains constant through the first decade of life (Shore, 1997). Examining toddler language development provides a window into this burst of developmental activity. At 18 months, most children begin learning an average of nine new words every day, through early childhood (Neurons, p. 127). Although the research on language acquisition specifically for toddlers experiencing homelessness is limited, we do know that children who grow up in households with high income and high parent education levels have more than double the expressive vocabulary at age 3 compared to children raised in low-income homes (Center for the Developing Child, 2007). In fact, by age 3, a low-income child has heard 30 million fewer words than her higher-income peers (Hart & Risley, 2003). Inability to communicate effectively may heighten the frustration a toddler feels, as he/she seeks more independence and tries to cope with stressful circumstances.

More broadly, children who are homeless during this period begin to display developmental delays. In a study conducted in Worcester, Massachusetts with homeless and housed children, researchers observed that children's developmental trajectories were normative until about 18 months, particularly on cognitive tasks. Using the Bayley Scales of Infant Development and the Vineland Screener—both rigorous measures—researchers examined sensory-perceptual acuities, memory, learning, problem-solving ability, vocalization, and early signs of the ability to form generalizations. After 18 months, children's scores decreased, leading researchers to conclude that "the significant decreases in scores with age may be due to the cumulative effect of an impoverished, high-risk environment, to which all these children were exposed, and the increasing cognitive and verbal demands with increasing age in developmental assessments" (Garcia Coll et al., 1998, p. 1372).

Toddlerhood is a sensitive period of development and the limited opportunities for exploration that come with being homeless may have a long-lasting impact. For example, in their study of third-graders, Fantuzzo et al. (2013) learned that children who were first homeless as toddlers were 60 % more likely to not meet math proficiency standards, compared to children who first experienced homelessness in elementary school. A study by Perlman and Fantuzzo (2010) showed similar results when examining the academic proficiency of second-graders who had experienced homelessness as toddlers. Students who had experienced homelessness as toddlers scored four to six points lower on standardized academic achievement outcomes (math, reading, language, and vocabulary) compared to those who had not experienced homelessness.

Social–Emotional Development

Toddlers look to their caregiver to provide a safe base from which they can explore the world and return for comfort, guidance, and regulation. Parents provide the scaffolding to help them grow their skills—from learning how to turn the pages of a book gently, to brushing their teeth, to letting them help with household tasks. "I do it" may be the sentence spoken most often by toddlers, who are eager to try out their newfound mobility and ever-expanding social abilities.

Research is limited on the social–emotional development of homeless toddlers specifically. In one study of young homeless mothers and their children, staff reported that mothers became more frustrated with their children's behavior at around 18 months (DeCandia, 2012). While this may be true for many parents of young children, the dynamic is likely exacerbated by the experience of homelessness. Toddlers crave routine, predictability, and reliable caregivers. The stress homeless toddlers are surrounded by, from their caregivers and the shelter environment, can impact their ability to regulate their emotions and may lead to regression and fight-flight-freeze responses, making a challenging stage of development all the more difficult.

Physical Development

Like in other areas of toddler development, children reach major physical milestones during this period. They learn to walk, run, jump, throw, and kick with intention. Their sleep–wake patterns become more stable. Their motor skills become sophisticated enough to hold a crayon and scribble on paper. They begin using utensils for eating. By the end of toddlerhood, potty training has begun.

Empirical research on the physical development of toddlers experiencing homelessness is particularly limited, but we do know that shelter environments often do not give toddlers the opportunities they need to move and explore. Children may have limited space to run and climb. Rules may dictate that children be kept quiet or be confined to a particular space. Opportunities to play outdoors may be limited at best. Parents may be hesitant to let their children be as active as they need and want to be, because of safety concerns and fear of getting in trouble with staff or other parents.

Early Childhood (3–6 Years)

As children move from toddlerhood to early childhood, they build on and weave together the developmental tasks of the prior 3 years; social–emotional skills begin to emerge more definitively, their cognitive skills are increasingly sophisticated, and their systems are physically stable and strong. They are preparing to individuate and assert their autonomy yet they need a safe, reassuring emotional and physical environment and caregiver relationship.

Strong attachment relationships established from birth to this point become protective factors that can buffer the negative impact of the shelter environment. However, given the tendency towards poor attachment in early years, children who are homeless may experience high levels of unregulated behavior, a lack of stimulating and developmentally appropriate toys, and limited access to literacy materials that foster language and academic development (David et al., 2012; The National Center on Family Homelessness, 2009). Additionally, when children have been exposed to high rates of toxic stress, their cognition, memory, and emotional regulation skills may be significantly impacted (National Scientific Council on the Developing Child, 2010).

Cognitive Development

Building on the bursts of language development that occurred in toddlerhood, preschool children begin to develop literacy and numeracy skills and simple problem-solving skills. Children's prekindergarten cognitive skills strongly predict later academic success (National Research Council and the Institute of Medicine, 2000). When Shinn and colleagues (2008) examined cognitive measures among 4–6 year olds, children who experienced homelessness were one standard deviation below normative ranges. Using a large administrative data set, Rouse and Fantuzzo (2008) examined academic achievement and behavioral outcomes in 10,300 second-graders. They examined risk factors including low birth weight, poor prenatal care, low maternal education, poverty, homeless experience, and child maltreatment. Homelessness was related to not meeting reading proficiency standards at end of second grade. The more risk factors the child had, the more likely she was to have poor reading and mathematical skills. The study also showed that low maternal education, homelessness, and biological birth risks (e.g., low birth weight) all increased the odds of poor learning behavior—that is, persistence, initiation, academic motivation, and positive interactions with teachers and peers during instruction.

Social–Emotional Development

Beginning around age 3, researchers have found that children who experience homelessness have mental health issues at greater rates than their housed peers. Approximately 20 % of homeless preschoolers demonstrate clinically significant emotional disturbances (The National Center on Family Homelessness, 1999). In a study of 5,000 homeless, doubled-up, and low-income housed children, Park and colleagues (2011) learned that the health, cognitive development, and health care use were similar among all subgroups, with the exception of mental health. At 3 years of age, 28 % of homeless children demonstrated clinically significant internalizing symptoms on the Child Behavior Checklist, compared to 19 % of low-income housed children. In Rouse and Fantuzzo's study (2008), controlling for all other risk factors, homelessness was one of the strongest indicators for high absenteeism, school suspensions, and teacher-rated low social skills. This likely has to do with the experience of homelessness itself, particularly the instability and high mobility.

Physical Development

Children who experience homelessness also tend to experience a number of chronic and acute health problems, and of those, asthma "has become a hallmark of poor health among homeless children" (The National Center on Family Homelessness, 2009). Exact figures vary by study. The National Center on Family Homelessness (2009) reports that one in nine children who are homeless has one or more asthma-related conditions. A study that exclusively focused on 4–7 year olds experiencing homelessness in Minnesota showed that 27.9 % had asthma—three times the state average (Cutuli, Herbers, Rinaldi, Masten, & Oberg, 2010). The condition seemed to be both "severe and poorly managed," (Cutuli et al., 2010, p. 150) which led to missed days of school, limited opportunities to play actively and with peers, and caused additional stress for parent and child (The National Center on Family Homelessness, 2009). Asthma also has the potential to negatively impact other areas of functioning, including hyperactivity/inattention, behavior problems, and lower academic functioning.

Strategies to Foster Normative Developmental Trajectories

To examine the developmental pathways for children experiencing homelessness is to examine the accumulation of risk. As developmental stages build on one another, so do experiences of trauma, hardship, and deprivation. The mother who is homeless and pregnant is at risk for negative prenatal experiences, which places the child at risk for future difficulties. That risk is the first layer, which may be compounded as the child moves through infancy, then toddlerhood, then the preschool years.

But, not all children experiencing risks evidence adverse outcomes—many evidence resilience. As Ann Masten (2001) writes, "resilience does not come from rare and special qualities, but from the everyday magic of ordinary, normative human resources in the minds, brains, and bodies of children, in their families and relationships, and in their communities" (235). In other words, we must nurture children's ordinary systems—their physical, cognitive, and social–emotional well-being. Strong attachment relationships, well-developed self-regulation skills, the presence of supportive adults, and opportunities to exercise their problem-solving skills are just a few of the ways we can support children.

The *Strengthening at Risk and Homeless Young Mothers and Children* Initiative, a collaboration among The National Center on Family Homelessness, the National Alliance to End Homelessness, and ZERO TO THREE, outlined three major goals to working with homeless and at-risk families (DeCandia, 2012). These goals, although focused on young families in particular, have broad applicability to families experiencing homelessness. They are as follows:

1. Stabilize Families in Housing. Working to eliminate poverty and prevent and end homelessness must be our ultimate goals. However, in the interim, we must work to find safe, stable housing for children and families as quickly as possible and then support families in creating stable lives in the community, connected to formal and informal supports that nurture caregivers and children alike.
2. Reduce Risk Factors. There are a number of ways to reduce the many risk factors facing children and their caregivers discussed in this Chapter. Here are just a few:

   (a) Improve access to routine medical care. One in ten children experiencing homelessness has not seen a doctor in the previous year. These children are using emergency rooms as their primary source of health care instead and seeking assistance only when problems are severe and urgent (Burt & Sharkey, 2002). Pediatricians have a prime opportunity to support and nurture these children's well-being across various developmental domains. The American Academy of Pediatrics has called on pediatricians to take a more ecological view of their role in the care of children (Shonkoff, J., Garner, A., and the Committee on Psychosocial Aspects of Child and Family Health, Committee on Early Childhood, Adoption, and Dependent Care, and Section on Developmental and Behavioral Pediatrics, 2012; Shonkoff et al., 2012) and to make the reduction of toxic stress in the lives of children a high priority.

   (b) Encourage enrollment in the Special Supplemental Nutrition Program for Women, Infants, and Children (WIC). WIC participation has been associated with beneficial maternal health behaviors, including initiation and duration of prenatal visits and infant health outcomes and initiation of breastfeeding (Richards et al., 2011, 2010).

   (c) Support/implement home visiting programs. Evidence-based home visiting programs have been shown to improve birth outcomes, child health and development, school readiness, and to reduce child abuse and neglect. These programs also are supportive of caregivers, reducing maternal stress and depression, improving parenting attitudes and knowledge, improving child–parent bonds, and increasing parent access to services (including education and employment resources). The Nurse–Family Partnership, Healthy Families America, Parents as Teachers, and Home Instruction Program for Preschool Youngsters are among the best-known and most thoroughly evaluated home visiting programs (McDonald & Grandin, 2009).

   (d) Provide training and other educational opportunities. Work with parents and program staff to become keen observers of child behavior. From infancy, children communicate with us. We must be highly attuned to messages they are sending.

3. Build Solid Foundations for Individual and Family Development.

(a) Utilize Early Intervention services and encourage participation in high quality early childhood programs. Early Intervention programs are aimed at enhancing the development of infants and young children and minimizing the risk of developmental delays. Some work intensively with the child, while others focus on both parent(s) and child (Goode, Diefendorf, & Colgan, 2011). They have been shown to benefit children across multiple domains of development, including cognition and academic achievement, behavioral and emotional competencies, educational progression and attainment, child maltreatment, health, delinquency and crime, social welfare program use, and labor market success (Rand, 2005).

(b) Create developmentally rich and appropriate environments. In organizations and in the child's home, ensure that there are developmentally appropriate toys and other materials, including access to books and word games to encourage literacy skills, adequate space to play, and materials that encourage creativity and imagination.

(c) Support breastfeeding whenever possible. Breastfeeding is good for babies, good for mothers, and an important tool in creating strong attachment and bonding between mother and child (see The National Center on Family Homelessness and the American Academy of Pediatrics for resources).

(d) Connect families to family-focused programs in the community. Community centers, libraries, and civic organizations often offer developmentally appropriate, free programming for young children and their caregivers.

(e) Support caregivers. Children's well-being hinges on their caregiver's well-being, especially when they are young. Supporting caregivers through peer groups, opportunities for respite, and other social supports ultimately creates better developmental outcomes for the child.

Given the prevalence of traumatic experiences in the lives of homeless children and families, adopting trauma-informed perspective is essential to working with them. Trauma-informed care is defined as a "strengths-based framework that is grounded in an understanding of and responsiveness to the impact of trauma, that emphasizes physical, psychological, and emotional safety for both providers and survivors, and that creates opportunities for survivors to rebuild a sense of control and empowerment" (Hopper, Bassuk, & Olivet, 2010). See Chap. 8 (Guarino), this volume for a full discussion of trauma-informed practices.

Studies of children experiencing homelessness do not seem to consistently deconstruct the developmental trajectories of young children at particular stages. It would be helpful and instructive for the research community to report their findings based on age groupings that are parallel to developmental stages rather than grouping all young children together. Additionally, much homelessness research compares homeless children to housed peers living in poverty, which often reveals minimal if any differences in the trajectories of these two groups. We must change our perspective. Homeless or housed, children living in poverty is not acceptable. As we work to end homelessness, so must we work to end poverty and nurture those "ordinary systems" that promote children's well-being.

References

Burt, M. R. & Sharkey, P. (2002). *The role of Medicaid in improving access to care for homeless people*. Washington, DC: The Urban Institute. Retrieved November 29, 2008, from Access to care report, Burt et al. www.urban.org/publications/410595.html.

Burt, M., et al. (1999). *Homelessness: Programs and the people they serve*. Washington, DC: The Urban Institute. Retrieved from www.urbaninstitute.org.

Center for the Developing Child at Harvard University. (2007). *In brief: The impact of early adversity on children's development*. Retrieved February 13, 2013, from http://developingchild.harvard.edu/index.php/resources/briefs/inbrief_series/inbrief_the_impact_of_early_adversity.

Cutuli, J., Herbers, J., Rinaldi, M., Masten, A., & Oberg, C. (2010). Asthma and behavior in homeless 4- to 7- year-olds. *Pediatrics, 125*, 145–151.

David, D., Gelberg, L., & Suchman, N. (2012). Implications of homelessness for parenting young children: A preliminary review from a developmental attachment perspective. *Infant Mental Health Journal, 33*, 1–9.

DeCandia, C. (2012). *Designing developmentally-based services for young homeless families*. Needham, MA: The National Center on Family Homelessness. Retrieved April 19, 2013, from http://www.familyhomelessness.org/media/313.pdf.

Easterbrooks, M. A., & Graham, C. A. (1997). Security of attachment and parenting: Homeless and low-income housed mothers and infants. *The American Journal of Orthopsychiatry, 69*, 337–346.

Fantuzzo, J., LeBoeuf, W., Brumely, B., & Perlman, S. (2013). A population-based inquiry of homeless episode characteristics and early education wellbeing. *Children and Youth Services Review, 35*, 966–972.

Friedman, D. H. (2000). *Parenting in public: Family shelter and public assistance*. New York: Columbia University Press.

Garcia Coll, C., Buckner, J. C., Brooks, M. G.,Weinreb, L. F., & Bassuk, E. L. (1998). The developmental status and adaptive behavior of homeless and low-income housed infants and toddlers. *American Journal of Public Health, 88*, 1371–1374.

Gerhardt, S. (2004). *Why love matters: How affection shapes a baby's brain*. New York: Routledge.

Gerson, J. (2006). *Hope springs maternal: Homeless mothers talk about making sense of adversity*. New York: Gordian Knot Books.

Giraud, J. M. (2013). *D.C.'s new status quo: Homeless families, children left in the cold. Huffington post*. Retrieved April 19, 2013, from http://www.huffingtonpost.com/jeanmichel-giraud/dcs-new-status-quo-homele_b_2735650.html.

Goode, S., Diefendorf, M., & Colgan, S. (2011). *The importance of early intervention for infants and toddlers with disabilities and their families*. National Early Childhood Technical Assistance Center. Retrieved April 19, 2013, from http://www.nectac.org/~pdfs/pubs/importanceofearly-intervention.pdf.

Guarino, K. & Bassuk, E. (2010). *Working with families experiencing homelessness: Understanding trauma and its impact*. ZERO TO THREE. Retrieved February 13, 2013, from http://main.zerotothree.org/site/DocServer/Working_With_Families_Experiencing_Homelessness.pdf?docID=10741.

Hart, B. & Risley, T. (2003). *The early catastrophe: The 30 million word gap by age three. Taken from an article excerpted with permission from meaningful differences in the everyday experiences of young American children, 1995, Brookes publishing*. Retrieved April 19, 2013, from http://www.gsa.gov/graphics/pbs/The_Early_Catastrophe_30_Million_Word_Gap_by_Age_3.pdf.

Hopper, E., Bassuk, E., & Olivet, J. (2010). Shelter from the storm: Trauma-informed care in homelessness service settings. *The Open Health Services and Policy Journal, 3*, 80–100. Retrieved from www.homeless.samhsa.gov/ResourceFiles/cenfdthy.pdf.

Knudsen, E. I. (2004). Sensitive periods in the development of the brain and behavior. *Journal of Cognitive Neuroscience, 16*, 1412–1425.

Knitzer, J., Theberge, S., & Johnson, K. (2008). *Project thrive issue brief number 2: Reducing maternal depression and its impact on young children: Toward a responsive early childhood policy framework.* National Center for Children in Poverty, Columbia University, Mailman School of Public Health. Retrieved February 13, 2013, from http://www.nccp.org/publications/pdf/text_791.pdf.

Malley, C. (1991). *Toddler development (family day care facts series).* National Network for Child Care. Amherst, MA: University of Massachusetts. Retrieved April 19, 2013, from http://www.nncc.org/child.dev/todd.dev.html.

Masten, A. (2001). Ordinary magic: Resilience processes in development. *American Psychologist, 56*, 235.

McDonald, S. & Grandin, M. (2009). *Early education home visiting: Supporting children experiencing homelessness.* Needham, MA: The National Center on Family Homelessness. Retrieved April 19, 2013, from http://www.familyhomelessness.org/media/184.pdf

National Research Council and the Institute of Medicine. (2000). *From neurons to neighborhoods: The science of early childhood development.* In J. P. Shonkoff & D. A. Phillips (Eds.), Committee on Integrating the Science of Early Childhood Development. Board on Children, Youth, and Families, Commission on Behavioral and Social Sciences and Education. Washington, DC: National Academy Press.

National Scientific Council on the Developing Child (2010). *Persistent fear and anxiety can affect young children's learning and development: Working paper no. 9.* Retrieved April 19, 2013, from http://www.developingchild.net.

Park, J., Fertig, A., & Allison, P. (2011). Physical and mental health, cognitive development, and health care use by housing status of low-income young children in 20 American cities: A prospective cohort study. *American Journal of Public Health, 101*, S255–S261.

Perlman, S., & Fantuzzo, J. (2010). Timing and influence of early experiences of child maltreatment and homelessness on children's educational wellbeing. *Children and Youth Services Review, 32*, 874–883.

Rand. (2005). *Proven benefits of early childhood interventions.* In L. A. Karoly, M. R. Kilburn, & J. S. Cannon (Eds.), *Early childhood interventions: Proven results, future promise.* Retrieved April 19, 2013, from http://www.rand.org/pubs/research_briefs/RB9145/index1.html.

Richards, R., Merrill, R., & Baksh, L. (2011). Health behaviors and infant health outcomes in homeless pregnant women in the United States. *Pediatrics, 128*, 438–446.

Richards, R., Merrill, R., Baksh, L., & McGarry, J. (2010). Maternal health behaviors and infant health outcomes among homeless mothers: U.S. Special supplemental nutrition program for women, infants, and children (WIC) 2000–2007. *Preventive Medicine, 52*, 87–94.

Rouse, H., & Fantuzzo, J. (2008). Multiple risks and educational well being: A population-based investigation of threats to early school success. *Early Childhood Research Quarterly, 24*, 1–14.

Shinn, M., Schteingert, J., Williams, N., Carlin-Mathis, J., Bialo-Karagis, N., Becker-Klein, R., et al. (2008). Long-term associations of homelessness with children's well-being. *American Behavioral Scientist, 51*, 789–809.

Shonkoff, J., Garner, A., & The Committee on Psychosocial Aspects of Child and Family Health, Committee on Early Childhood, Adoption, and Dependent Care, and Section on Developmental and Behavioral Pediatrics. (2012). Technical reports: The lifelong effects of early childhood adversity and toxic stress. *Pediatrics, 129*, e232–e246.

Shonkoff, J., Siegel, B., Dobbins, M., Earls, M., Garner, A., McGuinn, L., et al. (2012). Early childhood adversity, toxic stress, and the role of the pediatrician: Translating developmental science into lifelong health. *Pediatrics, 129*, e224–e231.

Shore, R. (1997). What have we learned? In *Rethinking the brain* (pp. 15–27). New York: Families and Work Institute.

The National Center on Family Homelessness. (1999). *Homeless children: America's new outcasts.* Newton, MA.

The National Center on Family Homelessness. (2009). *America's youngest outcasts: State report card on child homelessness.* Newton, MA: The National Center on Family Homelessness.

Weinreb, L., Buckner, J., Williams, V., & Nicholson, J. (2006). A comparison of the health and mental health status of homeless mothers in Worcester, Mass: 1993 and 2003. *American Journal of Public Health, 96,* 1444–1448.

Weinreb, L., Goldberg, R., Bassuk, E., & Perloff, J. N. (1998). Determinants of health and service use patterns in homeless and low-income housed children. *Pediatrics, 102,* 554–562.

Chapter 3
Trauma Exposures and Mental Health Outcomes Among Sheltered Children and Youth Ages 6–18

Beryl Ann Cowan

Abstract Children living in families without homes endure multiple risks associated with poor mental health and adaptive functioning. Research over a 20-year period has demonstrated that this growing population of vulnerable children is at risk for elevated rates of internalizing and externalizing disorders and symptoms associated with posttraumatic stress. School-age children also lag behind peers due to high rates of learning disabilities and cognitive delays. This chapter outlines research in the area and provides recommendations for promoting positive mental health outcomes in precariously housed children and families.

Families with children comprise almost 40 % of the population of persons without homes in the USA (National Alliance to Homelessness, 2010; National Center on Family Homelessness, 2012). Approximately 1.6 million children are reported to be homeless in the USA each year (National Law Center on Homelessness and Poverty, 2004). This is most likely an *underestimate* of the population; census data do not include families doubling up with relatives and friends, those living in hard to reach places, or those turned away from emergency homeless service centers (Gould & Williams, 2010; Samuels, Shinn, & Buckner, 2010; US Conference of Mayors, 2012). While other subpopulations of persons without homes have decreased in recent years, most notably single adults experiencing *chronic* housing instability (Annual Report on Homelessness, 2012), the numbers of families living without homes has risen and is expected to continue to increase due to economic conditions that most adversely affect those who are already poor (Culhane, Webb, Grimm, Metraux, & Culhane, 2003; Cunningham, 2009; Joint Center for Housing Studies of Harvard University, 2011; Nicols, 2012; Pelletiere, 2009; US Conference of Mayors, 2012). Structural conditions that increase the risk of housing instability are created

B.A. Cowan, J.D., Ph.D. (✉)
Clinical and Community Psychologist and Consultant, Boston, MA, USA
e-mail: berylanncowan@gmail.com

M.E. Haskett et al. (eds.), *Supporting Families Experiencing Homelessness: Current Practices and Future Directions*, DOI 10.1007/978-1-4614-8718-0_3, © Springer Science+Business Media New York 2014 by high rates of unemployment; the reduction of federal benefits and state subsidies for housing; the mortgage crisis with its attendant rise in foreclosures; and the influx of more consumers seeking low income and affordable rentals in markets already under-resourced to meet demand (Cronley, 2010; Cunningham, 2009; Joint Center for Housing Studies of Harvard University, 2011). As Buckner (Chap. 1 of this volume) and others have described, the prevalence of cumulative psychosocial risk factors in the lives of marginalized and poor families such as substance abuse, mental illness, and experiences of interpersonal violence, increases the likelihood that episodes of housing loss will occur (Bassuk et al., 1997; Browne, 1993; Caton et al., 2005; Haber & Toro, 2004; Koegel, Melamid, & Burnam, 1995; Lehmann, Kass, Drake, & Nichols, 2007; Shinn et al., 1998; Van den Bree et al., 2009).

While most families without homes are comprised of a mother with relatively young children, approximately 40 % of the children living in shelters are under age 6 (National Center on Family Homelessness, 2010). Recent trends reflect more two parent families with older children are in acute need of emergency housing and related services (US Conference of Mayors, 2012). Housing instability is highly stressful for *all* family members, yet the unique developmental needs of children and youth make the amalgam of homeless-related stressors particularly difficult and can lead to enduring ramifications for adjustment (Anooshian, 2005; Browne, 1993; Gewirtz, Hart-Shegos, & Medhanie, 2008; Goodman, Saxe, & Harvey, 1991; Masten, Miliotis, Graham-Bermann, Ramirez, & Neemann, 1993; McCaskill, Toro, & Wolfe, 1998; Muñoz, Vazquez, Bermejo, & Vazquez, 1999). Based on 20 years of scholarly investigations and a robust literature, this chapter focuses on risks to well-being of children who experience homelessness and on what is known about the mental health and adaptive functioning of school-age children without homes.

Stressors Associated with Homelessness

Events *leading up* to housing loss are often traumatic for parents and children and the increased stress can negatively impact the tenor of their interactions (Anooshian, 2005; Anderson, Stuttaford & Vostanis, 2006; Browne, 2003; Muñoz et al., 1999; Yo, North, LaVesser, Osborne, & Spitznagel, 2008). Such events are likely to include eviction, natural disasters, geographic moves, and flight from episodes of domestic violence (Anderson et al., 2006; Burt & Aron, 2000; Caton et al., 2005). Once displaced from their homes, adults and children alike experience the turmoil of housing uncertainty; the loss of personal possessions and a sense of place; and the fraying of bonds with neighborhood friends and extended family members (Cowan, 2007; Rafferty, Shinn, & Weitzman, 2004; Rog & Buckner, 2007). Housing loss often results in the separation of family members from each other (Barrow & Lawinski, 2009; Cowal, Shinn, Weitzman, Stojanovic, & Labay, 2002). Many shelters refuse to admit male caregivers and boys as well adolescent siblings of both genders. Other shelters have restrictions on the number of family members that may be served. Children who are separated from parents may end up living with friends or relatives or enter foster care (Cowal et al., 2002; Culhane et al., 2003; Park,

Metraux, Brodbar, & Culhane, 2004). The unnecessary separation of siblings, parents, and caregivers adds to the stress, anxiety, and loss felt by all family members.

Homelessness forces families to live under unsuitable conditions. Children without homes may spend days accompanying their parents to various social service agencies looking for a place to stay for the night, as well as for longer-term accommodations. Until stable housing is found, many families live in overcrowded motels without kitchen facilities, in congregant emergency shelters, or doubled up with family members and friends. Other families live in cars, train stations, parks, camp grounds, or empty buildings not meant for habitation. Leaving known surroundings and then moving from place to place, often among strangers, can frighten children as well as interrupt important family rituals and routines (Anooshian, 2005; Buckner, Bassuk, Weinreb, & Brooks, 1999; Cowan, 2007; Friedman, 2000; Goodman et al., 1991; Samuels et al., 2010). Children can be forced to undertake age-inappropriate caretaking with long-term negative consequences for their own adjustment (Byng-Hall, 2002; Jurkovic, 1997).

A significant stressor associated with homelessness is extreme and enduring poverty, a condition related to a host of negative outcomes for young children. A continuum of psychosocial stressors and destabilizing events that often occur in the context of poverty can alone and in combination interrupt emotional and behavioral trajectories during childhood (Attar, Guerra, & Tolan, 1994; Barrera et al., 2002; Conger, Ge, Elder, Lorenz, & Simmons, 1994; Garmezy, Masten, & Tellegen, 1984; Graham-Bermann, Coupet, Egler, Mattis, & Bayard, 1996; Masten et al., 1993; Rutter, 1987). Beginning at conception, socioeconomic disparities such as lack of health care access, poor nutrition, unsafe neighborhoods, and residential proximity to environmental toxins create conditions that deleteriously impact typical development and healthy functioning (Ratcliffe & McKernan, 2012; Shonkoff & Phillips, 2000). People living in poverty, when compared with the general population, are more often exposed to interpersonal and community violence, harming both victims and those that witness such events (Gorman-Smith & Tolan, 1998; Popkin, Acs, & Smith, 2009; Toth, Harris, Goodman, & Cicchetti, 2011). Child abuse and neglect exists at higher rates in poor families, creating lifelong scars and unhealthy patterns for interpersonal relationships (Anooshian, 2005; Ford et al., 2000). High rates of chronic illness, untreated mental illness, and substance abuse among poor parents inhibits functioning across domains, including the ability of parents to adequately care for and protect their children (Anderson et al., 2006; Buckner et al., 1999; Conger et al., 1994; Gravener et al., 2012). Social inequities that historically have impacted the poor, and especially ethnic minorities and persons of color, are translated into poor schools and inadequate training opportunities (Leventhal & Brooks-Gunn, 2000; Leventhal, Dupree, & Brooks-Gunn, 2009; Sampson, Morenoff, & Gannon-Rowley, 2002; Shinn, 2002). A majority of children born into poverty will remain so into their adulthoods (McDonald, 2012; Ratcliffe & McKernan, 2012; Van den Bree et al., 2009). Given the cumulative risks faced by children living in poverty, it is not surprising that disadvantaged children have higher rates of developmental delays, cognitive and physical disabilities, chronic illnesses, and emotional and behavioral disturbances than those raised in affluent communities (Toth, Harris, Goodman, & Cicchetti, 2012; Yo et al., 2008). High rates of unidentified or untreated learning disabilities impair academic success for many, and rates of truancy, grade retention, and dropout are high (Zima, Bussing, Forness, & Benjamin, 1997). Poor children are more likely to live with family members with mental illness and/or substance abuse, both of which are highly correlated with impaired social–emotional and behavioral functioning in youngsters (Gravener et al., 2012; Herring & Kaslow, 2002).

For some children, the stressors associated with homelessness and poverty discussed above are experienced as traumatic. Trauma occurs when an individual interprets an experience as posing an overwhelming threat to his or her own safety or to the safety of someone that he or she is close to (Briere & Spinnazzola, 2005). As described elsewhere in this volume (see Guarino, Chap. 8), traumatic experiences result in immediate physiological changes as well as longer-term biochemical, affective, cognitive, and behavioral manifestations. A robust literature describes the mental health presentation of children who have experienced traumatic exposures (Browne, 1993; Cloitre et al., 2009; Pynoos, Steinberg, & Piacentini, 1999). As with all adaptations to stress, genetic variables, age, developmental characteristics, cognitive skills, and the larger social context determine the type and degree of severity of mental health outcomes. Children who are exposed to traumatic events are likely to present a range of symptoms that include aggression, blunted affect, hypervigilance or hypovigilance, depersonalization, disorientation, fear, and nightmares and depression (Miller, 1999; Pynoos et al., 1999). As discussed in detail below, many children who are living without homes have been exposed to highly stressful and traumatic events—including those related to housing loss—and their cognitive, affective, and social–emotional needs may result from these singular and cumulative experiences (e.g., Cowan, 2007).

Child Development in Context

It is important to underscore that *all* children without homes are *not* alike, and that any conceptualization of this subpopulation as a monolithic composite of disturbed behaviors and emotions is without scientific support (Cowan, 2007; Douglass, 1996; Huntington, Buckner, & Bassuk, 2008; Masten, 2005). As with children everywhere, regardless of housing status, heterogeneity in mental health functioning exists within families as well as across age, racial, ethnic, and cultural groups. Each child presents with strengths and challenges that can manifest and then recede over time given a unique combination of risk and protective factors (Luthar, 2006; Masten, 2005). While some children function poorly in the face of adversity, others are resilient and manage to thrive (Luthar, 2006). The field of child development is expanding to build a better understanding of the mechanisms needed to support healthy functioning in at risk populations.

Children's mental health functioning is multi-determined by both nature or biological processes, *and* nurture, or environmental factors (Levy & Orlans, 2003; Shonkoff & Phillips, 2000). No single pathway underlies the development of psychopathology (Greenberg, 1999; Nader, 1997; Tyrka et al., 2012). An ecological–transactional framework is useful to understand how child development and physical and mental health unfolds in the context of biological and environmental experiences. Bronfenbrenner (1979), Lynch and Cicchetti (1998), and others describe development as shaped by the multiple transactions that take place at various levels of a child's ecology.

Although temperament and an increased vulnerability to certain behavioral and emotional disturbances are associated with genetic blueprints passed on at conception (Tyrka et al., 2012), the expression of maladaptive functioning is believed to be triggered by interrelated stress-mediated mechanisms (Cicchetti & Rogosch, 2012; Shonkoff & Phillips, 2000). From an ecological–transactional perspective, social-emotional, behavioral, and adaptive functioning is influenced by biological processes as well as bidirectional interactions that occur between children and their family members, peers, schools, neighborhoods, and the greater community (Bronfenbrenner, 1979; 2005; Brooks-Gunn, Johnson, & Leventhal, 2001; Lynch & Cicchetti, 1998; Shonkoff & Phillips, 2000). Culture, moreover, permeates the developmental experience through intertwined beliefs and practices that, for example, include behavioral norms and age-related expectations; parenting styles, and disciplinary measures (Carlson & Harwood, 2003; Ford et al., 2000; Shonkoff & Phillips, 2000; Toth et al., 2012). At a more distal level, social policies that favor economically advantaged families while burdening the poor translate into discrepant experiences during critical periods of child development (Conger et al., 1994; Gorman-Smith & Tolan, 1998; Shinn, 2002; Shonkoff & Phillips, 2000).

Children's development at each ecological level is shaped by an amalgam of risk and protective factors. While some risk factors directly affect a child's experience, for example, the loss of a parent or important caregiver during early childhood, others more indirectly impact children's lives, such as living in a neighborhood with high rates of unemployment and underfunded schools (Bronfenbrenner, 1979; Cicchetti & Lynch, 1993). Protective factors similarly can be proximate and integral to a child's everyday experience, such as a large extended family network or more distal, for example, the availability of an affordable, comprehensive afterschool program that supports working parents on a night shift.

In the absence of salient protective factors, exposures to significant stressors during childhood are strongly associated with poor mental health functioning (Gorman-Smith & Tolan, 1998; Lynch & Cicchetti, 1998; Haber & Toro, 2004; Masten & Garmezy, 1985; Toth et al., 2012). Moreover, the numbers, types, and chronicity of stressful exposures increases exponentially the likelihood and degree of cognitive, affective, behavioral, and health impairments (Briere, Kaltman, & Green, 2008; Briere & Spinnazzola, 2005; Cloitre et al., 2009; Felitti et al., 1998).

Nonetheless, as will be discussed in greater detail below, many children exposed to extreme adversity demonstrate resilience (Luthar, 2006; Masten, 2002; Masten & Garmezy, 1985). Protective factors that support resilience include children's intellectual abilities; strong parent–child bonds; parent, caregiver, or other adult involvement in children's activities; and positive peer affiliations (Douglass, 1996; Luthar, 2006; Masten, 2005; Masten & Garmezy, 1995; Milotis, Sesma, & Masten, 1999). A better understanding of the mechanisms of resilience is needed to target homeless individuals and families most at risk for adverse outcomes (Douglass, 1996; Hoge, Austin, & Pollack, 2007; Huntington et al., 2008; Obradovic, 2010; Samuels et al., 2010). Masten and others in a 10-year longitudinal study of urban youth found that person-centered variables, such as a child's IQ, along with the strength of the parent–child bond and quality of parenting practices, were associated with competence and well-being (Masten & Sesma, 1999; Milotis et al., 1999). Other research demonstrates that among children living in shelters and supportive housing, significant child–adult attachments with parents, teachers, and mentors were protective (Douglass, 1996; Gerwirtz, DeGarmo, Plowman, August, & Realmuto, 2009; Milotis et al., 1999; Obradovic, 2010). Further research is needed to identify protective processes and the mechanisms to bolster families at risk for housing loss as well as those living without homes.

Attachment and Mental Health Functioning

The type and tenor of human interactions from birth onward effect well-being and mental health development. Attachment theorists including Ainsworth and Bowlby (Ainsworth, 1973; Bowlby, 1988) posit that an infant's earliest interactions with primary caregivers creates an enduring template for interpreting human relationships and one's own efficacy (Levy & Orlans, 2003; Toth et al., 2011). Infants are born with a primitive ability to convey needs for sustenance, closeness, and protection in expectation that their needs will be provided for by their parents and caregivers. Parents and caregivers under the best circumstances have the requisite emotional capabilities to interpret and respond to their offspring through action and communication. The patterns by which children and caregivers interact have long lasting behavioral and emotional ramifications (Cummings, Davies, & Campbell, 2000; Greenberg, 1999; Levy & Orlans, 2003). Infants and young children who have relationships with adults that respond to their needs of care and continuity form secure attachments. Youngsters with secure attachments fare better across their lifetimes compared to children with insecure attachments; they are better able to form positive peer relationships, interact better with adults, have greater academic success, and experience fewer behavioral and emotional challenges (Fearon, Bakersman-Kranenburg, Van IJzendoorn, Lapsley, & Roisman, 2010; Toth et al., 2011). Adults who as a result of their own hardships, childhood histories, and mental health distress, including depression often have fewer emotional or care-related resources to bring to their caretaking role and may inconsistently or inappropriately respond to their children's needs for care, protection and guidance (Conger et al., 2004; Narayan, Herbers, Plowman, Gewirtz, & Masten, 2012; Gravener et al., 2012). In the presence of erratic caretaking, maltreatment, and neglect, children form insecure, avoidant, or disorganized attachment patterns (Ainsworth, 1973; Bowlby, 1988; Fearon et al., 2010; Toth et al., 2011). These patterns are associated with affective, behavioral, and cognitive difficulties, including internalizing and externalizing disorders, antisocial and deviant conduct; academic challenges and less positive relationships with adults and peers (Brumariu & Kearns, 2010; Fearon et al., 2010; Gravener et al., 2012; Greenberg, 1999; Levy & Orlans, 2003; Toth et al., 2012).

The elevated incidence of their own histories of neglect, maltreatment, and out of home placements, as well as mental illness and substance abuse among extremely poor parents is associated with suboptimal parenting practices, leading to cognitive, affective, and behavioral difficulties in their children (Byng-Hall, 2002; Gravener et al., 2012; Greenberg, 1999; Herring & Kaslow, 2002). Interventions in settings serving families without homes and other at risk populations that are targeted to parental support focusing on the parent, the child and their interactions present promise for breaking cycles of dysfunction across generations (Anderson et al., 2006;Gewirtz, 2007; Gerwirtz et al., 2009; Lee et al., 2010; Tischler, Edwards, & Vostanis, 2009).

Research on Adjustment of Children Who Are Homeless

Given the many homelessness-related disruptions and stresses that coincide with periods of development when children's needs for consistency and structure are considered critical, physicians, mental health clinicians and researchers, educators, and social scientists have sought to understand how this vulnerable population of children is affected by such episodes (Rog & Buckner, 2007; Rubin et al., 1996; Samuels et al., 2010; Shinn, 2002). High rates of behavioral and emotional distress have been found in children without homes, with older children exhibiting more symptoms than those who are younger (Bassuk, Weinreb, & Brooks, 1999; Brinamen, Taranta, & Johnston, 2012; Gewirtz et al., 2008; Haber & Toro, 2004; Lee et al., 2010). Posttraumatic distress, internalizing and externalizing disorders, disruptive behaviors, and poor social–emotional functioning as well as aggression affects many children both during episodes of homelessness and thereafter (Obradovic, 2010; Park, Metraux, Culhane, & Mandell, 2012; Zima et al., 1999). Many children who experience homelessness have been found to experience significant challenges in their social–emotional and behavioral functioning (Anooshian, 2005; Bassuk et al., 1997; Buckner et al., 1999; Davey, 2004; Donahue & Tuber, 1995; Goodman et al., 1991; Graham-Bermann et al., 1996; Lee et al., 2010; Haber & Toro, 2004; Masten et al., 1993; Park et al., 2012; Yu et al., 2008). Rates of emotional and behavioral disturbances are estimated to be higher in poor children when compared with the general population and even higher among children experiencing episodes of homelessness (Gewirtz et al., 2008; Lee et al., 2010; Park et al., 2012). Research findings over the past 20 years have demonstrated elevated rates of internalizing and externalizing disorders, disruptive and deviant behaviors, social challenges, and aggression among children living in families without homes (Bassuk & Gallagher, 1990; Menke & Wagner, 1998; McCaskill et al., 1998; Park et al., 2012).

School is the catalyst for the acquisition of cognitive and social skill building. Research has demonstrated that children's educational experiences are negatively impacted by housing instability (Masten et al., 1997; Milotis et al., 1999). Children living without homes are reported to experience elevated rates of developmental and cognitive delays, learning disabilities, and academic difficulties when compared to same age peers (Herbers et al., 2011; Masten et al., 1997; Milotis et al.,1999; Yamaguchi, Strawser, & Higgins, 1997) School-age children without homes fall behind same-age peers in the general population as measured by achievement indices, including math and language skills (Herbers et al., 2011; Lee et al., 2010; Obradovic et al., 2009; Rubin et al., 1996; Zima et al., 1997). Some studies have demonstrated that children who are or have been without homes do less well than their poor but housed peers, and continue to lag even after housing is restored (Obradovic et al., 2009; Rafferty et al., 2004). Despite educational guarantees incorporated into the McKinney–Vento Education Act, many children without homes attend numerous schools during the course of their public school educations, even when compared with housed low-income peers (Herbers et al., 2011; Obradovic et al., 2009; Yamaguchi et al., 1997). Rates of truancy, grade retention, and school dropout are high among children living without homes (Rafferty et al., 2004). Students without homes in need of individual education plans and other remedial services often do not receive them (Rafferty et al., 2004; Yamaguchi et al., 1997; Zima et al., 1997; Zima, Forness, Bussing, & Benjamin, 1998). Moreover, due to economic and transportation constraints, many students without homes are barred from participating in the afterschool and extracurricular activities that would provide them with protective experiences and prosocial ties to their peers and communities. Many students with precarious housing feel poorly about their school experiences (Cowan, 2007) and are cut off from the experiences of competency they might otherwise build.

Rates of mental health disturbances are believed to increase in older children living without homes (Gerwirtz et al., 2009; Park et al., 2012). Based on surveys completed by mothers and case managers at 18 supportive housing units in a major Midwestern metropolitan area, Gewirtz and others found that while 14 % of infants and toddlers met criteria for mental health services, the rate increased to 47 % among 5–11 year olds and was 67 % for adolescents (Gewirtz et al., 2008). Many agencies serving families without homes lack screening and assessment protocols, or procedures for referring youngsters in need to appropriate mental health providers (Brinamen et al., 2012; Lee et al., 2010). Because mental health difficulties in children without homes appear to become more pronounced as youngsters age, it is important to screen and identify those experiencing challenges as early as possible (Brinamen et al., 2012; Buckner, 2008; Lee et al., 2010). Buckner and others have underscored the importance of undertaking future research initiatives that identify the types of children most vulnerable for mental health functioning during homeless episodes and beyond (Buckner, 2008). Many researchers in the field are investigating interventions that can be brought to settings where families without homes live temporarily or receive services (see Gewirtz et al., 2008; Lee et al., 2010; Tischler et al., 2010). For a full discussion of research on programs for children experiencing homelessness, see Chap. 11 (Herbers and Cutuli) of this volume.

A majority of the research involving the functioning of precariously housed children focuses on sheltered populations and students without homes that are identified by schools. Many studies are based on archival data from longitudinal studies. Missing from the literature are findings that address the mental health functioning of the significant numbers of children in rural and suburban locales, those living doubled up with family members and friends, and those in settings that are hard to reach (e.g., in abandoned buildings, tent cities, and weekly motels). The transient and growing numbers of such children would suggest that they too are likely to experience significant hardship and mental health challenges. Efforts to identify children living "under the radar" of agencies that serve families without homes are needed in order to provide supportive mental health to what could be a significant proportion of children without homes.

While past and current research findings in the field have demonstrated elevated rates of emotional and behavioral disturbances among children living without homes, the mechanisms associated with poor mental health outcomes among this population of children are not uniformly agreed upon by researchers. Different research methodologies and targets of investigation have resulted in varied findings (Buckner et al., 1999; Huntington et al., 2008; Masten et al., 1993; Samuels et al., 2010). Because children without homes are exposed to numerous stressors and often experience trauma, it is can be difficult to determine whether a particular constellation of risk factors, not including homelessness, contributes to mental health challenges and/or whether homelessness itself contributes to or mediates dysfunction. Again, research findings are varied. For example, in a study of low-income school-age children in Minneapolis who were between the ages of 8 and 17, recent life events, parental distress, and a greater number of risks—not including homelessness, predicted mental health functioning (Masten et al., 1993). Buckner and colleagues in a study of 80 homeless and 148 never homeless school-age children found that housing status was associated clinical range scores on internalizing disorders, with 47 % of children without homes evidencing clinical range scores compared to 21 % of housed low-income youngsters. While children without homes scored higher on scales for externalizing disorders than housed peers, such differences were not statistically significant (Buckner et al., 1999).

A within-group study of 81 sheltered children measured the association between mental health functioning and children's lifetime traumatic events and homeless related stressors (Cowan, 2007). In this study of children ages 8–16, children and their mothers participated in structured interviews and completed self-report measures of highly stressful events that often occur in the context of poverty and homelessness, self-report measures of child aggression, and child- and mother-reports of trauma symptoms. Frequencies of lifetime traumatic events were high: 37 % of participants reported between 12 and 17 exposures. The chart below lists the most frequent types of exposures.

Nature of event	Percentage (%)
Death of parent or family member that child really loved	72
Lots of yelling, arguing, cursing at home	63
Child heard gunshots in neighborhood	63
Child was really sick and needed to go to the hospital	56
Child witnessed fights between *nonfamily* members	55
Parent became sick and could not care for the child	52
Mother or father arrested and/or jailed	48
Child stayed back in school	34
Child helped break up a fight between *parents or family members*	33
Parents called child names or put child down	29
Child witnessed parents hurting each other	28

As is evident in this data, the participants experienced traumatic events in three critical domains: in relationships with parents and caregivers (death, illness, domestic violence family discord, emotional abuse, and incarceration); interpersonal and community violence, and school failure. Additionally, 65 % of participants were separated from a sibling living outside of the shelter. Sixty-five percent of mothers reported living in two or more places besides a shelter in the past 12 months, with the mean number of residences being 3.4. Sixty-five percent of children attended two or more schools during the past academic year (Cowan, 2007).

The frequencies of homeless related stressors were high within this population, with 49 % of participants reporting between 6 and 10 experiences and 20 % endorsing 11–18 such events. The chart below lists the experiences that participants reported finding the most stressful aspect of living without homes. These data demonstrate that children endorsed the following as highly stressful: disconnection from important peers and family members; changes in roles within the child–parent relationship; concern about school; and difficulty adjusting to shelter rules and regulations.

Reported exposure to traumatic events	
Item reported	Percentage (%)
Had to learn new rules at shelter	80
Stopped seeing special friends	72
Changed schools	69
Had to help mom in new ways since becoming homeless	67
Loss of important toys and possessions	58
Missed a lot of school	47
Friends not allowed to visit at shelter	44
Stopped seeing aunts, cousins, grandparents	42
Mom behaved differently since becoming homeless	36
Teased by peers	33
Feels unsafe at shelter	22
Bullied by peers	21
Separated from family members not allowed to stay at shelter	20
Feels threatened at shelter	11

As expected, rates of negative mental health outcomes were high in this population: 40 % of minor participants scored in the clinical range on a self-report measure of aggression (Aggression Scale; Orpinas & Frankowski, 2001), while 43 % percent of mothers reported having a child with clinical range symptoms of posttraumatic distress (Cowan, 2007). Clinical ranges of symptoms of depression, anxiety, anger, and posttraumatic stress on the Trauma Symptom Checklist ranged from 12 to 17 %. Multiple regression analyses conducted in the context of this study found that exposures to lifetime traumatic experiences *and* homeless related stressors independently accounted for a significant amount of the variance in symptoms of depression, anxiety, aggression, and posttraumatic stress among this population of currently sheltered children. Lifetime trauma alone accounted for the variance in anger and anxiety related symptomatology. The numbers of lifetime trauma experienced were strongly associated with the posttraumatic behaviors observed by parents. A novel finding in this study was that stressors experienced in the context of being homeless contributed to parent observed symptomatology above and beyond the contributions of child age, gender, and lifetime trauma exposures. These varied research findings underscore the need for continued research efforts that target enhancing understanding of the underlying mechanisms associated with the disproportionately high rates of poor mental health among children experiencing homelessness. This understanding could help to strategically inform mental health interventions for children and families experiencing homelessness. Other areas of scholarly debate, involve the degree to which the mental health presentations of children without homes differ from those of poor housed children also at elevated risk for psychopathology. In a longitudinal study, Park and colleagues (2012) found that children without homes utilized more inpatient and community-based mental health resources than housed peers. In a study comparing youngsters living in permanent supportive housing following episodes of homelessness with a matched school-based sample of children considered at risk for disruptive behavior problems and enrolled in a prevention program, both groups scored below the general population on measures of academic skills. Furthermore, although children without homes had higher rates of internalizing and externalizing problems and academic challenges, group differences were not statistically significant (Lee et al., 2010). Mothers of the participants living in supportive housing reported significantly higher levels of psychological distress, utilized more mental health services, and engaged in less optimal parenting practices than mothers of at-risk children. These studies underscored the need to provide prevention services in community settings, including permanent supportive housing, where children without homes and their parents can receive needed services (Lee et al., 2010). Moreover, because of the fluidity between those who are precariously housed and those without homes, it is important to target at risk families with significant needs for mental health and other supportive services regardless of their housing status.

Another study with relevance to this debate is the investigation conducted by Monsoo Yu and colleagues (2007), who examined the association of homelessness and maternal factors with cognitive functioning and psychiatric disorders in a study of mothers and children living without homes and a matched housed sample.

Based on mothers' reports, one-third of the children met criteria for DISC diagnoses. Anxiety disorders were the most prevalent diagnostic category reported followed by disruptive disorders. Disruptive disorders were four times more prevalent among children living without homes than among their housed peers. With respect to children's intellectual functioning, there were no significant differences between groups on nonverbal and composite IQ scores, but verbal scores were statistically lower among youth without homes than among housed peers. An interesting finding of this study was that verbal scores of homeless mothers were lower than those of their housed peers. Maternal levels of education and specific types of maternal psychopathology were associated with disruptive behaviors in children. Homelessness was also found to be associated with children's behavioral disorders (Yu et al., 2007).

Several other have studies targeted the association between maternal variables and mental health outcomes among children living without homes (Haber & Toro, 2004; LaVesser, Smith, & Bradford, 1997). In study of children and mothers in a domestic violence shelter, Jarvis and colleagues found that children's PTSD symptomatology was associated with the extent of intimate partner violence they had witnessed while behavioral problems were associated with maternal anger and anxiety (Jarvis, Gordon, & Novaco, 2005). While this study involved a domestic violence shelter setting, the population of parents living without homes are ostensibly the same. Anooshian (2005) investigated the role of aggression and family violence in the lives of children living without homes. Extremely high rates of both childhood and adult victimization were found to have occurred in mothers. This study correlated family violence with children's behavior problems and associated difficulties in peer relationships. Aggression in this population of children was found to contribute to social isolation and avoidance behaviors in youngsters (Anooshian, 2005). Taken together these studies emphasize the need for interventions targeted to remediate the impact of violence on all family members.

Recommendations for Practice and Policy

Research findings over a 20 year period demonstrate without question the vulnerability of school-age children without homes to elevated risk of mental health distress. Episodes of homelessness during childhood are predictive of adult housing instability, and thus, it is imperative to break the cycles of emotional and behavioral disturbances, adaptive dysfunction and psychosocial risk that increase vulnerability across generations. In addition to support for policies that target the structural underpinnings of homelessness, the following recommendations, while not exhaustive, incorporate approaches to address mental health among families without homes:

- Early screening and assessment for mental health issues in all families seeking homelessness related services. Screening services should be available in communities of care and other settings frequented by families who are precariously housed or without homes. Screening measures must be culturally competent and appropriate to the developmental stages of each family member. Evaluation of need should incorporate parent and teacher observations when possible.

- Referral networks for *all* family members found to be in need of care or at risk for mental health disturbances. Levels of care should be appropriate to needs and should follow individuals and families when stable housing is resumed.
- Age-appropriate interventions focusing on trauma exposures, family violence and the stressors associated with homelessness. Services should target parental mental health, parent–child bonds, and psycho-education in the field of child development.
- Interventions should be available in the settings where families reside including emergency shelters, domestic violence programs, transitional housing, and permanent supportive housing.
- Research initiatives must be targeted on identifying best practices and empirically supported interventions for this high-risk population of children and families. Creating networks to share best practices among providers without cost should be a priority.
- Staff training in all settings serving homeless and at risk families should include information about the mental health and psychosocial presentations of this vulnerable population. Promoting positive parenting and strengthening child–parent bonds through culturally competent strategies should be a central part of every programmatic domain.
- Appropriate supervision, continuing education, and self-care opportunities should be made available to all staff and providers serving populations of families and children. Recognition among staff of the stressful nature of working with families in crisis and with multiple long-standing needs reduces staff burn out.
- School-based supportive services for children without homes. In addition to targeted remediation and IEPs, school communities should find mechanisms to engage students with pro-social extracurricular activities. Funding should incorporate transportation and participation fees.
- Case management services that link families or individuals with enduring communities of support. Focus on family strengths and interests with activities that promote protective bonds with individuals and communities. Such activities might include communities of faith, Foster Grandparent initiatives, scouting, Big Brother/Big Sister mentors, and Boys and Girls Club programming.

References

Ainsworth, M. D. S. (1973). The development of infant-mother attachment. In B. M. Caldwell & H. N. Ricciuti (Eds.), *Review of child development research* (Vol. 3, pp. 1–94). Chicago: University of Chicago Press.

Anderson, L., Stuttaford, M., & Vostanis, P. (2006). A family support service for homeless children and parents: User and staff perspectives. *Child and Family Social Work, 11*, 119–127.

Anooshian, L. J. (2005). Violence and aggression in the lives of homeless children. *Journal of Family Violence, 20*, 373–387.

Attar, B. K., Guerra, N. G., & Tolan, P. H. (1994). Neighborhood disadvantage, stressful life events, and adjustment in urban elementary school children. *Journal of Clinical Child Psychology, 23*, 391–400.

Barrera, M., Prelow, H. M., Dumka, L. E., Gonzales, N. A., Knight, G. P., Michaels, M. L., et al. (2002). Pathways from family economic conditions to adolescents' distress: Supportive parenting, stressors outside the family and deviant peers. *Journal of Community Psychology, 30*, 135–153.

Barrow, S. M., & Lawinski, T. (2009). Contexts of mother child separations in homeless families. *Analyses of Social Issues and Public Policy, 9*, 157–176.

Bassuk, E. L., Buckner, J. C., Perloff, J. N., & Bassuk, S. S. (1998). Prevalence of mental health and substance use disorders among homeless and low-income housed mothers. *The American Journal of Psychiatry, 155*, 1561–1564.

Bassuk, E. L., Buckner, J. C., Weinreb, L. F., Browne, A., Bassuk, S. S., Dawson, R., et al. (1997). Homelessness in female-headed families: Childhood and adult risk and protective factors. *American Journal of Public Health, 87*, 241–248.

Bassuk, E. L., Weinreb, L., Buckner, J. C., Browne, A., Salomon, A., & Bassuk, S. S. (1996). The characteristics and needs of sheltered homeless and low-income sheltered mothers. *Journal of the American Medical Association, 276*, 640–646.

Bowlby, J. (1988). *A secure base: Parent–child attachment and healthy human development.* New York: Basic Books.

Briere, J., Kaltman, S., & Green, B. (2008). Accumulated stress and symptom complexity. *Journal of Traumatic Stress, 21*, 223–226. doi:10.1002/jts20317.

Briere, J., & Spinnazzola, J. (2005). Phenomenology and psychological assessment of complex posttraumatic states. *Journal of Traumatic Stress, 18*, 401–402.

Brinamen, C. F., Taranta, A. N., & Johnston, K. (2012). Expanding early childhood mental health consultation to new venues: Serving infants and young children in domestic violence and homeless shelters. *Infant Mental Health Journal, 33*, 283–293.

Brooks-Gunn, J., Johnson, A. D., & Leventhal, T. (2001). Disorder, turbulence and resources in children's neighborhoods. In G. W. Evans & T. D. Watts (Eds.), *Chaos and its influence on children's development: An ecological perspective.* Washington, DC: APA.

Bronfenbrenner, U. (1977). Toward an experimental ecology of human development. *American Psychologist, 32*, 513–531.

Bronfenbrenner, U. (1979). *The ecology of human development.* Cambridge, MA: Harvard University Press.

Bronfenbrenner, U. (1986). Ecology of the family as a context for human development: Research perspectives. *Developmental Psychology, 22*(6), 723–742.

Browne, A. (1993). Family violence and homelessness: The relevance of trauma histories in the lives of homeless women. *American Journal of Orthopsychiatry, 63*, 370–384.

Brumariu, L. E., & Kearns, K. A. (2010). Parent–child attachment and internalizing symptoms in childhood and adolescence: A review of empirical findings and future directions. *Development and Psychopathology, 22*, 177–203. doi:10.1017/S0954579409990344.

Buckner, J. C. (2008). Understanding the impact of homelessness on children: Challenges and future research directions. *American Behavioral Scientist, 51*, 721–736.

Buckner, J. C., Bassuk, E. L., Weinreb, L. F., & Brooks, M. G. (1999). Homelessness and its relation to the mental health and behavior of low income school age children. *Developmental Psychology, 35*, 246–257.

Burt, M., & Aron, L. Y. (2000). *America's homeless II: Populations and services.* Washington, DC: The Urban Institute.

Byng-Hall, J. (2002). Relieving parentified children's burdens in families with insecure attachment patterns. *Family Process, 41*, 375–388.

Carlson, V. J., & Harwood, R. L. (2003). Alternate paths to competence: Culture and early attachment relationships. In S. M. Johnson & V. E. Wiffen (Eds.), *Attachment processes in couple and family therapy* (pp. 85–99). New York: The Guilford Press.

Caton, C. L. M., Boanerges, D., Schaner, B., Hasin, D. S., Shrout, P. E., Felix, A., et al. (2005). Risk factors for long-term homelessness: Findings from a longitudinal study of first-time homeless single adults. *American Journal of Public Health, 95*, 1753.

Chiu, S., & DiMarco, M. A. (2010). A pilot study comparing two developmental screening tools for use with homeless children. *Journal of Pediatric Health Care, 24*, 73–80. doi:10.1016/j.pedhc.2009.01.003.

Cicchetti, D., & Lynch, M. (1993). Towards an ecological/transactional model of community violence and child maltreatment: Consequences for children's development. *Psychiatry, 56*, 96–118.

Cicchetti, D., & Rogosch, F. A. (2012). Gene x environment interaction effects of child maltreatment and serotonin corticotropin releasing hormone, dopamine and oxycotin genes. *Development and Psychopathology, 24*, 411–427.

Cloitre, M., Stolbach, B., Herman, J. L., van der Kolk, B., Pynoos, R. W., & Jing-Petkova, E. (2009). A developmental approach to complex PTSD, childhood and adult cumulative trauma as predictors of symptom complexity. *Journal of Traumatic Stress, 22*, 399–408.

Community Planning and Development. Retrieved from http://www.huduser.org/portal.publications/povsoc/ahar

Conger, R. E., Ge, X., Elder, G. H., Lorenz, F. O., & Simmons, F. L. (1994). Economic stress, coercive family process, and developmental problems of adolescents. *Child Development, 65*, 541–561.

Cowal, K., Shinn, M., Weitzman, B. C., Stojanovic, D., & Labay, L. (2002). Mother–child separations in homeless and housed families receiving public support in New York city. *American Journal of Community Psychology, 30*, 711–730.

Cowan, B. A., (2007). *Trauma exposure and behavioral outcomes in sheltered homeless children: The moderating role of perceived social support.* Retrieved from http://digitalarchive.gsu.edu.

Cowan, B. A., Jurkovic, G. J., & Kuperminc, G. P. (2005). *The ASTEQ—Brief version (ASTEQ-lite).* Unpublished measure.

Cowan, B. A., Kuperminc, G. P., & Jurkovic, G. J. (2005). The homeless experiences questionnaire for children (HEQC).

Cronley, C. (2010). Unraveling the social construction of homelessness. *Journal of Human Behavior in the Social Sciences, 20*, 2. doi:10.1080/10911350903269.

Culhane, J. F., Webb, D., Grimm, S., Metraux, S., & Culhane, D. P. (2003). Prevalence of child welfare services among homeless and low income mothers: A five year birth cohort study. *Journal of Sociology and Social Work, 30*, 3.

Cummings, E. M., Davies, P. T., & Campbell, S. B. (2000). *Developmental psychopathology and family process.* New York: The Guilford Press.

Cunningham, M. (2009). *Preventing and ending homelessness - The next steps.* Washington, DC: The Urban Institute.

Davey, T. L. (2004). A multiple family group intervention for homeless families: The weekend retreat. *Health and Social Work, 29*, 326–329.

Donahue, P. J., & Tuber, S. B. (1995). The impact of homelessness on children's level of aspiration. *The Bulletin of the Menninger Clinic, 59*(1), 1–10.

Douglass, A. (1996). Rethinking the effects of homelessness on children: Resiliency and competency. *Child Welfare, 75*, 741–751.

Fearon, R. P., Bakersman-Kranenburg, M. J., Van IJzendoorn, M. H., Lapsley, A. M., & Roisman, G. I. (2010). The significance of insecure attachment and disorganization in the development of children's externalizing behavior: A meta-analytic study. *Child Development, 8*, 435–456.

Felitti, V. J., Anda, R. F., Nordenberg, D., Williamson, D. F., Spitz, A. M., Edwards, V., et al. (1998). Relationship of childhood abuse and household dysfunction to many leading causes of death in adults. *American Journal of Preventive Medicine, 14*, 245–258.

Ford, J. D., Racusin, R., Ellis, C. G., Davis, W. B., Reiser, J., Fleisher, A., et al. (2000). Child maltreatment, other trauma exposure and posttraumatic symptomatology among children with oppositional defiant and attention deficit disorder. *Child Maltreatment, 5*, 205–217.

Friedman, D. H. (2000). *Parenting in public.* New York, NY: Columbia University Press.

Friedman, D. H., Meschede, T., & Hayes, M. (2003). Surviving against the odds: Families' journeys off welfare and out of homelessness. *Cityscape: A Journal of Policy Development and Research, 6*, 187–206.

Gerwirtz, A. H., DeGarmo, S., Plowman, E. J., August, G., & Realmuto, G. (2009). Parenting, parental mental health and child functioning in families residing in supportive housing. *The American Journal of Orthopsychiatry, 79*, 336–347.

Gewirtz, A. H. (2007). Promoting children's mental health in family supported housing: A community–university partnership for formerly homeless children and families. *The Journal of Primary Prevention, 28*, 359–374.

Gewirtz, A. H., Hart-Shegos, E., & Medhanie, A. (2008). Psychosocial status of children and youth in family supported housing. *American Behavioral Scientist, 51*, 810–823.

Goodman, L., Saxe, L., & Harvey, M. (1991). Homelessness as psychological trauma: Broadening perspectives. *American Psychologist, 46*, 1219–1225.

Gorman-Smith, D., & Tolan, P. (1998). The role of exposure to community violence and developmental problems among inner city youth. *Development and Psychopathology, 10*, 101–116.

Gould, T. E., & Williams, A. R. (2010). Family homelessness: An investigation of structural effects. *Journal of Human Behavior in the Social Sciences, 2*, 170–192. doi:10.1080/10911350903269765.

Graham-Bermann, S. A., Coupet, S., Egler, L., Mattis, J., & Banyard, V. (1996). Interpersonal relationships and adjustment of children in homeless and economically distressed families. *Journal of Clinical Child Psychology, 25*, 250–261.

Gravener, J. A., Rogosch, F. A., Oshri, A., Narayan, A. J., Cicchetti, D., & Toth, S. L. (2012). The relations among maternal depressive disorder, maternal expressed emotion, and toddler behavior problems and attachment. *Journal of Abnormal Child Psychology, 40*(5), 803–813.

Greenberg, M. T. (1999). Attachment and psychopathology in childhood. In J. Cassidy & P. R. Shaver (Eds.), *Handbook of attachment* (pp. 469–496). New York, NY: The Guildford Press.

Haber, M. G., & Toro, P. A. (2004). Homelessness among families, children and adolescents: An ecological-developmental perspective. *Clinical Child and Family Psychology Review, 7*, 123–164.

Herbers, J. E., Cutuli, J. J., Lafavor, D., Vrieze, C. L., Obradovic, J., & Masten, A. S. (2011). Direct and indirect effects of parenting on the academic functioning of young homeless children. *Early Education and Development, 22*, 77–104.

Herring, M., & Kaslow, N. (2002). Depression and attachment in families: A child-focused perspective. *Family Process, 41*, 494–518.

Hoge, E. A., Austin, E. D., & Pollack, M. H. (2007). Resilience: Research evidence and conceptual considerations for posttraumatic stress disorder. *Depression and Anxiety, 24*, 139–152.

Huntington, N., Buckner, J. C., & Bassuk, E. L. (2008). Adaptations in homeless children: An empirical examination using cluster analysis. *American Behavioral Scientist, 51*, 737–755.

Jarvis, K. L., Gordon, E. E., & Novaco, R. W. (2005). Psychological distress of children and mothers in domestic violence emergency centers. *Journal of Family Violence, 20*, 389–402.

Joint Center for Housing Studies of Harvard University. (2011). *Rental market stresses impact of the great recession on affordability and multifamily lending*. Washington, DC: The Urban Institute.

Jurkovic, G. J. (1997). *Lost childhoods: The plight of the parentified child*. New York: Brunner/Mazel.

Koegel, P., Melamid, E., & Burnam, M. A. (1995). Childhood risk factors for homelessness among homeless adults. *American Journal of Public Health, 85*, 1642–1649.

Kuehn, D., Pergamit, M., & Vericker, T. (2011). *Vulnerability, risk and the transition to adulthood*. Washington, DC: The Urban Institute.

LaVesser, P. D., Smith, E. M., & Bradford, S. (1997). Characteristics of homeless women with dependent children: A controlled study. *Journal of Prevention and Intervention in the Community, 15*, 37–52.

Lee, S. S., August, G. J., Gewirtz, A. H., Klimes-Dougan, B., Bloomquist, M. L., & Realmuto, G. (2010). Identifying unmet mental health needs of children of formerly homeless mothers living in a supportive housing community sector of care. *Journal of Abnormal Child Psychology, 38,* 421–432.

Lehmann, E. R., Kass, P. H., Drake, C. M., & Nichols, S. B. (2007). Risk factors for first time homelessness in low income women. *The American Journal of Orthopsychiatry, 77,* 20–28.

Leventhal, T., & Brooks-Gunn, J. (2000). The neighborhood they live in: The effect of neighborhood residences on child and adolescent outcomes. *Psychological Bulletin, 126*(2), 309–337.

Levy, T. M., & Orlans, M. (2003). Creating and repairing attachments in biological foster and adoptive families. In S. M. Johnson & V. E. Whiffen (Eds.), *Attachment processes in couple and family therapy* (pp. 165–190). New York: The Guildford Press.

Low income families (Working Paper 21). Washington, DC: The Urban Institute.

Luthar, S. S. (2006). Resilience in development: A synthesis of research across five decades. In D. Cicchetti & D. J. Cohen (Eds.), *Developmental Psychopathology* (Vol. 3). Hoboken, NJ: Wiley.

Lynch, M., & Cicchetti, D. (1998). An ecological-transactional analysis of children and contexts: The longitudinal interplay among child maltreatment, community violence, and children's symptomatology. *Development and Psychopathology, 10,* 235–237.

Lynch, M., & Cicchetti, D. (2002). Links between community violence and family systems: Evidence from children's feelings of relatedness and perceptions of parent behavior. *Family Process, 41,* 519–532.

Masten, A. (2002). Ordinary magic: Resilience processes in development. In M. E. Hertzig, & E. A. Farber (Eds.), New York: Routledge, Taylor & Francis.

Masten, A. S. (2005). Ordinary magic: Resilience processes in development. American Psychologist, 56, 227 – 238. Reprinted in M. E. Hertzig & E. A. Farber (Eds.), *Annual progress in child psychiatry and child development 2002.* New York, NY: Routledge.

Masten, A. S., & Garmezy, N. (1985). Risk, vulnerability protective factors in developmental psychopathology. In B. B. Lahey & A. E. Kazdin (Eds.), *Advances in clinical child psychology* (Vol. 8, pp. 1–52). New York, NY: Plenum.

Masten, A. S., Miliotis, D., Graham-Bermann, S. A., Ramirez, M., & Neemann, J. (1993). Children in homeless families: Risks to mental health and development. *Journal of Consulting and Clinical Psychology, 61,* 335–333.

Masten, M. S., Sesma, A., Si-Asar, R., Lawrence, C., Milotis, D., & Dionne, J. A. (1997). Educational risks for children experiencing homelessness. *Journal of School Psychology, 35,* 27–46.

McCaskill, P. A., Toro, P. A., & Wolfe, S. M. (1998). Homeless and matched housed adolescents: A comparative study of psychopathology. *Journal of Clinical Child Psychology, 27,* 306–319.

McDonald, S. (2012). *Children in poverty: A census update.* Retrieved from http://blog.endhomelessness.org/children-in-poverty-a-census-update/.

Menke, E. M., & Wagner, J. D. (1998). A comparative study of homeless, previously homeless and never homeless school age children's health. *Issues in Comprehensive Pediatric Nursing, 20*(3), 153–173.

Miller, L. (1999). Treating post-traumatic stress disorder in children and families: Basic principles and clinical applications. *American Journal of Family Therapy, 27,* 21–34.

Milotis, D., Sesma, A., & Masten, A. S. (1999). Parenting as a protective process for school success in children from homeless families. *Early Education and Development, 10,* 111–133.

Muñoz, M., Vazquez, C., Bermejo, M., & Vazquez, J. J. (1999). Stressful life events among homeless people: Quantity, types, timing and perceived causality. *Journal of Community Psychology, 27,* 73–90.

Nabors, L., Proescher, E., & DeSilva, M. (2001). School based mental health prevention activities for homeless and at risk youth. *Child and Youth Forum, 30,* 3–18.

Nader, K. (2011). Trauma in children and adolescents: Issues related to age and complex trauma reactions. *Journal of Child and Adolescent Trauma, 4,* 161–180.

Nader, K. O. (1997). Assessing traumatic experiences in children. In T. M. Wilson & J. Pike (Eds.), *Assessing psychological trauma and PTSD* (pp. 291–348). New York, NY: Guilford Press.

National Center on Family Homelessness. (2011). *The characteristic and needs of families experiencing homelessness.* MA: Needham.

Narayan, A. J., Herbers, J. E., Plowman, E. J., Gewirtz, A. H., & Masten, A. S. (2012). Expressed emotion in homeless families: A methodological study of the five-minute speech sample. *Journal of Family Psychology, 26*, 648–653.

Nicols, A. (2012). *Poverty in the United States*. Washington, DC: The Urban Institute.

Obradovic, J. (2010). Effortful control and adaptive functioning of homeless children: Variable focused and person focused analyses. *Journal of Applied Developmental Psychology, 31*, 109–117.

Obradovic, J., Long, J. D., Cutuli, J. J., Chan, A., Hinz, E., & Heisted, D. (2009). Academic achievement of homeless and highly mobile children in an urban school district: Longitudinal evidence of risk, growth and resilience. *Journal of School Psychology, 42*, 1.

Orpinas, P., & Frankowski, R. (2001). The aggression scale: A self report measure of aggressive behavior for young adolescents. *Journal of Early Adolescence, 21*(1), 50–67.

Orpinas, P., Parcel, G. S., McAlister, A., & Frankowski, R. (1995). Violence prevention in middle schools: A pilot evaluation. *Journal of Adolescent Health, 17*(6), 360–371.

Park, J. M., Metraux, S., Brodbar, G., & Culhane, D. (2004). Child welfare involvement among children in homeless families. *Child Welfare, 83*, 423–436.

Park, J. M., Metraux, S., Culhane, D., & Mandell, D. (2012). Homelessness and children's use of mental health services: A population based study. *Children and Youth Services Review, 34*, 261–265.

Pelletiere, D. (2009). Preliminary assessment of American Community Survey Data shows housing affordability gap worsened for lowest income households from 2007–2008. *The national low-income housing coalition*. Retrieved from www.nlihc.org.

Popkin, S., Acs, G., & Smoth, R. (2009). *The Urban Institute's Program on Neighborhoods and Youth Development: Understanding how place matters for kids*. Washington, DC: The Urban Institute.

Pynoos, R. S., Steinberg, A. M., & Piacentini, J. C. (1999). A developmental psychopathology model of childhood traumatic stress and intersection with anxiety disorders. *Biological Psychiatry, 46*, 1542–1554.

Rafferty, Y., Shinn, M., & Weitzman, B. C. (2004). Academic achievement among formerly homeless adolescents and their continuously housed peers. *Journal of School Psychology, 42*, 179–199.

Ratcliffe C. & McKernan, M. (2012). *Child poverty and its lasting consequences*.

Rog, D. J. & Buckner, J. C. (2007). Homeless families and children. *Presented at the National Symposium on Homeless Research*. Washington, DC.

Rubin, D. H., Erickson, C. J., Augustin, M. S., Cleary, S. D., Allen, J. K., & Cohen, P. (1996). Cognitive and academic functioning of homeless children compared with housed children. *Pediatrics, 97*, 289–294.

Rutter, M. (1987). Psychosocial resilience and protective mechanisms. *American Journal of Orthopsychiatry, 57*(30), 16.

Sampson, R. J., Morenoff, J. D., & Gannon-Rowley, T. (2002). Assessing "neighborhood effects": Social process and new directions in research. *Annual Review of Sociology, 28*, 443–478. doi:28.110601.14114.

Samuels, J., Shinn, M., & Buckner, J. C. (2010). *Homeless children: Update on research, policy, programs and opportunities*. Washington, DC: U.S. Department of Health and Human Services, Office for Planning and Evaluation.

Shinn, M. (2002). Homelessness: What is a psychologist to do? In T. A. Revenson et al. (Eds.), *A quarter century of community psychology: Readings from the American journal of community psychology* (pp. 1–10). New York: Kluwer Academic/Plenum Publishers.

Shinn, M., Weitzman, B. C., Stojanovic, D., Knickman, J. R., Jimenez, L., Duchon, L., et al. (1998). Predictors of homelessness among families in New York City: From shelter request to housing stability. *American Journal of Public Health, 88*, 1561–1657.

Shonkoff, J. P., & Phillips, D. A. (Eds.). (2000). *From neurons to neighborhoods: The science of early childhood development*. Washington, DC: National Academy Press.

Tischler, V., Edwards, V., & Vostanis, P. (2009). Working therapeutically with mothers who experience the trauma of homelessness: An opportunity for growth. *Counseling and Psychotherapy Research, 9*(1), 42–46.

Toth, S. L., Harris, L. S., Goodman, G. S., & Cicchetti, D. (2011). Influence of violence and aggression on children's psychological development: Trauma, attachment and memory. In P. Shaver & M. Mikulincer (Eds.), *Human aggression and violence, causes and manifestations.* Washington, DC: APA.

Tyrka, A. R., Lee, J. K., Graber, J. A., Clement, A. M., Kelly, M. M., DeRose, L., et al. (2012). Neuroendocrine predictors of emotional and behavioral adjustment in boys: Follow up of a community sample. *Psychoneuroendocrinology, 37*(12), 2042–2046. doi:10.1016/j.psyneuen.2012.04.004.

U.S. Conference of Mayors. (2012). *Report on hunger and homelessness.*

U.S. Conference of Mayors (2012) *Hunger and homelessness survey, A status report on Hunger and Homelessness in America. A 25 City Survey.* Washington, D.C.: The United States Conference of Mayors.

U.S. Department of Housing and Urban Development. (2012). *6th Annual Homelessness Report.* Washington, DC: HUD.

U.S. Government, Department of Housing: Vol 1, 2012 Annual Homelessness Assessment Report.

Van den Bree, M., Shelton, K., Bonner, A., Moss, S., Thomas, H., & Taylor, P. J. (2009). A longitudinal population based study of factors in adolescence predicting homelessness in young adulthood. *Journal of Adolescent Health, 45,* 571–578.

Yamaguchi, B. J., Strawser, S., & Higgins, K. (1997). Children who are homeless: Implications for educators. *Intervention in School and Clinic, 33,* 90–97.

Yo, M., North, C. S., LaVesser, P. E., Osborne, V. A., & Spitznagel, E. L. (2008). A comparison of psychiatric and behavior disorders and cognitive ability among homeless and housed children. *Community Mental Health Journal, 44,* 1–11.

Yu, M., North, C. S., LaVesser, P. E., Osborne, V. A., & Spitznagel, E. L. (2008). A comparison of psychiatric and behavior disorders and cognitive ability among homeless and housed children. *Community Mental Health Journal, 44*(1), 1–11.

Zima, B. T., Bussing, R., Bystritsky, M., Widawski, M. H., Belin, T. R., & Benjamin, B. (1999). Psychosocial stressors among sheltered homeless children: Relationship to behavior problems and depressive symptoms. *American Journal of Orthopsychiatry, 69,* 127–133.

Zima, B., Bussing, R., Forness, S., & Benjamin, B. (1997). Sheltered homeless children: Their eligibility and unmet need for special education evaluations. *American Journal of Public Health, 87*(2), 236–240.

Zima, B., Forness, S. R., Bussing, B., & Benjamin, B. (1998). Homeless children in emergency shelters: Need for pre-referral intervention and potential eligibility for special education. *Behavioral Disorders, 23,* 98–110.

Zlotnick, C., Kronstadt, D., & Klee, L. (1998). Foster care and family homelessness. *American Journal of Public Health, 88*(9), 1368–1370.

Zlotnick, C., Tam, T., & Zerger, S. (2012). Common needs but divergent interventions for U.S. homeless and foster care children: Results from a systematic review. *Health and Social Care in the Community, 20*(5), 449–476.

Chapter 4
Parenting in the Face of Homelessness

Staci Perlman, Sandy Sheller, Karen M. Hudson, and C. Leigh Wilson

Abstract The number of families with children experiencing homelessness increased by over 30 % from 2007 to 2011 (U.S. Department of Housing and Urban Development (2012). 6th Annual Homelessness Report. Washington DC: HUD. Of the more than 300,000 children within these families, it is estimated that 40–50 % are under age 6 National Center on Family Homelessness (2011). America's youngest outcasts 2010: State report card on child homelessness. National Center on Family Homelessness. These young children and their families are disproportionately more likely to experience a myriad of other structural, economic, social, and health stressors. Left unaddressed, these stress experiences can adversely influence children's short- and long-term growth, development, and well-being (Shonkoff, 2011). Recent research demonstrates the protective influence that positive parent–child relationships can exert on children's development (Shonkoff, J. P. (2011). Protecting brains, not simply stimulating minds. Science, 333, 982–98. This chapter provides an overview of parenting within the context of homelessness, followed by practice and policy suggestions for promoting positive parent–child relationships among families experiencing homelessness.

S. Perlman, M.S.W., Ph.D. (✉)
Department of Human Development and Family Studies/Delaware Education Research & Development Center, University of Delaware, 4425 Spruce Street, Apt. 1, Newark, DE 19104, USA
e-mail: sperlman@udel.edu

S. Sheller, M.A., A.T.R.-B.C., L.P.C.
The Salvation Army, Drexel University, Philadelphia, PA, USA

K.M. Hudson, M.S.W., L.S.W.
The Children's Hospital of Philadelphia, Philadelphia, PA, USA

C.L. Wilson, M.S.W.
People's Emergency Center, Philadelphia, PA, USA

M.E. Haskett et al. (eds.), *Supporting Families Experiencing Homelessness: Current Practices and Future Directions*, DOI 10.1007/978-1-4614-8718-0_4, © Springer Science+Business Media New York 2014

Families Experiencing Homelessness

Estimates on the number of families with children experiencing homelessness vary greatly. The most recent national data indicate that more than 172,000 families with children (more than 537,000 people) were served by emergency/transitional (EH/TH) housing providers in 2011 (US Department of Housing and Urban Development, 2012). Data suggest that children under age 6 are disproportionately represented among people experiencing homelessness—with up to 30 % of people in these families being comprised of children ages 5 and younger (National Coalition for the Homeless, 2009; US Department of Housing and Urban Development, 2012). As large as these numbers are, they likely underestimate the true number of families and children experiencing homelessness. These estimates only include families served by EH/TH providers—and not families who have been turned away from shelter, have stayed in hard to access locations, or who lived doubled-up with family or friends. A more inclusive count conducted by the National Center on Family Homelessness (2010) estimated that nearly 1,000,000 families experienced homelessness in 2010, and that 1.55 million children were homeless.

Among families, the experience of homelessness is often not an isolated stressor. Rather, family homelessness occurs within the context of structural, economic, health, and social stressors. Structural stressors, including diminished economic conditions and reduced federal and state support for new or subsidized housing (Grant et al., 2007) contribute to the lack of available affordable housing (Grant et al., 2007) and the increased risk of experiencing homelessness. From 2007 to 2010, the number of families entering EH/TH programs increased by 38.5 % (US DHUD, 2012) likely due, in part, to the influence of the economic recession and a decrease in the availability of affordable housing (Mierzwa, Nelson, & Newburger, 2010). Families experiencing homelessness are also likely to have had more limited educational and employment opportunities and thus are less buffered from fluctuations in the economy (Averitt, 2003; Gewirtz, 2007; Grant et al., 2007). For instance, findings from a recent study demonstrate that among children experiencing homelessness, over 35 % had been born to a mother with less than a high school education (Perlman & Fantuzzo, 2013). This vulnerability can contribute to an increased risk of poverty, food insecurity, and housing instability (Averitt, 2003; Gewirtz, 2007; Grant et al., 2007).

In terms of health, families and children experiencing homelessness are more likely than other families to receive poor health care and to be diagnosed with chronic health conditions (Cutuli, Herbers, Rinaldi, Masten, & Oberg, 2009; Healing Hands, 2000; Perlman & Fantuzzo, 2013). For very young children, poor health care can start even before birth. One study found that more than 50 % of children in emergency housing received inadequate prenatal care (Perlman & Fantuzzo, 2013) and other studies indicate homeless children were disproportionately more likely to be born at low birth weight or prematurely (Merrill, Richards, & Sloan, 2011; Stein, Lu, & Gelberg, 2000). Children experiencing homelessness also less likely than their housed peers to receive health care through a primary care physician (30 % compared to just over 60 %) (Shinn et al., 2008). Additionally, children experiencing homelessness were more likely than their peers to be diagnosed with chronic health conditions, such as asthma, chronic ear infections, and iron deficiency anemia (Cutuli et al., 2009; Grant et al., 2008; Weinreb, Goldberg, Bassuk, & Perloff, 1998).

Finally, children and families experiencing homelessness are more likely than housed children to have experienced family violence (Gewirtz, 2007; Guarino, Rubin, & Bassuk, 2007; Swick, 2008; Tischler, Rademeyer, & Vostanis, 2007; Zlotnick, Tam, & Bradley, 2007). A study by Bassuk and colleagues (1996) found that over 60 % of women in emergency housing had experienced domestic violence. Another study found that most women who had experienced domestic violence and who utilized emergency or domestic violence shelters had one or more children with them (Thomas, 2011). Furthermore, most of these children were under age 6, indicating a high prevalence of children experiencing homelessness who have witnessed domestic violence (Thomas, 2011). In addition to witnessing violence, children experiencing homelessness are more likely than their peers to have experienced child maltreatment. A recent study found that almost 40 % of children who had lived in emergency housing had also experienced substantiated child abuse or neglect (Perlman & Fantuzzo, 2013).

Over time, if left unaddressed, these stress experiences can result in a "toxic stress response" (National Scientific Council on the Developing Child, 2011). Toxic stress is defined as, "strong, frequent or prolonged activation of the body's stress management system" (National Council on the Developing Child, 2011, p. 1). Prolonged exposure to toxic stress can adversely influence children's development and well-being. In the case of homelessness, children who have experienced homelessness are more likely than their peers to evidence poor social–emotional, behavioral, and academic outcomes (Buckner, Beardslee, & Bassuk, 2004; Gewitz, 2007; Perlman & Fantuzzo, 2010, 2013; Rafferty & Shinn, 1991). For summaries of research on children and adolescents, see Cowan (Chap. 3, this volume) and Volk et al. (Chap. 2 this volume). This increased risk for poor outcomes underscores the importance of identifying strategies that promote the development and well-being of children experiencing homelessness.

Positive Parent–child Relationships

While toxic stress experiences such as homelessness can exert an adverse influence on children's growth and development, researchers have identified protective factors that can mitigate against these adverse influences. Chief among these are positive parent–child relationships (Appleyard & Berlin, 2007; Bowlby, 1969; Hackman, Farah, & Meaney, 2010; Herbers, Cutuli, Lafavor, Vrieze, Leibel, Obradovic, & Masten, 2011; Shonkoff, 2011). Positive parent–child relationships are characterized by "sensitive and responsive care; [...] developmentally appropriate expectations and supervision; warm, positive, and responsive verbal interaction; and seeing the child as a unique individual" (Appleyard & Berlin, 2007, p. 2). Positive early relationships can serve as a buffer against the adverse effects of exposure to risk factors, such as childhood homelessness, by helping children learn to manage their emotions and to self-regulate (Appleyard & Berlin, 2007; Gewirtz, DeGarmo, Plowman, August, & Realmuto, 2009; Hackman et al., 2010; Shonkoff, 2011).

Furthermore, positive parent–child relationships have been demonstrated to be associated with enhanced brain development and children's development of executive function (Center on the Developing Children at Harvard University, 2011; Herbers et al. 2011; Shonkoff, 2011). Executive function is associated with the development of learning behaviors and social skills that are necessary for children's academic achievement and development of future competencies (Center on the Developing Children at Harvard University, 2011).

Parenting in Emergency/Transitional Housing

While positive parent–child relationships can promote child development, as documented above, parents' own experiences of stress can adversely influence the quality of parent–child interactions (Hackman et al., 2010; Herbers et al., 2011). In addition to the stress associated with unstable housing, the experience of living in EH/TH can inadvertently contribute to challenges in the development of these relationships. Among the challenges facing families living in EH/TH are disconnects in: family routines; disciplinary strategies; children's needs; family separations; culture; and social isolation. The following section provides an overview of each of these challenges.

Disconnects in family routines. Families living in EH/TH may experience a disruption in their typical routines (Friedman, 2000; Schultz-Krohn, 2004). Family routines, including mealtimes, nap schedules and bedtime routines are essential for healthy family functioning (Schultz-Krohn, 2004) and the very experience of living in EH/TH often disrupts these routines (Friedman, 2000; Schultz-Krohn, 2004: Torquati, 2002). For example, mealtimes and menus may not account for eating habits, work habits, cultural needs, or taste preferences. Meals are often served during set times and are frequently made from institutionalized menus. Furthermore, families often are not allowed to supplement meals with their own foods and snacks (Hudson, Bourjolly, & Frasso, 2013). This can contribute to parents' perceptions that they failed to be effective providers for their children or that they are being displaced (Averitt, 2003; Meadows-Oliver, 2003; Mothers in emergency housing. Personal communication, 2010–2012).

Disciplinary strategy disconnects. Friedman (2000) maintains that parents living in EH/TH are "parenting in public". This public exposure of their parenting places them under scrutiny, redirection, and criticism by staff and other residents whose views on discipline and appropriate childhood behavior may differ (Lindsey, 1998; Meadows-Oliver, 2003; Tischler et al., 2007). For parents who have been active caretakers of their children prior to living in EH/TH, this public exposure can erode their authority and impact how their children listen and respond to parental directives, wishes, and commands (Paquette & Bassuk, 2009). Additionally, most EH/TH programs prohibit corporal punishment. For parents who do not have other disciplinary strategies, this may be frustrating and heighten concerns about being reported to child welfare authorities (Lindsey, 1998; Swick, 2008; Swick & Williams, 2010).

Parents living in EH/TH may feel pressured to be in charge of their children at all times, regardless of the children's ages, parents' schedules, or developmental needs of both (Choi & Snyder, 1999; Swick, 2008). Over-crowded conditions of many EH programs and inadequate spaces for children to play may heighten tensions within and among families residing in shelter. Additionally, some EH programs still require families to leave the shelter every morning and remain out of the shelter until the traditional "end of the working day" just prior to dinner. As a result, children who are too young to be enrolled in school may be on the street with their parent for the whole day.

Disconnects in children's needs. Meeting the needs of children at multiple developmental stages also represents a challenge in the EH/TH environment (Schultz-Krohn, 2004; Lindsey, 1998). Very young children require space to be able to explore and play—while school-age children and youth require quiet spaces to complete homework/study. Public spaces with EH/TH programs can be limited, crowded, and noisy (Tischler et al., 2007). Competing demands for this space can sometimes result in acting-out behaviors—producing high levels of mistrust or lack of safety among staff and families. In response to these experiences, children may evidence increased behavioral or academic difficulties (Bassuk et al., 1996; Buckner et al., 2004).

Parent–child separations. Parents experiencing homelessness also experience high rates of separation from their children. Children experiencing homelessness are disproportionately more likely than their housed peers to be separated from their mothers due to placement in foster care (Barrow & Lawinski, 2009; Perlman & Fantuzzo, 2013). However, placement into foster care is not the only reason for parent–child separations. Many EH/TH programs have strict rules regarding the age limits for male children (i.e., male children over age 14 may not be permitted to be in shelter with their mothers) (Thomas, 2011). This can result in mothers being separated from their adolescent male children, who must seek shelter through the adult system or live doubled-up with family or friends. Additionally, the recent increase in demand for EH/TH services by families may also contribute to families separating in order to access services (Paquette & Bassuk, 2009). Mothers and young children may seek services through family EH/TH providers, while fathers and older children seek shelter elsewhere. This can result in young male children being raised in environments that are predominantly female and without positive male role models. Additionally, these separations not only strain family relationships in the short-term, but they may also have long-term negative implications for when families are eventually reunified.

Cultural disconnects. The strict rules and regulations associated with living in EH/TH may exacerbate feelings of frustration, guilt, anger, depression, loss, and powerlessness (Averitt, 2003; Choi & Snyder, 1999; Finfgeld-Connett, 2010). This can result in cultural disconnects. For instance, among African American families, the rules and regulations of EH/TH programs may erode a strong ethic and desire to maintain personal power to determine their own destiny (Temple & Diamond-Berry, 2010; Tischler et al., 2007). Furthermore, parents' efforts to exert their will may be misunderstood for disrespect or acting-out—which can result in them being disciplined or chastised by EH/TH staff. For a more detailed discussion of culture, see Garrett-Akinsaya, Chap. 8 of this volume.

Social isolation. Research demonstrates that families experiencing homelessness are more likely than non-homeless families to face social isolation (Howard, Cartwright, & Barajas, 2009; Vostanis, Tishler, Cumella, & Bellerby, 2001). Low social support is associated with an increased likelihood of employing maladaptive parenting strategies (MacKenzie, Kotch, & Lee, 2011; Oravecz, Osteen, Sharpe, & Randolph, 2011) and is a risk factor for child maltreatment. While mothers may have extended family support in the community, these relationships may not be embraced or fostered during the time that they are living in EH/TH. For instance, extended family or kinship networks are rarely invited or encouraged to visit families living in EH/TH, even though these networks provide the kind of intergenerational teaching, comfort, and support that have been so crucial for this group's survival (Pasquette & Bassuk, 2009). Furthermore, while many African American families come from a culture that teaches, "It takes a village to raise a child," living within the context of EH/TH may implicitly or explicitly make parents feel that they must not trust or depend on each other for support in parenting or raising their children (Temple & Diamond-Berry, 2010). Missed opportunities abound when connections to extended families and communities are not encouraged and facilitated on behalf of families living in EH/TH. Helping families reconnect with family and other social supports can help build and sustain the sense of village.

Parenting in the Context of Homelessness: Specific Subpopulations

The parenting challenges associated with living in EH/TH may be exacerbated for specific subpopulations of families experiencing homelessness, including teenage parents and fathers. Also see DeCandia, Chap. 5 of this volume, for a discussion of issues facing special populations facing homelessness.

Teenage parents. Single young women with young children are considered the fastest growing segment of those experiencing homelessness (Choi & Snyder, 1999; Guarino et al., 2007). A recent study found that over 30 % of young children living in emergency housing had been born to a mother under the age of 19 (Perlman & Fantuzzo, 2013). These young mothers face the developmental challenges of adolescence while simultaneously learning how to be a parent in an unstable living situation. Adolescence represents a development period of rapid physical, social, and emotional changes. During adolescence, youth must master the developmental tasks of establishing a sense of identity, personal values, and competency through trying different roles. He or she must also successfully individuate from caregivers and form new give-and-take attachment relationships (Erickson, 1968; Scharf, Mayseless, & Kivenson-Baron, 2004). During this time, adolescents still rely on the support of parents, caregivers, and other adults to assist with resolving developmental tasks. Young parents experiencing homelessness may face the stressors of adolescence without those supports.

For young women growing up in poverty and lacking social, educational, and/or vocational experiences and opportunities, early motherhood may hold a promise of comfort from the emotional upheaval involving these changes (Cohler & Musick, 1996). Motherhood may represent a viable and appealing identity that will offer the youth someone to love, status as an adult, and a place in the world (Cohler & Musick, 1996; Stevens, 1995). However, becoming a parent requires that the adolescent relinquish her own developmental needs to prematurely assume the adult responsibilities of caring and being responsible for a dependent child or children (Hans, Bernstein, & Percansky, 1991). While early childbearing may provide a valued social role, the additional stress it produces may negatively impact parenting practices, parent–child relationships, and the overall well-being and long-term outcomes of both mother and child (Larson, 2004).

Young mothers who have experienced significant conflict and/or pain associated with their own upbringing may view having a child as providing the mothers with someone of their very own who will return their love (Cohler & Musick, 1996; Stevens, 1995). The conflict between the teen's own needs and her young child's needs places her at risk for either being intrusive and overprotective in her parenting, or lacking warmth and being dismissive (Hans et al., 1991; Mayers & Siegler, 2004). There is an additional risk that the child will be viewed as an extension of the teen instead of an independent person (Mayers & Siegler, 2004). The teen may hold distorted and unrealistic expectations that the child can and will fulfill her unmet needs and when the child's own complicated needs interfere, disappointment and despair can lead to maltreatment (Mayers & Siegler, 2004).

Teenage mothers may not have an understanding of early childhood development, nor what parenting behaviors best promote early development. They may have unrealistically high expectations for their children's developmental abilities which can lead to frustration, disappointment, and harsh or even harmful parent–child interactions (Cohler & Musick, 1996; Mayers & Siegler, 2004; Osofsky, Hann, & Peebles, 1993). In addition, teenage parents tend to be less verbally expressive and sensitive to their young children, express more negative affect and punitive child-rearing attitudes, and experience more instances of depression affecting the well-being and development of their children (Hans et al., 1991; Mayers & Siegler, 2004; Osofsky et al., 1993). These challenges may contribute to the increased likelihood that children born to teenage mothers will evidence disproportionately higher rates of insecure attachments and other psychosocial challenges (Kelly, Buehlman, & Caldwell, 2000; Osofsky et al., 1993; Rafferty & Shenn, 1991).

Fathers. Fathers experiencing homelessness face a unique set of challenges. Although most families experiencing homelessness are female-headed, many have male partners/fathers who remain involved with the family (Barrow &

Lawinski, 2009; Paquette & Bassuk, 2009). In some cases, intact families may be separated because many family EH/TH programs do not serve men; in other cases, there simply may not be enough space available to accommodate the father in a family (Pasquette & Bassuk, 2009). In these instances, adult men and often adolescent boys are served by EH programs for single men—while women and girls are served by family programs (Barrow & Lawinski, 2009; Choi & Snyder, 1999; Zlotnick, Tam, & Bradley, 2007). In some families, the father may not live with the family (prior to entry to EH/TH), but still remain involved through emotional or material supports (Barrow & Lawinski, 2009). These separations result in fathers being rendered invisible in their children's lives.

Similarly, single, custodial fathers living in EH/TH are an emerging group whose needs have not been directly understood, supported, or addressed (McArthur, Zubrzycki, Rochester, & Thomson, 2006; Schindler & Coley, 2007). The programming in EH/TH programs for single custodial fathers may prohibit male participation or be overly focused the needs of mothers (Pasquette & Bassuk, 2009; Schindler & Coley, 2007). These restrictions may reduce fathers' access to programming that promotes positive parental involvement and thereby diminishes fathers' attempts to be "responsible parents" (Schindler & Coley, 2007).

Societal expectations about what constitutes masculine behavior may adversely influence fathers' capacities to meet the needs of their children (Pasquette & Bassuk, 2009). Preconceived notions that asking for social support is not manly can contribute to the stressors, burdens, isolation and demands of single fathers parenting (Levy-Shiff, 1999; Summers, Boller, & Raikes, 2004). For instance, fathers experiencing homelessness are less likely to receive public assistance benefits such as childcare subsidies, which can reduce their availability to work or participate in rehabilitation programs (Schindler & Coley, 2007). This, coupled with a lack of male gender-specific services for fathers in shelter settings and negative stereotypes that men experiencing homelessness are substance-abusing irresponsible fathers with criminal records, can adversely influence how these men are treated (Fathers in shelter personal communication, 2008–2012; Schindler & Coley, 2007).

Parenting Interventions

Given the importance and protective benefits of positive parent–child relationships, interventions that address the specific needs and experiences of families experiencing homelessness are needed. These parent–child interventions must be culturally competent in order to be effective. Additionally, trauma and attachment issues must be taken into consideration when developing interventions or parenting programs with families in EH/TH. Finally, parent training programs need outcome measurement that addresses both parental attitudes as well as child and/or parent behaviors.

Parenting interventions targeting the needs of families experiencing homelessness must be informed by the realities of EH/TH programs. Currently, most effective parenting interventions are likely to be too lengthy and/or intensive to be successfully implemented in shelters, especially when families are encouraged to move through the EH/TH system within weeks or months. Many of these interventions also require involvement of highly experienced and educated clinicians, and thus might be too expensive to be considered within the tight economic budgets EH/TH programs are forced to operate within. Given these constraints, few EH/TH programs have implemented evidence-based parenting programs to date, and there is limited research identifying which parenting interventions are effective for parents living in EH/TH settings (Haskett, Burkhart, & Loehman, under review) (see Gewirtz et al., 1998; Chap. 9 of this volume, for a more extensive discussion). Thus, there is limited empirical basis for recommendations about approaches to strengthen families and improve parenting quality of mothers and fathers without homes. Instead, our recommendations are based on knowledge of the needs of these families and results of approaches and interventions designed for parents whose needs are similar to those of families without homes. Our recommendations are grounded in attachment theory and recent research on early parent–child relationships and trauma.

Many interventions in shelter settings intended to strengthen families focus narrowly on the urgent and immediate needs of the caregiver and lose sight of the well-being of the child and the importance of building nurturing relationships (Bernstein, Campbell, & Akers, 2001). As a result, interventions have not resulted in the desired level of positive improvement in parenting practices, parent–child relationships, or outcomes for children that were anticipated (Egeland, Weinfield, Bosquet, & Cheng, 2000). Supporting nurturing relationships and healthy secure attachments between the parent and child is especially critical for breaking maladaptive cycles and strengthening child well-being (Erickson, Egeland, & Pianta, 1989; Egeland et al., 2000). As noted earlier in this chapter, many mothers entering EH/TH do so with their own histories of childhood abuse. These experiences may make it more challenging for parents to develop healthy attachment relationships with their children. Given the powerlessness and stigma associated with homelessness, parenting interventions must be done in a way that does not further stigmatize, disrespect, undermine, demean, or attempt to control parents who are likely to feel overwhelmed and highly stressed (Averitt, 2003). Programmatic emphasis should be placed on supporting and helping parents find strength and enhance their capacity to parent rather than focusing exclusively on reprimanding or pointing out the shortcomings of the parent or child. Creating an accepting, supportive climate in which parents are free to honestly express their own views and beliefs about parenting practices becomes that "secure base" or "holding environment" that allows them to articulate their struggles, test out new ways of thinking and behaving, and then grow in their relationship with their children. Additionally, establishing trusting meaningful relationships is a critical ingredient to well-being and healing in general. Programs in shelters could benefit parents by the presence of supportive well-trained staff who can continue relationship-building with parents even after time-limited parenting programs and interventions are completed by the parents.

Parents are more at-risk of repeating harsh parenting behaviors if they split-off or idealize (either all good or all-consuming bad) their own past, and then do not see connections between their childhood histories and how they are raising their children (Egeland & Erickson, 1990; Fraiberg, Adelson, & Shapiro, 1980). Cooper and Murray (1997) found that programs focusing on understanding parents' own early attachment histories as it related to current parenting behaviors were more effective in improving parent–child relationships than were programs based on cognitive-behavioral interventions alone. In order for parents to alter negative intergenerational patterns and pathways, they must themselves experience relationship-based sensitive and responsive nurturance—"mothering the mother" (Bernstein et al., 2001; Fraiberg, 1987). As such, parenting the parents as they parent their children should be viewed as a parallel process.

In caring for the caregiver, the conditions are created for parents to be able to better understand and monitor their reactions and become more reflective about their children's feelings and needs. Insensitivity and misinterpretation of a child's signals and cues can result in viewing that child as all-bad, purposely demanding, willful, or controlling, and may lead to harsh parental treatment (Cohler & Musick, 1996). The developers of Circle of Security report that, with support, parents can learn to identify and override perceived threats and inaccurate perceptions that would interfere with being available, responsive, sensitive, and nurturing to their children (Cooper, Hoffman, Powell, & Marvin, 2005; Marvin, Cooper, Hoffman, & Powell, 2002).

Adopting a Trauma-Informed Perspective

The role trauma plays in parenting is often not understood by well-meaning social service providers whose sometimes critical attitudes can be perceived by parents to be uncaring (Shelter mothers communication, 2008–2010). Unresolved trauma, social isolation, loss of control over one's life, and the stress of experiencing homelessness can negatively influence parenting capacities (Bassuk, Perloff, & Dawson, 2001; Choi & Snyder, 1999). As a result, a key component of parenting interventions for families living in EH/TH programs is that they be trauma-informed. Trauma-informed care endeavors to avoid re-traumatizing or blaming people for their efforts and circumstances, however maladapted, to manage traumatic triggers and reenactments (Prescott & National Center on Family Homelessness, 2007). Preliminary research suggests that children and families residing in EH/TH programs that employ trauma-informed perspectives and services have better outcomes than programs that do not incorporate these principles (Cocozza et al., 2005; Morrissey & Ellis, 2005; Rog, Holupka, & McCombe-Thornton, 1995).

Trauma-informed care enhances healing and well-being (Bassuk, Weinreb, Browne, & Bassuk, 1996). However, it requires a paradigm shift in which the emphasis is on understanding, awareness, and the ability to respond to the unique and complex challenges, issues, and special needs of those experiencing traumatic stress.

A commitment is made to facilitate recovery by creating a strength-based, empowering, predictable environment that allows people to rebuild personal control and efficacy over their lives. Rules and protocols are rewritten with more realistic expectations to encourage self-reflection, personal responsibility, and community buy-in. Mutual trust, respect, and collaboration are enhanced as staff and consumers together are taught about the effects of trauma and learn new coping and self-care skills (National Center on Family Homelessness, 2009). For those needing more attention, trauma-specific and other behavioral health services are offered in ways that empower and do not further stigmatize. See Guarino, Chap. 7 of this volume, for a full discussion of trauma-informed practices and policies.

More than teaching skills. Successfully changing parenting behavior is a challenging, complex, and often lengthy process, because of the many conscious and unconscious factors and emotional processes coalescing together that make-up how parents understand and experience themselves and their children (Egeland et al., 2000). Teaching skills through direct instruction may not be enough to change parental behaviors, especially when parents are under chronic and enduring stress. If parents are consumed with their own trauma and stressors, they may not be able to be emotionally available or sensitive to their children's needs. When faced with family and peer pressure, they may easily revert back to unconscious and familial parenting patterns and behaviors.

Parents' unconscious emotional experiences associated with negative and painful childhood memories, if not examined on a conscious emotional level, may continue to behaviorally affect and reinforce negative parenting behaviors over generations (Cooper et al., 2005; Fraiberg et al., 1980). Lessons gleaned from childhood experiences of being parented oneself (sometimes called, "Ghosts from the Nursery," "Voices from the Past," "Shark Music"), are the strongest of the influences leading to reenactment of maladapted parenting behavioral patterns (Fraiberg et al., 1980; Marvin et al., 2002). If parents are preoccupied with their own harsh past experiences and are caught in both rage and shame about how they perceive their child is acting, they are not likely to respond sensitively and appropriately in the moment. Without awareness, parents are at-risk for reacting to their children as if they were participants in the parent's memory (Mayers & Siegler, 2004).

Reflective thinking can help parents to identify triggers associated with past emotional pain and then challenge and change associated reactive parenting behaviors (Bernier & Dozier, 2003; Mayers & Siegler, 2004). Growing this ability is also important because reflective thinking or the capacity to envision and think about the mental state of self and other is significant for healthy social–emotional functioning (Mayers & Siegler, 2004). Marvin et al. (2002) claim that parenting interventions purposed to help parents become more consistently sensitive, available, and responsive to their children's needs and cues by altering behavioral reactions stemming from early emotional experiences, best predict positive changes in parenting behaviors (Marvin et al., 2002). Altering and changing internal cognitions that drive behavior results in a deeper and more lasting change (Bernier & Dozier, 2003; Marvin et al., 2002).

With the capacity to perceive, understand, and consider the underlying motives and emotions driving their children's behaviors, parents can naturally become more appropriate and responsive to their cues and needs and derive more pleasure in the relationship (Bernier & Dozier, 2003; Cooper et al., 2005). Cooper et al. (2005) posit that with repeated interactions of sensitivity and responsiveness, young children will develop internal frameworks of security in which caregivers are seen as safe havens for protection and comfort, and secure bases from which to explore the world, learn, and grow. These inner models then will guide their emotions, behaviors, and expectations in all their relationships throughout their lives, even their own future parenting behaviors (Cooper et al., 2005).

Example of a promising parenting intervention. The Family Care Curriculum (FCC), developed in 2009, is a train-the-trainer parenting program that combines best practices from attachment and trauma theory, and principles of Effective Black Parenting and self-care. FCC was designed to shift parental attitudes, so that the natural tendency parents have to love their children and act on that love in consistent and nurturing ways can be actualized. The program is designed for practitioners (including paraprofessionals and skilled clinicians) to learn how to help parents become more receptive, sensitive, and responsive to their children's developmental, emotional, and cultural needs even while experiencing homelessness and/or other stressors.

Attachment theory and research serves as the basis for several parenting interventions (e.g., Cooper et al., 2005; Kelly et al., 2000; Marvin et al., 2002) but has only recently been incorporated into nonclinical parenting interventions for at-risk populations, and has not been used in shelters with paraprofessional trainers or facilitators. In FCC, unskilled trainers learn how to provide nurturing attachment-based experiences for parents who are coached to explore how their background histories, the "Ghosts in the Nursery," have prevented them from being able to optimally meet their children's deeper developmental and emotional needs. FCC focuses on bringing to the forefront the historical cultural context that perpetuates certain behaviors and parents learn how important it is to understand and resolve historical life issues and past trauma in order to enhance their capacity to parent.

This 6-week curriculum, standardized with a manual and developed for families in transition, is designed to be easily understood and implemented and relevant to parents' experiences so they can embrace the training in the midst of experiencing homelessness. Parents learn to reframe their children's behaviors through a lens of understanding attachment and developmental needs. Along with teaching new information and behaviors, FCC helps parents develop reflective capacities that drive behaviors (thinking about what they and their children are thinking and feeling). By acquiring mental flexibility and self-reflection it is expected that parents will become more mindful about the thoughts and emotions that lead to certain behaviors and this will enable a deep and lasting change. Parents also learn how to provide for their own needs for rest, respite, creativity, and self-enhancement, in order to better care for their children's needs.

A preliminary evaluation of FCC supports its use with families experiencing homelessness. Preliminary findings from a mixed methods evaluation demonstrate a positive shift in parenting attitudes for mothers who participated in the intervention. Quantitative analyses demonstrate a positive shift in parenting attitudes from beginning to end of the interventions. Qualitatively, parents reported better understanding their children's behaviors, and learning different disciplinary methods. Additionally, results of self-evaluations of staff trained in the FCC suggest that the transfer of knowledge enhanced their relationship skills both at work and in their personal life. Feedback from all the trainers presently using FCC have been that group facilitation has gone surprisingly well and trainers are seeing a difference in the parents and their interactions with their children weeks and months after the training. An unanticipated positive effect has also been the observation that parents are being supportive of one another outside of the FCC sessions by continuing to encourage and support one another in solidifying parental attitude and behavioral changes. Literature substantiates that building social support networks to encourage and support positive changes in parenting behavior has resulted in enhanced parent well-being and satisfaction with parenting, along with, improved parent–child relationships (Jacobson & Frye, 1991; Osofsky et al., 1993).

Policy Interventions

Policy and practice interventions that address the complex challenges and risks families experiencing homelessness face are necessary to promote positive parent–child relationships. In 2010, the United States Interagency Council on Homelessness (USICH) developed a strategic plan for ending homelessness that prioritized the needs of families with children (United States Interagency Council on Homelessness, 2010). Consistent with the most recent federal legislation, USICH's primary policy recommendation for families experiencing homelessness was funding for homelessness prevention and rapid-rehousing (HPRP). Homelessness prevention focuses on providing families with short-term assistance to maintain them in their own homes. For individuals and families who enter into the EH/TH system, rapid-rehousing is focused on rapidly transitioning them back into independent housing (National Alliance to End Homelessness, retrieved from http://www.endhomelessness.org/pages/prevention-and-rapid-re-housing). This recommendation was based largely on research on the needs of single, mentally ill, chronically homeless adult males (Culhane & Metraux, 2008). The success of this approach, in particular rapid rehousing, is highly contingent on both the availability and accessibility of permanent housing *and* the capacity of individuals/families to remain stably housed once housing is secured.

While HPRP has been shown to be effective with individuals who are chronically homeless, research evaluating the effectiveness of this approach for families with children is still being conducted (Bassuk & Geller, 2006). An early study evaluating rapid rehousing in New York City found that participation in rapid rehousing was associated with increased recidivism rates and lengths of stay for families (da Costa Nunez, Anderson, & Bazerjian, 2013). These findings suggest that rapid-rehousing may not result in long-term housing stability for families. Thus, while the needs of *some* families may be met by prevention and rapid rehousing, addressing the complex array of risks faced by many families experiencing homelessness—and addressing the stressors that adversely influence parent–child relationships among families experiencing homelessness—may require a more comprehensive response.

Promoting positive parent–child relationships among families experiencing homelessness likely requires strategies that ensure (1) that the basic needs of families are met; (2) that efforts be made to maintain and, as necessary, restore and heal family relationships; (3) that capacity-building opportunities are available to both parents and social service staff working with young children; and (4) that families have access to needed physical and mental health resources (National Scientific Council on the Developing Child, 2011; Shonkoff, 2011). The following provides an overview of these strategies.

Ensure that the basic needs of families are met. As noted previously in this chapter, the stress associated with unstable housing and food insecurity can adversely influence parent–child relationships (Averitt, 2003; Gewirtz, 2007; Grant et al., 2007). Addressing families' most basic needs is a first step towards promoting positive parent–child relationships. A recent study by Richards and colleagues (2011) found that among mothers experiencing homelessness, those who participated in the Special Supplemental Nutrition Program for Women, Infants, and Children (WIC) had better maternal and infant outcomes (including higher rates of prenatal care in the first trimester and increased infant birth weights), than those who did not. Consistent with these findings, national advocacy organizations have prioritized increased funding and access to housing and food supplements for families experiencing homelessness. For instance, the National Center on Family Homelessness (NCFH, 2011) has emphasized the importance of maintaining/strengthening funding for and increasing family/provider knowledge about the Supplemental Nutrition Assistance Program (SNAP) (http://www.familyhomelessness.org/media/364.pdf). Similarly, the National Law Center on Homelessness and Poverty (NLCHP, 2013) has advocated for increases in funding for affordable housing (http://www.nlchp. org/content/pubs/HAG%20priorities%2020132.pdf). Increasing families' access to shelter and nutritious food should contribute to stabilizing families and promote more positive parent–child relationships by minimizing stressors.

Maintaining, restoring, and healing family relationships. As noted earlier in this chapter, many families experiencing homelessness have also experienced domestic violence (Gewirtz, 2007; Guarino et al., 2007; Swick, 2008; Tischler et al., 2007; Zlotnick et al., 2007). Witnessing domestic violence can adversely influence parent–child relationships and children's development (Bogat, DeJonghe, Levendosky, Davidson, & von Eye, 2006; Scheeringa & Zeanah, 1995). Several national organizations have developed policy responses that address domestic violence. Among these recommendations are increasing funding and access to emergency and transitional housing for women experiencing domestic violence

(NLCHP, 2013). Additionally, the National Center on Family Homelessness rec-
ommends that women who have experienced domestic violence should have
access to cash assistance to facilitate being economically able to remain safely in
their homes (NCFH, 2011). Finally, as noted throughout the chapter, given the
high prevalence of domestic violence experiences among families experiencing
homelessness, service delivery should be trauma-informed. Training and professional development opportunities can be offered to housing provider staff to
increase the use of trauma-informed practices.

Individuals in families experiencing homelessness may be separated due to EH/
TH restrictions and/or availability of space. As noted previously these separations
can take a toll on family and child well-being both during and after the separation
occurs. Several strategies could be used to address the difficulties associated with
these separations. For adolescent boys separated from their families due to age
restrictions, housing providers can engage in outreach to include these youth in
services such as family counseling. Additionally, efforts should be made by providers to ensure that the needs of youth are being addressed—even if they are not residing within the EH/TH program. Inclusion of adolescent males will not only promote
their well-being while they are separated from their families, but may also help
enable a smoother transition when the family is able to be reunified. Additionally,
the most recent federal legislation, the Homeless Emergency Assistance and Rapid
Transition to Housing [HEARTH], prohibits denial of services by EH programs due
to children's ages. These regulations were recently implemented, and thus little is
known about how agencies are adjusting their services in response to these changes.

Efforts could also be made to encourage engagement of noncustodial fathers (as
is safe and appropriate), as well as other extended family members. Inclusion of
fathers may provide a means of both emotional and economic support to children
and their mothers (Schindler & Coley, 2007). The presence of a positive male role
model, either a father or other male relative/kin should also be supported for young
boys experiencing homelessness. Notably, the identification of extended family/kin
requires giving families without homes the opportunity to define for themselves
who constitutes extended family/kin (Gasker & Vafeas, 2010). Opportunities and
access to these extended family relationships can facilitate positive parent–child
relationships through the development of social supports and the reduction of social
isolation often experienced during episodes of homelessness.

Capacity-building opportunities. Capacity building opportunities for parents and
social services staff working with young children should be made available.
Shonkoff (2011) notes that young mothers of young children may benefit from
interventions that promote executive function and address mental health issues.
These interventions could be offered in combination with or separately from targeted parenting interventions. Furthermore, for pregnant women entering into or
residing with EH/TH programs, these interventions should begin prior to the child's
birth (Shonkoff, 2011). Providing these services can not only increase the caregivers' own capacities for parenting—but also potentially have a ripple effect to other
areas of the caregivers' life (including employment and education). However,

providing these opportunities to caregivers alone is not adequate. Shonkoff (2011) also argues that similar opportunities should be offered to social services and child care staff working with very young children. These professional development opportunities should focus on normative child development, "executive function skills, and self-regulation" (Shonkoff, 2011, p. 983). Participation in these types of trainings can not only reduce the risk of burnout among these social service professionals but also improve the quality of interactions between staff/providers and families.

Access to physical and mental health care. As noted throughout the chapter, families experiencing homelessness face a complex array of risks. In addition to accessing services that address families' basic needs, many families with children will also benefit from access to mental health, substance abuse, and other health care services (NCFH, 2011). As noted in Bray, Chap. 6 of this volume, an integrated service delivery approach could ensure that families are connected to these services as necessary. Among these services, access to prenatal care for pregnant women, primary health care providers, and mental health professionals should be prioritized (NCFH, 2011). Services could be provided through community-based centers or within the context of the emergency/transitional housing environment. For example, the Homeless Healthcare Initiative (HHI) of the Children's Hospital of Philadelphia (http://www.chop.edu/about/chop-in-the-community/homeless-health-initiative/) provides free, monthly "health and health-related programs" in EH/TH programs serving women and children.

Although positive parent–child relationships can help buffer young children from the adverse effects of toxic stress, quality early childhood experiences can help promote early learning and academic success. Young children experiencing homelessness are disproportionately more likely than their housed peers to experience developmental delays (Garcia, Coll, Buckner, Brooks, Weinreb, & Bassuk, 1998). Current early intervention policy emphasizes the importance of identifying developmental delays among children experiencing homelessness and making referrals to early intervention as necessary (US Department of Education, 2008). Families with young children should be prioritized for access to early intervention and quality early childhood education (National Scientific Council on the Developing Child, 2004). Routine developmental screenings of young children entering EH/TH programs would be the first step toward promoting early development, as well as positive parent–child interactions by ensuring that children and families receive necessary developmental supports. In concert with positive parent–child relationships, quality early childhood education experiences are paramount for promoting positive early childhood development—especially among vulnerable young children (for more discussion, see Chap. 2). Efforts should be made to connect young children experiencing homeless with quality early childhood education programs. This could include increased funding for programs such as Early Head Start and Head Start. But it could also include increasing the availability and access to subsidized child care and increasing the number of available slots in non-federally funded high-quality child care programs.

Conclusion

Positive parent–child relationships can serve as a protective factor for children and youth experiencing homelessness. Supporting these relationships requires a comprehensive, integrated approach that focuses on addressing the needs of both parents and children. Though parents experiencing homelessness often face numerous challenges, many are committed to meeting their children's physical, emotional, educational, and social needs. Ensuring access to services that can meet the basic needs of their families in combination with other educational and social supports, can help increase parents' capacity to have the positive, nurturing relationships with their children that they desire—and ultimately promote more positive parent and child outcomes.

References

Appleyard, K. & Berlin, L. J. (2007). *Supporting healthy relationships between children and their parents: Lessons from Attachment Theory and Research*. Report prepared for Center for Child and Family Policy.

Averitt, S. S. (2003). "Homelessness is not a choice!" The plight of homeless women with preschool children living in temporary shelters. *Journal of Family Nursing, 9*, 79–100.

Barrow, S. M. & Lawinski, T. (2009). Contexts of mother-child separations in homeless families. *Analyses of Social Issues and Public Policy, 00*, 1–20.

Bassuk, E.L. & Geller, S. (2006). The role of housing and services in ending family homelessness. *Housing Policy Debate, 17*, 781–806.

Bassuk, E. L., Perloff, J., & Dawson, R. (2001). Multiplying homeless families: The insidious impact of violence. *Housing Policy Debate, 12*, 299–320.

Bassuk, E. L., Weinreb, L. F., Buckner, J. C., Browne, A., Salomon, A., Bassuk, S.S. (1996). The characteristics and needs of sheltered homeless and low-income housed mothers. *Journal of the American Medical Association, 276*(8), 640–646.

Bernier, A., & Dozier, M. (2003). Bridging the attachment transmission gap: The role of maternal mind-mindedness. *International Journal of Behavioral Development, 27*, 355–365.

Bernstein, A., Campbell, S., & Akers, A. (2001). Caring for the caregiver: Supporting the well-being of at-risk parents and children through supporting the well-being of the programs that serve them. In J. N. Hughes, A. M. La Greca, & J. C. Conoley (Eds.), *Handbook of psychological services for children and adolescents* (pp. 107–131). Oxford: Oxford University Press.

Bernstein, V. J., Hans, S. L., & Percansky, C. (1991). Advocating for the young child in need through strengthening the parent–child relationship. *Journal of Clinical Child Psychology, 20*(1), 28–41.

Bogat, G. A., DeJonghe, E., Levendosky, A. A., Davidson, W. S., & von Eye, A. (2006). Trauma symptoms among infants exposed to intimate partner violence. *Child Abuse & Neglect, 30*(2), 109–125.

Bowlby, J. (1969). *Attachment and loss, Vol 1: Attachment*. New York: Basic Books.

Buckner, J. C., Beardslee, W. R., & Bassuk, E. L. (2004). Exposure to violence and low-income children's mental health: Direct, moderated, and mediated relations. *American Journal of Orthopsychiatry, 74*, 413–423.

Choi, N. G., & Snyder, L. (1999). Voices and homeless parents: The pain of homelessness and shelter life. *Journal of Human Behavior in the Social Environment, 2*, 55–77.

Cocozza, J. J., et al. (2005). Outcomes for women with co-occurring disorders and trauma: Program-level effects. *Journal of Substance Abuse Treatment, 28*, 109–119.

Cohler, B. J., & Musick, J. S. (1996). Adolescent parenthood and the transition to adulthood. In J. A. Graber, J. Brooks-Gunn, et al. (Eds.), *Transition through adolescence: Interpersonal domains and context* (pp. 201–231). Hillsdale, NJ: Lawrence Erlbaum Associates.

Cooper, G., Hoffman, K., Powell, B., & Marvin, R. (2005). The circle of security intervention: Differential diagnosis and differential treatment. In L. J. Berlin, Y. Ziv, L. Amaya-Jackson, & M. T. Greenberg (Eds.), *Enhancing early attachments: Theory, research, intervention, and policy* (pp. 127–151). NY: The Guilford Press.

Cooper, P. J., & Murray, L. (1997). The impact of psychological treatments of postpartum depression on maternal mood and infant development. In L. Murray & P. J. Cooper (Eds.), *Postpartum depression and child development* (pp. 201–220). NY: Guilford.

Culhane, D. P. & Metraux, S. (2008). Rearranging the deck chairs or the lifeboats? Homelessness assistance and its alternatives. *Journal of the American Planning Association, 74*, 111–121.

Cutuli, J. J., Herbers, J. E., Rinaldi, M. M, Masten, A. S., & Oberg, C. N. (2009). Asthma and behavior in homeless 4- to 7-year olds. *Pediatrics, 10*, 145–151.

da Costa Nunez, R., Anderson, D., & Bazerjian, L. (2013). *Rapidly rehousing homeless families: New York City – A case study*. Institute for Children, Poverty, and Homelessness. Retrieved from http://www.icphusa.org/filelibrary/ICPH_brief_RapidlyRehousingHomelessFamilies.pdf.

Egeland, B., & Erickson, M. F. (1990). Rising above the past: Strategies for helping new mothers break the cycle of abuse and neglect. *Zero to Three, 11*(2), 29–35.

Egeland, B., Weinfield, N. S., Bosquet, M., & Cheng, V. K. (2000). Remembering, repeating, and working through: Lessons from attachment-based interventions. In J. D. Osofsky & H. E. Fitzgerald (Eds.), *Handbook of infant mental health* (pp. 36–89). NY: Wiley.

Erickson, E. H. (1968). *Identity, youth, and crisis*. NY: Norton.

Erickson, E. H., Egeland, B., & Pianta, R. C. (1989). The effects of maltreatment on the development of young children. In D. Cicchetti & V. Carlson (Eds.), *Child maltreatment: Theory and research on the causes and consequences of child abuse and neglect* (pp. 647–684). Cambridge, MA: Cambridge University Press.

Finfgeld-Connett, D. (2010). Becoming homeless, being homeless, and resolving homelessness among women. *Issues in Mental Health Nursing, 31*, 461–469.

Fraiberg, S. (1987). Ghosts in the nursery. In L. Fraiberg (Ed.), *Selected writings of Selma Fraiberg* (pp. 100–136). Columbus, Ohio: Ohio State University Press.

Fraiberg, S., Adelson, E., & Shapiro, V. (1980). Ghosts in the nursery: A psychoanalytic approach to the problems of impaired mother-infant relationships. In S. Fraiberg (Ed.), *Clinical studies in infant mental health: The first year of life* (pp. 164–196). NY: Basic Books.

Friedman, D. (2000). *Parenting in public: Family shelter and public assistance*. NY: Columbia University Press.

Garcia Coll, C., Buckner, J. C., Brooks, M. G., Weinreb, L. F., & Bassuk, E. L. (1998). The developmental status and adaptive behavior of homeless and low-income housed infants and toddlers. *American Journal of Public Health, 88*, 1371–1374.

Gewirtz, A. H., DeGarmo, D. S., Plowman, E., August, G.J., & Realmuto, G. (2009). Parenting, parental mental health, and child functioning in families residing in supportive housing. *American Journal of Orthopsychiatry, 79*, 336–347.

Gewirtz, A. H. (2007). Promoting children's mental health in family supportive housing: a community-university partnership for formerly homeless children and families. *Journal of Primary Prevention, 28*(3–4), 359–374.

Grant, R., Shapiro, A., Joseph, S., Goldsmith, S., Rigual-Lynch, L., & Redlener, I. (2008). The health of homeless children revisited. Advances in Pediatrics, 54, 173–187.

Guarino, K., Rubin, L., & Bassuk, E. (2007). Trauma in the lives of homeless families. In E. K. Carll (Ed.), *Trauma psychology: Issues in violence, disaster, health and illness* (pp. 231–258). Westport, CT: Praeger.

Hackman, D. A., Farah, M. J., Meaney, M. (2010). Socioeconomic status and the brain: mechanistic insights from human and animal research. *Nature Review, 11*, 651–659.

Hans, S. L., Bernstein, V. J., & Percansky, C. (1991). Adolescent parenting programs: Assessing parent-infant interaction. *Evaluation & Program Planning, 14*, 87–95.

Haskett, M. E., Burkhart, K. & Loehman, J. (under review). Parenting interventions in shelter settings: A review of the literature.

Healing Hands (December, 2000). *Short of breath: A winter's tale of asthma, COPD, & homelessness*. Retrieved February 26, 2013 from http://www.nhchc.org/wp-content/uploads/2012/03/Dec2000HealingHands.pdf.

Howard, K.S., Cartwright, S., & Barajas, R.G. (2009). Examining the impact of parental risk on family functioning among homeless and housed families. *American Journal of Orthopsychiatry, 79*, 326–335.

Hudson, K., Bourjolly, J., & Frasso, R. (2013). *CHOP night evaluation*. Presented at HHI team meeting. Philadelphia, PA.

Institute for Children & Poverty (April, 2003). *Children having children: Teen pregnancy and homelessness in New York City*. A Report for the Institute for Children and Poverty, pp. 1–4.

Jacobs, F., Little, P. M., & Almeida, C. (1993). Supporting family life: A survey of homeless shelters. *Journal of Social Distress and the Homeless, 2*, 269–288.

Jacobson, S. W., & Frye, K. F. (1991). Effect of maternal social support on attachment: Experimental evidence. *Child Development, 62*, 572–582.

Kelly, J. F., Buehlman, K., & Caldwell, K. (2000). Training personnel to promote quality parent–child interaction in families who are homeless. *Topics in Early Childhood Special Education, 20*, 174–185.

Larson, N. C. (2004). Parenting stress among adolescent mothers in transition to adulthood. *Child and Adolescent Social Work Journal, 21*, 457–476.

Levy-Shiff, R. (1999). Fathers' cognitive appraisals, coping strategies, and support resources as correlates of adjustment to parenthood. *Journal of Family Psychology, 13*, 554–567.

Lindsey, E. W. (1998). The impact of homelessness and shelter life on family relationships. *Family Relations, 47*, 243–252.

MacKenzie, M. J., Kotch, J. B., & Lee, L. C. (2011). Toward a cumulative ecological risk model for the etiology of child maltreatment. *Children and Youth Services Review, 33*, 1638–1648.

Marvin, R., Cooper, G., Hoffman, K., & Powell, B. (2002). The Circle of Security project: Attachment-based intervention with caregiver-pre-school child dyads. *Attachment and Human Development, 4*, 107–124.

Mayers, H., & Siegler, A. L. (2004). Finding each other: Using a psychoanalytic-developmental perspective to build understanding and strengthen attachment between teenaged mothers and their babies. *Journal of Infant, Child, and Adolescent Psychotherapy, 3*, 444–465.

McArthur, M., Zubrzycki, A., Rochester, A., & Thomson, L. (2006). 'Dad, where are we going to live now?' Exploring fathers' experiences of homelessness. *Australian Social Work, 59*, 288–300.

Meadows-Oliver, M. (2003). Mothering in public: A meta-synthesis of homeless women with children living in shelters. *Journal for Specialists in Pediatric Nursing, 8*(4), 130–136.

Merrill, R. M., Richards, R., & Sloan, A. (2011). Prenatal maternal stress and physical abuse among homeless women and infant health outcomes in the United States. *Pediatrics, 128*, 438–446.

Mierzwa, E., Nelson, K. P., & Newberger, H. (2010). *Affordability and availability of rental housing in Pennsylvania*. Pennsylvania: Federal Reserve Bank of Philadelphia.

Morrissey, J. P., & Ellis, A. R. (2005). Outcomes for women with co-occurring disorders and trauma: Program and person-level effects. *Journal of Substance Abuse Treatment, 28*, 121–133.

National Center on Family Homelessness. (2009). *America's youngest outcasts: State report card on child homelessness*. National Center on Family Homelessness.

National Center on Family Homelessness. (2010). *America's youngest outcasts: State report card on child homelessness*. National Center on Family Homelessness.

National Center on Family Homelessness. (2011). *America's youngest outcasts 2010: State report card on child homelessness*. National Center on Family Homelessness.

National Coalition for the Homeless. (July, 2009). *Minorities and homelessness*. Retrieved February 11, 2013 from http://www.nationalhomeless.org/factsheets/minorities.pdf.

National Law Center on Homelessness and Poverty. (2013). *The impact of the Violence Against Women Reauthorization Act of 2013 on the housing rights of survivors of domestic violence.* Retrieved from http://www.nlchp.org/content/pubs/VAWA%202013%20Fact%20Sheet%20 FINAL%205%2023%2013.pdf.

National Scientific Council on the Developing Child. (2011). *Building the Brain's "Air Traffic Control" System: How Early Experiences Shape the Development of Executive Function: Working Paper No. 11.* Retrieved from http://www.developingchild.harvard.edu; www.developingchild.harvard.edu.

National Scientific Council on the Developing Child. (2004). *Young Children Develop in an Environment of Relationships: Working Paper No. 1.* Retrieved from http://www.developingchild.harvard.edu; www.developingchild.harvard.edu.

Oravecz, L., Osteen, P.J., Sharpe, T., & Randolph, S. (2011). Assessing low-income African American preschoolers' behavior problems in relationship to community violence, interpartner conflict, parenting, social support, and social skills. *Child & Family Social Work, 16.*

Osofsky, J. D., Hann, D. M., & Peebles, C. (1993). Adolescent parenthood: Risks and opportunities for mothers and infants. In C. H. Zeanah (Ed.), *Handbook of infant mental health* (pp. 106–119). New York: Guilford Press.

Paquette, K. & Bassuk, E. L. (2009). Parenting and homelessness: Overview and introduction to the special section. *American Journal of Orthopsychiatry, 79,* 292–298.

Perlman, S. & Fantuzzo, J. (2013). Predicting risk of placement: A population-based study of out-of-home placement, child maltreatment, and emergency housing. *Journal of the Society for Social Work and Research, 4,* 99–113.

Perlman, S., & Fantuzzo, J. (2010). Timing and influence of early experiences of child maltreatment and homelessness on children's educational well-being. *Children and Youth Services Review, 32,* 874–883.

Prescott, L. & National Center on Family Homelessness. (2007). *A long journal home: A guide for creating trauma-informed services for homeless mothers and children.* Newton: MA: National Center on Family Homelessness. Unpublished manual.

Rafferty, Y., & Shinn, M. (1991). The impact of homelessness on children. *American Psychologist, 46*(11), 1170–1179.

Richards, R., Merrill, R. M., Baksh, L., & McGarry, J. (2011). Maternal health behaviors and infant health outcomes among homeless mothers: U.S. Special supplemental nutrition program for women, infants, and children. *Preventive Medicine, 52,* 87–94.

Rog, D., Holupka, S., & McCombe-Thornton, K. (1995). Implementation of the homeless family project: 1. Service models and preliminary outcomes. *American Journal of Orthopsychiatry, 65,* 514–528.

Scharf, M., Mayseless, O., & Kivenson-Baron, I. (2004). Adolescents' attachment representations and developmental tasks in emerging adulthood. *Developmental Psychology, 40,* 430–444.

Schindler, H. S., & Coley, R. L. (2007). A qualitative study of homeless fathers: Exploring parenting and gender role transitions. *Family Relations, 56*(1), 40–51.

Schultz-Krohn, W. (2004). The meaning of family routines in a homeless shelter. *The American Journal of Occupational Therapy, 58,* 531–542.

Scheeringa, M. S., & Zeanah, C. H. (1995). Symptom expression and trauma variables in children under 48 months of age. *Infant Mental Health Journal, 16*(4), 259–270.

Shinn, M., Rog, D. J., & Culhane, D. P. (2006). *Family homelessness: Background research findings and policy opinions.* Washington, DC: Interagency Council on Homelessness.

Shinn, M., Schteingart, J. S., Chioke Williams, N., Carlin-Mathis, J., Bialo-Karagis, N., Becker-Klein, R., et al. (2008). Long-term associations of homelessness with children's well-being. *American Behavioral Scientist, 51,* 789–809.

Shonkoff, J. P. (2011). Protecting brains, not simply stimulating minds. *Science, 333,* 982–983.

Stevens, J. W. (1995). Adult status negotiation among poor urban African American pregnant and nonpregnant late age adolescent females. *Journal of Applied Social Science, 20*(1), 39–50.

Stein, J. A., Lu, M. C., & Gelberg, L. (2000). Severity of homelessness and adverse birth outcomes. *Health Psychology, 19,* 524–534.

Summers, J. A., Boller, K., & Raikes, H. (2004). Preferences and perceptions about getting support expressed by low-income fathers. *Fathering: A Journal of Theory, Research, and Practice about Men as Fathers, 2*, 61–82.

Swick, K. J. (2008). Empowering the parent–child relationship in homeless and other high-risk parents and families. *Early Childhood Education Journal, 36*, 149–153.

Swick, K. J. & Williams, R. (2010). The voices of single parent mothers who are homeless: Implications for Early Childhood Professionals. *Early Childhood Education Journal, 38*, 49–55.

Temple, T., & Diamond-Berry, K. (2010). The strength of a people: Exploring the impact of history and culture on African American families who are homeless. *Zero to Three, 30*(3), 46–51.

Tischler, V., Rademeyer, A., & Vostanis, P. (2007). Mothers experiencing homelessness: Mental health, support, and social care needs. *Health and Social Care in the Community, 15*, 246–253.

Thomas, K. A. (2011). Homelessness and domestic violence: Examining patterns of shelter use and barriers to permanent housing. *Dissertations available from ProQuest.* Paper AAI3485625. http://repository.upenn.edu/dissertations/AAI3485625.

Torquati, J. C. (2002). Personal and social resources as predictors of parenting in homeless shelters. *Journal of Family Issues, 23*, 463–485.

U.S. Department of Education. (2008). *Questions and answers on special education and homelessness.* Retrieved from http://www2.ed.gov/policy/speced/guid/spec-ed-homelessness-q-a.pdf.

U.S. Department of Housing and Urban Development. (2012). *6th Annual Homelessness Report.* Washington DC: HUD.

United States Interagency Council on Homelessness [USICH]. (2010). *Opening Doors: Federal Strategic Plan to End Homelessness.* Author.

Vostanis, P., Tishler, V., Cumella, S., & Bellerby, T. (2001). Mental health problems and social supports among homeless mothers and children victims of domestic and community violence. *International Journal of Social Psychiatry, 47*, 30–40.

Weinreb, L., Goldberg, R., Bassuk, E., & Perloff, J. (1998). Determinents of health and service use patterns in homeless and low-income housed children. *Pediatrics, 102*, 554.

Zlotnick, C. (2009). What research tells us about the intersecting streams of homelessness and foster care. *American Journal of Orthopsychiatry, 79*, 319–325.

Zlotnick, C., Tam, T., & Bradley, K. (2007). Impact of adulthood trauma on homeless mothers. *Community Mental Health Journal, 43*(10), 13–32.

Chapter 5
Needs of Special Populations of Families Without Homes

Carmela J. DeCandia, Christina M. Murphy, and Natalie Coupe

Abstract Although people experiencing homelessness all face the loss of their homes, the population is comprised of many diverse subgroups with unique needs, challenges, and strengths. Military families; lesbian, gay, bisexual, and transgender (LGBT) families; and immigrant and refugee families are all part of the homeless family population, but each subgroup faces its own unique set of challenges in addition to the common structural factors that lead most families into homelessness. Recognizing the needs of special groups within the homeless population is critically important for designing programs and services responsive to their unique challenges. Permanent housing is an essential part of the solution, but must be combined with adequate services and supports. Policymakers must attend to both the housing and income needs of these special populations as well as the social factors that increase the likelihood that a family might lose their home. The purpose of this chapter is to explore the needs of three special populations of people without homes: military, LBGT, and immigrant and refugee families. For each subgroup, we describe their needs and some of their unique challenges, and conclude by discussing directions for research, practice, and policy.

Introduction

Homelessness remains a tragic social problem endured by single adults, families, and unaccompanied youth. Although people experiencing homelessness all face the loss of their homes, the population is comprised of many diverse subgroups with unique needs, challenges, and strengths (Rosenheck, Bassuk, & Salomon, 1999). Families with children are the fastest growing subgroup (The National Center on

C.J. DeCandia, Psy.D. (✉) • C.M. Murphy, M.M. • N. Coupe
The National Center on Family Homelessness, Needham, MA, USA
e-mail: CarmelaDeCandia@familyhomelessness.org

M.E. Haskett et al. (eds.), *Supporting Families Experiencing Homelessness:*
Current Practices and Future Directions, DOI 10.1007/978-1-4614-8718-0_5,
© Springer Science+Business Media New York 2014

Family Homelessness, 2011a; US Department of Housing and Urban Development, 2012b), and within this subgroup, there is much variability. Military families; lesbian, gay, bisexual, and transgender (LGBT) families; and immigrant and refugee families are all part of the homeless family population, but each subgroup faces its own unique set of challenges in addition to the common structural factors (e.g., poverty, lack of affordable housing) that lead most families into homelessness.

Homelessness is primarily caused by structural factors including poverty, the gap between median rents and income, the lack of affordable housing, and limited job opportunities. See Chap. 1 (Buckner), for a discussion of structural challenges facing the homeless. The groups most vulnerable to these market forces are those with compromised economic and social resources. As the numbers of families headed by women parenting children alone have increased over the last decades, so have the numbers of homeless families. Currently, families headed by single mothers comprise 42 % of the overall homeless population (The National Center on Family Homelessness, 2011a, 2011b)—a dramatic increase over the last few decades. Female-headed families are among the poorest of all families. In addition, other factors contributing to homelessness among families include high rates of domestic violence, traumatic stress, maternal depression, and substance abuse (The National Center on Family Homelessness, 2011b), any one of which can overwhelm a family's ability to maintain housing.

Families who are compromised by both economic and social factors are at the highest risk for experiencing homelessness. Among these are military, LGBT, and immigrant and refugee families (The National Center on Family Homelessness, 2011b). Each group struggles with high rates of poverty and difficulty obtaining affordable housing and jobs that pay livable wages. In addition, these subgroups have experienced disproportionately high rates of traumatic stress. Researchers have documented the prevalence of trauma among homeless mothers (Bassuk et al., 1996, 1997; Bassuk, Buckner, Perloff, & Bassuk, 1998; Browne & Bassuk, 1997; Shinn & Bassuk, 2004), homeless veterans (Tanielian & Jaycox, 2008; United States Department of Veterans Affairs, 2004), immigrants and refugees (Beckerman & Corbett, 2008; Perez-Foster, 2001), and LGBT individuals and families (Kenney, Fisher, Grandin, Hanson, & Winn, 2012). Specifically, many veterans suffer from post-traumatic stress disorder (PTSD) and traumatic brain Injury (TBI), while immigrants, refugees, and LGBT families experience high rates of interpersonal violence, discrimination, and lack of access to services.

Recognizing the needs of special groups within the homeless population is critically important for designing programs and services responsive to their unique challenges. However, this recognition should be balanced with an understanding that structural issues, especially extreme poverty, lack of affordable housing, and limited job opportunities set the stage for homelessness. Permanent housing is an essential part of the solution, but must be combined with adequate services and supports. Policymakers must attend to both the housing and income needs of these special populations as well as the social factors that increase the likelihood that a family might lose their home (Rosenheck et al., 1999). Refer to Chap. 11 (da Costa Nunez & Adams), for a comprehensive presentation of these issues.

The purpose of this chapter is to explore the needs of three special populations of people without homes: military, LBGT, and immigrant and refugee families. For each subgroup, we describe their needs and some of their unique challenges, and conclude by discussing directions for research, practice, and policy.

Military Families

Overview

The combination of high unemployment rates, low-wage jobs, and a shortage of decent affordable housing increases the risk for homelessness among veterans and their families. In 2012, the US Department of Housing and Urban Development (HUD) and the Veterans Administration (VA) estimated there were 62,619 homeless veterans, a 17 % decline since 2009 (US Department of Housing and Urban Development, 2012c). While the overall number of homeless veterans is declining, the number of veterans of recent conflicts who are homeless is increasing. Veterans of recent conflicts are becoming homeless at a faster rate than during previous wars. After the Vietnam War, it generally took 9–12 years for veterans' circumstances to deteriorate to the point of homelessness. Today, Operation Enduring Freedom/Operation Iraqi Freedom (OEF/OIF) veterans are seeking housing services just months after returning home (Fairweather, 2006).

Women veterans are the fastest growing segment of the homeless population and are at higher risk of homelessness than their male counterparts (United States Department of Veterans Affairs, 2012). Women comprise an increasing number of active duty service members and veterans. It is estimated that the number of female veterans will increase from 1.8 million (8.2 % of all veterans) in 2010 to 2.1 million (15.2 %) in 2036. Female veterans of recent conflicts and deployments are more likely than female vets in prior conflicts to be between the ages of 18 and 25 years, to be divorced, and are three times as likely to be single parents (Foster & Vince, 2009; Joint Economic Committee, 2007; Street, Vogt, & Dutra, 2009). Women often struggle against gender-based discrimination both in the military and in civilian life, which can have a negative impact on their employment status, income levels, and ability to provide for their families. Unemployment for all veteran women is 9.1 % compared to 8.2 % among civilians and it is even higher for young women veterans between the ages of 18 and 24 years. For this young adult group, unemployment is staggering at 36.1 % compared to 14.5 % among same-aged civilians (United States Bureau of Labor Statistics, 2012). While women veterans tend to have higher education levels when compared to their male counterparts, their incomes are lower and unemployment rates are higher (BPW Foundation, 2007; Foster & Vince, 2009; United States Department of Veterans Affairs, 2006).

Military families face challenges associated with deployment and reintegration. Stressors during deployment include worries about the safety of the service member and a need for the family to adapt to changing situations and increased responsibilities at home. When service members return, often recovering from physical and psychological injuries, the challenge of reintegrating into family life, reconnecting to social supports, finding civilian employment, and redefining their roles in the community can be overwhelming. Spouses of veterans frequently find themselves in a caregiver role, often living with someone who is physically disabled and/or emotionally withdrawn or aggressive. This can cause stress between spouses. High divorce rates that result from family stress among service members can increase the risk of homelessness.

Challenges

Structural and psychosocial factors contribute to the high rates of homelessness among military families. Structural factors include lack of affordable housing, low wages, and unemployment. Psychosocial factors include a lack of work experience outside the military, PTSD or TBI and associated difficulties with self-regulation and self-control, substance abuse, and medical problems (Blanton & Foster, 2012).

The unemployment rate for veterans is consistently higher than the rate for civilians. Many veterans have difficulty translating the skills and experience they acquired during service into civilian employment. In particular, women and minority soldiers are more likely to develop general rather than specialized skills that are less transferable to the civilian workforce. This places minorities and women returning from service at a considerable economic disadvantage once home (Herbert, 1994).

Spouses of active duty service members are also less likely to be employed than spouses of civilians. They regularly report difficulty finding employment because of frequent moves, lack of child care if not living on a military installation, and stigma against employing military spouses (Weber Castaneda & Harrell, 2008). Military spouses that are employed earn significantly less than civilian spouses (Kniskern & Segal, 2010). As a result of unemployment and low-wage jobs for both veterans and their spouses, military families often struggle to cover the costs of living. Over half of families of active duty service members report occasional or frequent difficulty paying bills (Mancini & Archambault, 2000). These financial problems are often exacerbated by frequent moves and family separations (Booth et al., 2007).

Active duty members of the military separating from service leave a world in which their housing was either supplied or subsidized, only to find a shortage of affordable housing awaiting them. As civilians, veterans and their families struggle to find decent, affordable housing. Earning minimum wage in today's economy, a veteran cannot earn enough to pay for a two-bedroom apartment anywhere in the USA (Wardrip, Pelletiere, & Crowley, 2009). Currently, nearly four million veteran households spend more than 30 % of their income on housing.

While structural factors increase the risk of homelessness, many veterans also find their wounds, both visible and invisible, challenging when trying to achieve long-term stability for themselves and their families. Heavy burdens are placed on all members of a military family in and after separation from military service.

A growing body of research shows the negative impact of these burdens on the children, youth, and families of service members (Sogomonyan & Cooper, 2010). PTSD, TBI, family violence, and other mental health issues are associated with increased rates of homelessness among veterans and their families (Clervil, Grandin, & Greendlinger, 2010).

High rates of mental health conditions are prevalent among returning veterans, making them and their families more vulnerable to marital strain, family violence, and homelessness. More than two-thirds of homeless veterans suffer from mental health, alcohol, or substance use challenges (Substance Abuse and Mental Health Services Administration [SAMHSA], 2011). An estimated one-third of troops report symptoms of a mental health condition (Tanielian & Jaycox, 2008) and female veterans suffer from poorer mental health than civilian women or male veterans (Sadler, Booth, Mengeling, & Doebbeling, 2004; Tsai, Rosenheck, & McGuire, 2012). Substance abuse is a significant challenge for returning veterans. Alcohol and drug abuse among veterans impedes the ability to resolve traumatic issues, and become employed, maintain stable housing, and successfully reintegrate into civilian life. Although numerous substance abuse programs exist in communities and through the VA, the majority of veterans do not receive treatment (Hankin et al., 1999). Service members are often ingrained in a military culture that promotes strength, self-reliance, and independence. Because of this culture and the stigma and fear of repercussion, many do not access needed health care and mental health treatment (Hoge et al., 2004). Reluctant to ask for help or pursue mental health treatment, male and female veterans' needs may go unmet for years following reintegration into civilian life.

PTSD as a result of active military duty is a significant problem for many returning veterans; it impacts family functioning, employment, and residential stability. Recent research indicates that nearly 19 % of service members returning from OEF/OIF have symptoms of PTSD or major depression, and another 7 % suffer from traumatic brain injury (TBI) (Tanielian & Jaycox, 2008). Considered the signature injuries of OEF/OIF (Clervil et al., 2010), these disorders cause significant emotional, cognitive, and behavioral problems for returning veterans and increase the likelihood of substance abuse, family stress, and intimate partner violence (IPV) (American Psychological Association [APA], 2007). Rates of PTSD and TBI for veterans of OEF/OIF are higher than other wars (Bender, 2009). Male veterans with PTSD are more likely to engage in interpersonal violence (IPV) as compared to those without PTSD at a rate up to six times higher than the civilian population (Blue Shield, 2011). Once home, a veteran's PTSD reactions to triggers or "flashbacks", or the loss of impulse control common among TBI survivors, can lead to recurrent episodes of family violence.

Women's roles have expanded in military operations, and more and more women are being exposed to combat situations (Alvarez, 2009; LaBash, Vogt, King, & King, 2009), placing them at risk for developing combat related PTSD. In addition, it is estimated that 16–23 % of service members have experienced Military Sexual Trauma (MST) (United States Department of Veterans Affairs, 2004). While MST is not a female-specific issue, women are disproportionately affected (Sadler et al., 2004; United States Department of Labor, Women's Bureau, 2011). MST, which includes sexual harassment and assault during service, is associated with PTSD, depression, anxiety disorders, substance use disorders, and physical health problems (Sadler, Booth, Nielson, & Doebbeling, 2000; Street et al., 2009). MST compounds previous traumatic experiences and can have many long-term adverse impacts. People who have experienced MST typically have low rates of housing stability and poor economic and educational outcomes.

Female veterans are also less likely to be integrated into supportive networks when they return home after separation from the service than their male counterparts (Fontana, Rosenheck, & Desai, 2010). For military families, strong social networks often make the difference between a productive life in the community or one of social isolation and homelessness. Female veterans have gender specific needs that are not well understood by service providers. This lack of understanding often results in allegations that the VA fails to address the needs of women veterans (MacGregor, Hamilton, Oishi, & Yano, 2011). As a result, they are less likely to access needed medical and mental health services and are less likely to receive benefit entitlements (Blanton & Foster, 2012).

Family violence is also a concern for military families. Veteran status has been associated with three times the rates of IPV as compared to civilians (Sayers, Farrow, Ross, & Oslin, 2009) and IPV increases the risk for homelessness among families (Bassuk et al. 1997, 1996). In the military, and especially in combat situations, veterans are exposed to and must engage in a high degree of violence. After leaving the service, this high exposure to violence can manifest in the family as marital disputes and family violence (Marshall, Panuzio, & Taft, 2005). IPV within military families can largely be attributed to combat-related PTSD or a prior history of trauma (Marshall et al., 2005), and is associated with significant victim injury, negative child outcomes, substance use, and severe antisocial characteristics (Marshall et al., 2005).

Children in military families also face significant challenges. Many of these children demonstrate behavioral issues, anxiety, nightmares, and difficulties in school as they are separated from their parent upon deployment, worry about their safety, and take on increased responsibilities at home (National Center for Mental Health Promotion and Youth Violence Prevention, 2010). As parents return from war, it can be difficult to reintegrate into the daily routines of child rearing. Trauma reactions and the stress of reintegration can lead to increased rates of child maltreatment within military families. For service members with at least one dependent, the rate of child maltreatment increases by approximately 30 % for every 1 % increase in the number of active duty military who depart or return from combat deployment (Rentz et al., 2007).

Opportunities

Tackling the problem of homelessness among military families requires addressing the structural barriers related to unemployment, low-wage jobs, and the availability of decent, affordable housing, as well as family issues related to the stress of deployment and subsequent challenges such as PTSD, IPV, mental health and substance abuse disorders, and MST. Research, practices, and policies need to be developed with the unique needs of military and veteran families in mind.

Like other families at risk of and experiencing homelessness, homeless veteran families need services to increase access to safe and stable housing and employment opportunities that pay a living wage. Housing vouchers and job training programs have been effective in increasing stability and income and lowering the rates of veteran homelessness. The VA's homeless program is one of the largest networks of homeless programs in the country. Some of its many programs include the VA Health Care for Homeless Veterans (HCHV) program and the National Call Center for Homeless Veterans (NCCHV). In addition, the Housing and Urban Development-Veterans Affairs Supported Housing (HUD-VASH) program provides housing choice vouchers for permanent housing and case management for eligible homeless veterans and their families (United States Department of Veterans Affairs, 2013).

Community-based service providers play a significant role in ending veteran family homelessness; however, they must adapt services to meet the unique needs of military families. Military culture is significantly different than civilian culture, with different values, attitudes, goals, and terminology. Frequent moves, nontraditional work hours, and long absences of the deployed parent are common among military families. Today's civilian population knows less about military culture than in years past (Clervil et al., 2010). To effectively engage returning veterans and their families at risk of and experiencing homelessness, community service providers should have military cultural competency. Military cultural competency means understanding the issues, problems, values, and language associated with the military. Community based organizations can attract veterans and ease their concerns by understanding the barriers to accessing community services, becoming knowledgeable about the norms of military culture, and the impact of combat trauma, IPV, and MST on military families. All providers treating military families should be trained to implement trauma-informed services. A trauma-informed service system is "a human service or health care system whose primary mission is altered by virtue of knowledge about trauma and the impact it has on the lives of [veterans] receiving services" (United States Department of Labor, Women's Bureau, 2011). Providing a trauma informed service requires looking at all aspects of the service through the lens of trauma and understanding how traumatic experiences impact veterans and their families. See Chap. 7 (Guarino), for a review of trauma-informed practices and policies.

Veterans returning to their families require access to quality health and mental health service and programs, without stigma, to successfully reintegrate and maintain a stable home life. Many homeless programs focus on housing, benefits, assessment, and referral for mental health problems, and generally do not provide therapeutic services. Strong collaborations between homeless providers, the VA, and community-based service agencies are required to effectively treat service members suffering from mental health issues. In addition, maintaining family and community supports facilitates veterans' transitions home. Preliminary research findings suggest that highly developed networks of ongoing supports are available for some veterans with PTSD, and that veterans in these networks are at substantially lower risk for becoming homeless (Clervil et al., 2010).

In recent years, the US Department of Veterans Affairs (VA) has undertaken a campaign to increase awareness of and services for veterans experiencing homelessness and meet the federal government's goal of ending veteran homelessness by 2015. Policies that increase federal funding for VA services encourage collaboration between VAs and community service providers, and expand eligibility for services to all military family members are key to ending homelessness among military families.

Finally, research needs to be directed towards identifying empirically based treatment strategies to address the impact of military deployments, combat, and reintegration on veterans; housing and employment initiatives; and the unique needs of female veterans. Considering the expanding role of women in the military, research aimed at understanding the impact of PTSD on female veterans is needed. The confluence of IPV, MST, and health and mental health problems among military families and female veterans is not yet fully understood. As many women veterans are single mothers, the connection between their health and their child's well-being must be addressed in research, policy, and practice. Looking more closely at the characteristics of female veterans and their military families will enable the VA and community providers to collaborate more effectively, and design interventions and services to improve the quality of their lives.

LGBT Families

Overview

Within the broad group of homeless families are lesbian, gay, bisexual, and transgender (LGBT) families who have particular challenges based on their status as a sexual minority. However, very little data and information exist about LGBT families who are homeless. While most research looks at the number, types, and characteristics of LGBT families living in the USA, there is much less data about homelessness among LGBT families. Approximately nine million LGBT people live in the USA (Sears & Badgett, 2012). An analysis of 2010 US Census data found 646,464 same-sex couples (including those who identified themselves as husband/wife and as unmarried partners). Approximately 111,000 same-sex couples are raising their own children (e.g., sons or daughters of one partner or spouse by birth, marriage, stepchild, or adoption who are under the age of 18 and not married) (Gates & Cooke, 2010). Between two and three million children are being raised by LGBT parents, and this number is expected to grow in the coming years (Movement Advancement Project, Family Equality Council & Center for American Progress, 2011). Families with LGBT parents live in every state in the country (Gates & Cooke, 2010) and in 96 % of all US counties (Gates, 2011).

LGBT families are more likely to live in poverty—and even more so if they belong to a racial or ethnic minority group. According to the Williams Institute at UCLA School of Law, lesbian, gay, and bisexual adults experience higher poverty rates than heterosexual adults after controlling for a number of factors associated with poverty. Children of same-sex couples have twice the poverty rates of children in heterosexual married couples. African-American same-sex couples are significantly more likely to be poor than African-American married heterosexual couples and are three times more likely to live in poverty than white same-sex couples. Transgender people are four times more likely to have a household income of less than $10,000 and twice as likely to be unemployed compared to the typical person in the USA. Transgender people of color have four times the unemployment rate of the national average (Sears & Badgett, 2012).

A family living in poverty is at risk for becoming homeless (Bassuk et al., 1996). Data do not exist about the number of LGBT families who are homeless in the USA; however, the Williams Institute reports that approximately one in five transgender people are homeless at some point in their lives. Additionally, approximately 1.6 million youth experience homelessness in the USA each year, 20–40 % of whom identify as LGBT (Sears & Badgett, 2012).

Challenges

LGBT families experiencing homelessness face many challenges including discrimination; family separation; unfriendly shelter environments; and traumatic events and stressors. LGBT people encounter the socioeconomic challenges experienced by others of the same sex, race, ethnicity, age, and disability. In addition, many LGBT people face challenges based on their status as a sexual minority, including stigma, harassment, discrimination at school and in the workplace, and the inability to take advantage of the economic benefits of marriage. Discrimination has a negative impact on the health, wages, job opportunities, workplace productivity, and job satisfaction of LGBT people, making it more challenging to achieve financial stability and success (Sears & Badgett, 2012).

There is evidence of housing discrimination and homelessness in the LGBT community. Recent reports suggest that 38 % of same-sex couples were discriminated against when attempting to buy or rent property (Burns & Ross, 2011). Findings of a 2007 Michigan study indicate that same-sex couples face bias and discriminatory treatment based on sexual orientation when trying to access rental housing (Fair Housing Center of Metropolitan Detroit, Fair Housing Center of Southeastern Michigan, Fair Housing Center of Southwest Michigan & Fair Housing Center of West Michigan, 2007). In a survey of transgender and gender nonconforming people, 19 % had been refused housing or an apartment and 19 % became homeless as a result of their gender identity (Grant et al., 2011).

Families who experience homelessness have much higher rates of separation than other low-income families (Culhane, Webb, Grimm, Metraux, & Culhane, 2003). Some separations are dictated by the shelter system. About 55 % of cities surveyed by the US Conference of Mayors report that families may have to break up in order to enter shelter (The United States Conference of Mayors & Sodexho, Inc., 2006).

Homeless shelters often have rules that define what constitutes a family who is eligible for services. Because of guidelines from government programs and other funders, boards of directors, religious dictates, and other organizational practices, same-sex couples who are not legally married may not be eligible to enter all shelters together and receive services as a family unit. This could force one parent in a LGBT couple to separate from the rest of the family to gain access to shelter and services for the majority of family members. Separation from a parent during an already stressful period can have negative consequences for children (Guarino, Rubin, & Bassuk, 2007).

When in shelter, homeless families live among strangers—a double burden for LGBT families who are faced with deciding whether to be open about their status. Some may hide their LGBT status for fear of being discriminated against by service providers, volunteers, and other residents. If known as a LGBT family, some may face discrimination based on bias, stereotypes, and religious beliefs that could lead to unequal treatment or harassment. Many homeless service providers lack training in cultural competency and professional development opportunities to build the knowledge, skills, and language needed to identify LGBT youth and provide them with effective services and supports (Kenney et al., 2012). The same is likely true for LGBT families in the homeless service system. As a result, service providers may feel uncomfortable or unable to adequately identify and care for the needs of LGBT families who are homeless (Kenney et al., 2012).

In shelter, families must often adjust to overcrowded, difficult, and uncomfortable circumstances. Despite the efforts of dedicated service providers, many shelters are noisy, chaotic, unsafe, and lacking privacy (The National Center on Family Homelessness, 2011b). Some shelters do not have separate living and sleeping quarters or bathroom facilities for individual families, requiring all residents to live and sleep in communal spaces and use communal bathrooms/showers. This can be challenging to LGBT families, especially those with transgender members, for whom privacy is important.

The prevalence of traumatic stress in the lives of families experiencing homelessness is high. For many families, the experience of homelessness is often another major stressor among already complicated and traumatic experiences. For LGBT families, the traumatic experiences of being homeless are often compounded by traumatic experiences that stem from LGBT identity. For example, LGBT youth face many difficulties while homeless, including high rates of physical, sexual, and emotional abuse, conduct disorder, suicidal behavior, PTSD, and substance use. While homeless, LGBT youth are also at high risk for engaging in survival sex which often results in sexual assault; contracting sexually transmitted diseases including HIV; being bullied; and dropping out of school (Kenney et al., 2012). As youth, many LGBT people face harassment, victimization, violence, social stigma, rejection, and discrimination in their families, schools, employment, and social settings (Quintana, Rosenthal, & Krehely, 2010). When people are homeless as children and youth, it is likely that their risk for homelessness as an adult is increased. As adults, LGBT people can have similar traumas, and their children—regardless of

LGBT status—can experience these traumas alongside them. Whether homeless as children, youth, or adults, LGBT people and children of LGBT parents live with the effects of traumatic experiences and stressors.

Opportunities

The needs of LGBT families experiencing homelessness are similar to those of other homeless and low-income families, but because of the challenges previously discussed, they can be more complex. The implementation of targeted strategies in policy, research, and service delivery could help set LGBT families who are homeless on the path to long-term stability.

The US Department of Housing and Urban Development (HUD) took important steps in 2011 and 2012 to ensure that LGBT people have equal access to housing and HUD programs. In a final rule published in the Federal Register in February 2012 and effective in March 2012, HUD implemented policy to ensure that its core programs are open to all eligible individuals and families regardless of sexual orientation, gender identity, or marital status. It also clarified that the terms "family" and "household" as used in HUD programs include persons regardless of actual or perceived sexual orientation, gender identity, or marital status. Through this ruling, HUD stated its hope that these policies and programs will serve as models for equal housing opportunity (US Department of Housing and Urban Development, 2012a). Implementation of this rule at the federal, state, and local levels is critical to ensure that LGBT families have access to services free of discrimination and to keeping LGBT families together in the homeless shelter system. All homeless shelters and programs for homeless families, regardless of whether they are funded by HUD or not, should use this rule as a defining and guiding principle of care to ensure equal access and opportunity.

As noted above, data are sparse about LGBT families who are homeless. There is a great deal to be learned about this population and how to address their housing and service needs. For example, research is needed to study the implementation of the HUD equal access policies and strategies for addressing other structural factors impacting LGBT family homelessness. Prevalence data and information about the individual characteristics, pathways, and needs of homeless LGBT families will help increase understanding of the scope of the problem, support necessary resources, and foster positive outcomes. Documentation of effective housing and service practices for LGBT families is also needed. Steps must be taken to learn how homeless service providers can best identify LGBT families who are homeless and collect information about them in a safe, confidential way. Governing programs, funders, and organizations should use any data and information gained about LGBT families experiencing homelessness to develop and implement supportive policies and practices.

Programs that serve families who are homeless should include LGBT-friendly hiring and professional development practices, intake and assessment procedures, and safe spaces as well as trauma-informed policies. As previously described, many homeless service providers lack training in LGBT cultural competencies, and some may feel uncomfortable or unable to work with LGBT families. Culturally competent, formal training and professional development opportunities are necessary for service providers to gain the knowledge, skills, and language to respond to the needs of LGBT families. Further, hiring LGBT people and staff who are willing to learn about and work with LGBT families is critical. Including LGBT people on advisory and governing boards is important as is providing information and training to volunteers about the need for practices and policies of acceptance and non-discrimination. These recommendations also are discussed by Garret-Akinsanya (Chap. 8).

LGBT families should be accepted into programs and sheltered together. During intake procedures at homeless shelters and related programs, learning about a family's LGBT status is important in providing appropriate and effective services. Many LGBT families are likely to feel uncomfortable identifying themselves for fear of discrimination. Therefore, asking questions during intake processes that do not assume heterosexuality is key. In addition, regularly assessing homeless families is a practice that leads to improved outcomes (DeCandia, 2012). Assessment procedures must be LGBT-friendly and include referrals to LGBT-specific resources and services to be most effective.

LGBT families who are homeless need safe spaces where they will not face separation, discrimination, or harassment from service providers and other shelter residents and program participants. Safe spaces help LGBT families stay together, feel comfortable identifying and providing information about themselves, and engage in services that will foster positive outcomes. Homeless service agencies and providers can create safe spaces by facilitating a program culture that is inclusive and accepting of all forms of diversity, displaying posters or flyers that demonstrate LGBT acceptance in public spaces and in case manager and service provider office spaces, and implementing non-discrimination policies with grievance procedures. Service providers can also serve as models of acceptance and equal opportunity for other residents and participants to follow, and agencies can develop program rules that enforce these values. The physical shelter environment is also important—it is important to consider how to provide safe living spaces and sleeping quarters as well as bathroom facilities within the confines of program infrastructure and building space.

Because the traumatic experiences of being homeless are often compounded by traumatic experiences that stem from LGBT identity, LGBT families who are homeless need trauma-informed services. Becoming trauma-informed is a process that includes a way of understanding people and providing services and supports that integrates trauma concepts and trauma sensitive responses into daily practice. How to become trauma-informed varies from program to program and involves trauma training and the identification of specific changes in attitudes and practices (Guarino, Soares, Konnath, Clervil, & Bassuk, 2009). Two resources to help programs learn about trauma and begin to develop trauma-informed procedures in homeless service settings include: *A Long Journey Home: A Guide for Creating Trauma-Informed Services for Mothers and Children Experiencing Homelessness* (Prescott, Soares, Konnath, & Bassuk, 2008) and the *Trauma-Informed Organizational Toolkit for Homeless Services* which includes an organizational self-assessment (Guarino et al., 2009). Policies and procedures that acknowledge the effects of traumatic events and stress on families and that seek to lessen the impact of these stressors can help families recover and regain and maintain stability (Guarino & Bassuk, 2010).

Immigrant and Refugee Families

Overview

Immigrants

Immigrant and refugee families are growing in numbers as millions migrate across borders in search of a new home. In the USA and globally, immigrant and refugee families experiencing homelessness remain largely hidden from researchers and policymakers, and their unique service needs are not fully understood. Many immigrants and refugees do not access the homeless shelter or public benefit system, making their exact numbers unknown.

The US Census Bureau uses the term *foreign-born* to refer to "anyone who is not a US citizen at birth," including naturalized citizens, lawful permanent residents, temporary migrants, refugees, and undocumented immigrants (American Community Survey [ACS], 2012). Measuring the population of the foreign born is difficult due to a lack of reliable data. Based on US Census estimates (ACS, 2012; Bhaskar, Scopilliti, Hollmann, & Armstrong, 2010; US Census Bureau, 2011), the number of foreign-born in the USA is estimated to be nearly 40 million, or 13 % of the total population. Immigrants who are homeless often live with family or friends rather than entering the public shelter system. They are difficult to identify and recognize, falling beyond the scope of researchers, policy makers, and service providers (Joint Center for Housing Studies of Harvard University, 2010).

Racial and cultural diversity is hallmark of US society. Currently, immigrants inhabit every state in the USA and come from an estimated 125 countries (Matthews & Jang, 2007). Newcomers to the USA used to migrate to several traditional gateway cities in New York, New Jersey, and California. Today, immigrants enter through new gateway cities in southern and western states including Arizona, Colorado, North Carolina, and Oklahoma (Hernandez, Denton, & Macartney, 2007; Matthews & Jang, 2007), and homeless immigrants and refugees are found in both traditional and new gateway regions.

Historically, racial and ethnocultural minorities have been at a serious economic and social disadvantage in the USA, contributing to their disproportionate representation in the homelessness population (Rosenheck et al., 1999). Poverty and lack of access to affordable housing are significant factors leading to homelessness among these subgroups. According to the 2010 US Census, 19 % of immigrants live below the poverty line compared to 15 % of US born individuals. Currently, the highest rates of poverty are for immigrants from Latin America (24 %) and Africa (21 %).

Among Latin American immigrants, those from Mexico represent the highest poverty group (28 %) (ACS, 2012). These groups face more obstacles to accessing affordable housing, are more likely to live in overcrowded situations out of sight of the public system, and spend over half of their monthly income on housing costs (Capps, Fix, Ost, Reardon-Anderson, & Passel, 2004). They are also less likely to access public and private benefits including Temporary Assistance for Needy Families (TANF), the Supplemental Nutrition Assistance Program (food stamps), or private health insurance (ACS, 2012; Capps et al., 2004; Matthews & Jang, 2007).

Gender is an important contributing factor when understanding the problem of immigrant and refugee homelessness. Sikich (2008) argues that female homelessness is a global problem and often takes on a different form than male homelessness. Issues of domestic violence and sexual violence are major contributors to female homelessness in both developing and industrialized countries. Globally, female homelessness remains less visible, and trauma and economic disempowerment appear to be major contributing factors. In many countries, women have less economic or educational resources to sustain themselves independently. They may face societal restrictions or cultural pressures to remain in an abusive situation, and if they do leave, they may double-up or resort to prostitution in exchange for a place to live. This combination of economic and social factors makes immigrant and refugee women, many of whom are mothers, highly vulnerable to becoming homeless yet largely invisible to service providers, researchers, and policy makers.

Immigrants face many complex emotional and physical tasks as they leave their homelands and struggle to find their place in a new world. It can take between 10 and 20 years to adjust when immigrating to the USA (Clark, 2003; National Association for the Education of Homeless Children & Youth [NAEHCY], 2006, 2007). Immigrants are challenged with adapting to a new culture, possibly adopting a new language, adjusting to a new climate or environment, and learning new customs while maintaining their own family and cultural traditions. For many, this process of adaptation and acculturation, while stressful, is not traumatic (Perez-Foster, 2001). For others, trauma is central to their immigration experience (Yakushko, Watson, & Thompson, 2008).

Trauma can occur at three stages in an immigrant's journey: premigration, during migration, or post-migration (Beckerman & Corbett, 2008; Perez-Foster, 2001). Premigration refers to traumas immigrants may have experienced in their homeland prior to leaving. This may include experiences of extreme poverty, war, exposure to violence, natural disasters, or persecution. During migration, immigrants may be separated from loved ones or actually lose loved ones who are too weak to survive the journey. Throughout migration, the transition is marked by uncertainty and fear. Once arrived, many immigrants experience unexpected new traumas in their host country. This may include discrimination, loss of employment and poverty, living in substandard living conditions, and homelessness. An ever-present fear of deportation, especially for those who are undocumented, can cause enormous anxiety for families (Yakushko et al., 2008).

Children of immigrant parents are a highly diverse group with strong ties and roots in American society. Today, they comprise over one-fifth of the US population.

Twenty-two percent are young children under age 6 (Matthews & Jang, 2007). Eighty-one percent of children in immigrant families live in mixed status families, defined as those with one foreign-born and one native-born parent. Of this group, 68 % live with parents who had been in the USA for more than 10 years. While 26 % of immigrant children have at least one undocumented parent, approximately 93 % are US citizens (Capps, 2001; Capps et al., 2004; Hernandez et al., 2007; Matthews & Jang, 2007). Sixty percent live with a parent who is bilingual and 74 % of these children are fluent in English and another language, an incredible asset in an increasingly global economy. A smaller percentage, 26 %, live in families with no English-speaking parent and struggle with full integration into society (Hernandez et al., 2007). This group is most at risk for social isolation, poverty, and homelessness.

Refugees

Refugees are a subgroup within the immigrant or foreign-born population with a unique set of characteristics due to their legal status and reason for immigrating. The Office of the United Nations High Commissioner for Refugees (UNHCR, 2013) defines a refugee as someone who "owing to a well-founded fear of being persecuted for reasons of race, religion, nationality, membership of a particular social group or political opinion, is outside the country of his nationality, and is unable to, or owing to such fear, is unwilling to avail himself of the protection of that country." An asylum-seeker is someone who says he or she is a refugee, but whose claim has not yet been definitively evaluated. If someone is determined not to be a refugee or in need of international protection, he or she can be sent back to their country of origin (UNHCR, 2013).

There are more than 20 million people in the world who have fled to another country seeking asylum (Perez-Foster, 2001). Some are driven by poverty or persecution, and others are displaced by natural disasters (UNHCR, 2006). They flee their homelands in search of safety; however, in their host country, many are confronted with significant challenges as they resettle. They may be detained for months or even years in a state of limbo with no legal status in their host country and no ability to safely return home.

Since 1975, the USA has resettled nearly three million refugees. Once arrived, an unknown number of refugees migrate within the country due to the precariousness of their resettlement (UNHCR, 2011). In the USA, refugees struggle with an alarmingly high rate of food insecurity and unemployment (UNHCR, 2013). International research indicates high rates of chronic malnutrition and limited opportunities for employment that produces livable wages. Women's livelihoods are especially precarious, which places them and their children at high risk for poverty and homelessness (UNHCR, 2006).

Refugees' economic and psychosocial integration needs are considered much greater than those of the general population (UNHCR, 2011). Refugee families are often separated during the migration process and tend to suffer great loss and trauma (Perez-Foster, 2001). Resettlement agencies are designed to help refugees meet basic needs during their initial months in their host country. These services are not long-term however, and refugees soon find themselves on their own in a community unable to meet their complex needs. The United States' integration of immigrants in general, and refugees in particular, remains fragmented due to government policies, public attitudes towards the reception of these groups, and racial and ethnocultural discrimination (UNHCR, 2011). Local community agencies, including the homeless service system, often find themselves confronted with serving this subgroup without understanding their unique cultural, legal, and mental health needs. As a result, immigrants and refugees often contend with ongoing poverty, poor living conditions, economic exploitation, and discriminatory treatment. Their needs can go unmet for years as they struggle to resettle and establish a home in their new country.

Challenges

Homeless is a significant issue for immigrant and refugee families coming to the USA, yet very little attention has been paid to their needs. Poverty, low wages, unemployment, lack of affordable housing, experiences of trauma, discrimination, language barriers, and social isolation are all significant challenges for this subgroup.

Most homeless families who enter shelter report that they often moved multiple times prior to becoming literally homeless (The National Center on Family Homelessness, 2011a). Those living in doubled-up situations are sometimes referred to as the "hidden homeless" (Haan, 2011; Murdie, Preston, Ghosh, & Chevalier, 2006; Tanasescu et al., 2009). Doubled-up homelessness refers to those who lose their housing and consequently stay at the homes of others because they have no other place to live. For economic reasons, many immigrant or refugee families double-up to share housing (Joint Center for Housing Studies of Harvard University, 2010). For some newly arrived immigrants or refugees, doubling up may be more in line with familiar cultural practices. However, for many it is a result of lack of access to affordable housing and essential supports.

Although little is known about profiles of families who are doubled-up in the USA, evidence from Canadian literature suggests that there may be an over-representation of immigrants and refugees among the hidden homeless (Preston et al., 2011). Research indicates that Canadian immigrant and refugee families are more likely to live with family or friends than to stay in shelters (Haan, 2011; Murdie et al., 2006, Tanasescu et al., 2011). Staying temporarily with family or friends while trying to adjust to a new country can be immensely helpful. The informal social networks provide needed support and a sense of familiarity to the newly arrived. However, this living situation is not without stress. Overcrowding, a sense of burdening their host, and financial tensions strain these important relationships (Tanasescu et al., 2011).

Immigrants and refugees experiencing homelessness face significant losses that threaten their ability to become stably housed and self-sufficient. Loss of gainful employment and a meaningful work identity are not uncommon, leading to a downturn in socioeconomic status (Foster, 2001; Perez-Foster, 2001). Many new immigrants work in the service industries and struggle with being underemployed. Often parents' educational degrees and employment backgrounds are unrecognized in their new homeland, causing a sudden decline in standard of living and a higher risk of becoming homeless. Strong social support networks are protective and enhance individual and family resiliency (Center for the Study of Social Policy, 2011) and housing stability (Cohen, 2011; Lubell, Crain, & Cohen, 2007). Newcomer families who are non-English-speaking often lose these protective social support networks and are at highest risk of housing instability, social isolation, and lower integration into the host society. For immigrant and refugee families who are homeless, the loss of these networks is also a loss of connection to one's cultural group, a possible protective factor against later illness (Grant et al., 2004).

Despite the many challenges faced by immigrants experiencing homelessness, they initially demonstrate better physical and mental health than their US counterparts (Breslau et al., 2007; Chiu, Redelmeier, Tolomiczenko, Kiss, & Hwang, 2009). Research suggests that homeless immigrants who were in their new country for less than 10 years demonstrated less physical and mental health problems than those who had been in the country for more than 10 years. It is speculated that the multiple challenges faced by homeless immigrants and refugees—poverty, unemployment, social isolation, and migration—coupled with the normative acculturation process to Western society, act as accumulative stressors and take a toll on one's physical and mental well-being (Breslau et al., 2007; Chiu et al., 2009; Grant et al., 2004).

Finally, it is important to consider the challenges faced by immigrant and refugee children who are homeless. Medically, immigrant and refugee children, especially those who are homeless, are often lacking immunizations, preventive dental care, and screenings for developmental delays and post-traumatic stress responses (American Academy of Pediatrics, 2005). Educationally, homeless immigrant or refugee students tend to be highly mobile, which places them at risk for gaps in schooling and learning difficulties (NAEHCY, 2006; The National Center for Homeless Education, 2006). While their bilingual fluency is a strength, this skill is often not formally recognized by school systems who may be unprepared to provide bilingual instruction (NAEHCY, 2007). The majority of immigrant parents—homeless or not—have a strong desire to support their children's education so they may have a better future in America (Ariza, 2000); however, parental involvement (especially of those who are undocumented or not English-speaking) is sometimes lacking. The most common reasons parents cite for not being more involved with their children's school include language barriers, lack of translation services, a lack of understanding by school personnel of their cultural needs, and lack of knowledge regarding how to navigate the school systems (NAEHCY, 2007).

Opportunities

There is no doubt that understanding the special needs of immigrant and refugee families experiencing homelessness is essential for service providers. Similar to all homeless families, poverty and difficulty accessing affordable housing are the two primary barriers to be addressed. Immigrant and refugee families, depending on their legal status, may also face additional barriers related to eligibility for benefits, shelter services, and housing. In addition, experiences of discrimination due to race and culture add to the stress of acculturation and can be accompanied by experiences of immigration or refugee trauma. There are many opportunities to address the needs of homeless immigrants and refugees. These include improving access to housing and other social supports; designing programs and services to better meet the needs of this subgroup; and conducting research and evaluation to better inform policy and practice.

Access to affordable housing is a necessary first step in an immigrant's integration process (Murdie et al., 2006). Reestablishing a safe home is essential for homeless immigrant and refugee families to stabilize, heal from their journeys, and move forward with their lives. Immigrant and refugees' legal status directly impacts their access to housing and services. The longer families remain homeless or precariously housed, the higher the risk for an array of poor developmental and functional outcomes. Targeting services to address structural factors responsible for homelessness are critical, especially for new immigrants. This includes securing proper documentation, safe and affordable housing, access to benefits, job skills training, education and employment.

Services designed to meet the needs of homeless immigrant families should address housing and basic needs, while also assessing migration and trauma history. Not all families will experience immigrant or refugee trauma, but without an assessment of premigration and post-migration experiences, service providers will remain in the dark about how these experiences may be impacting family functioning. Recognizing the high rates of trauma in the homeless population, the homeless service system is steadily adapting a trauma-informed approach to delivering services (Guarino & Bassuk, 2010). This approach is well suited to addressing the needs of immigrant homeless families as well.

Immigrants and refugees often face discrimination from service systems and providers who are unfamiliar with their unique cultural/ethnic/racial backgrounds, language, and needs (Yakushko et al., 2008). Services for homeless immigrant and refugee families need to be provided by culturally and linguistically competent providers who understand different eligibility requirements related to refugee status, immigration status, and how to access legal resources for this subgroup. Providers must also be sensitive to the stress of acculturation (Martin, 2009). Staff's ability to recognize discrimination will validate an immigrant or refugee's experience and lend much needed support during a difficult time of adjustment. Finally, it is recommended that providers focus on strengthening and building connections to social networks to help buffer newcomer families from the stress associated with migration. Helping families stay connected to what is meaningful and relevant to them, within their culture framework, may act as a protective factor from future mental and physical stress-related illness.

Effective practices and policies are built upon a sound base of research. There remains a gap in the literature on the prevalence, characteristics, and service needs of immigrant homeless families. Research is necessary to ensure immigrant and refugee homelessness does not remain invisible and families are not hidden. To best meet the needs of this subgroup, we need to better understand who and where they are, and we must identify the characteristics of immigrants who are in shelter settings as well as those who are in doubled-up situations. In both groups, researchers need to look across cultures to assess how families may be differentially impacted by homelessness, and if they have unique service needs based on culture, immigration status, or duration in this country.

Immigrants and refugees are resilient. They possess a strong work ethic and desire to contribute to the American economy. We can support their integration into society through a better understanding of the factors that protect new immigrants from later stress-related illness. As global female homelessness increases, women and mothers with trauma histories migrate in search of a safe home for themselves and their children. Research is needed to better understand the impact of premigration and post-migration trauma on homeless women's mental health and on their children's development. With this knowledge we can design policies and practices to support parenting so they may provide their children with the healthy futures of their dreams.

Conclusion

Military, LBGT, and immigrant and refugee families represent three subgroups of the homeless population with unique characteristics and service needs. Despite their differences, they share much in common. They are geographically diverse and live in cities and suburbs across the USA; they are more likely than the general population to live in poverty and face obstacles to affordable housing, low wages, and unemployment; and they demonstrate high rates of past and current traumatic experiences. When homeless, these families face many challenges. They are impacted by discrimination and family separations, and are often met by programs and systems not designed to meet their unique needs. Housing alone will not solve all the problems faced by families who experience homelessness. While affordable housing, education, and employment can create pathways out of homelessness, understanding the context within which homelessness occurs enables providers to deliver targeted services. To best address the challenges that families face when homeless and foster sustained stability and positive outcomes, solutions must address both the common structural factors leading to homelessness and tailor services to meet the unique needs of various subgroups. For some it is related to their military experience, while for others it is related to their race, culture, or sexual orientation. For all, trauma-informed care delivered by culturally and linguistically competent staff is essential. Within this framework, research, policies, and practices should be tailored to the unique needs of each group to improve outcomes and ensure healthier generations to come.

References

Alvarez, L. (2009, August 16). GI Jane breaks the combat barrier. *New York Times*. Retrieved from www.nytimes.com/2009/08/16/us/16women.html

American Academy of Pediatrics. (2005). Providing care for immigrant, homeless, and migrant children. *Pediatrics, 115*, 1095–1100.

American Community Survey. (2012). *The foreign-born population in the United States: 2010*. U.S. Census Bureau. Retrieved from http://www.census.gov/prod/2012pubs/acs-19.pdf

American Psychological Association, Presidential Task Force on Military Deployment Services for Youth, Families and Service Members. (2007). *The psychological needs of U.S. military service members and their families: A preliminary report*. Retrieved from http://www.ptsd. ne.gov/publications/military-deployment-task-force-report.pdf

Ariza, E. N. (2000). Actions speak louder than words—or do they? Debunking the myth of apathetic immigrant parents in education. *Contemporary Education, 71*, 36–38.

Bassuk, E. L., Buckner, J. C., Perloff, J. N., & Bassuk, S. S. (1998). Prevalence of mental health and substance use disorders among homeless and low-income housed mothers. *American Journal of Psychiatry, 155*, 1561–1564.

Bassuk, E. L., Buckner, J., Weinreb, L., Browne, A., Bassuk, S., Dawson, R., et al. (1997). Homelessness in female-headed families: Childhood and adult risk and protective factors. *American Journal of Public Health, 87*(2), 241–248.

Bassuk, E. L., Weinreb, L., Buckner, J., Browne, A., Soloman, A., & Bassuk, S. S. (1996). The characteristics and needs of sheltered homeless and low-income housed mothers. *Journal of the American Medical Association, 276*, 640–646.

Beckerman, N. L., & Corbett, L. (2008). Immigration and families: Treating acculturative stress from a systemic framework. *Family Therapy, 35*(2), 63–81.

Bender, B. (2009, August 24). Veterans forsake studies of stress: Stigma impedes search for remedies. *Boston Globe*. Retrieved from http://www.boston.com/news/nation/washington/articles/2009/08/24/few_iraq_afghanistan_veterans_willing_to_take_part_in_boston

Bhaskar, R., Scopilliti, M., Hollmann, F., & Armstrong, D. (2010). *Plans for producing estimates of net international migration for the 2010 demographic analysis estimates*. U.S. Census Bureau Population Division, Working Paper No. 90, U.S. Census Bureau.

Blanton, R. E., & Foster, L. K. (2012, July). *California's women veterans: Responses to the 2011 survey*. Retrieved Aug 27, 2012, from California Research Bureau, California State Library http://www.library.ca.gov/crb/12/12-004.pdf

Blue Shield of California. (2011). *Preventing violence in the homes of military families. Issue brief*. Retrieved from http://www.familyhomelessness.org/media/241.pdf

Booth, B., Wechsler Segal, M. W., Bell, D. B., Martin, J. A., Ender, M. G., Rohall, D. E., et al. (2007). *What we know about army families: 2007 Update*. Fairfax, VA: Caliber Associates.

BPW Foundation. (2007). *Women veterans in transition*. Retrieved from http://www.bpwfoundation.org/

Breslau, J., Aguilar-Gaxiola, S., Borges, G., Kendler, K. S., Su, M., & Kessler, R. C. (2007). Risk for psychiatric disorder among immigrants and their US-born descendants: Evidence from the national comorbidity survey replication. *Journal of Nervous and Mental Disease, 195*, 189–195.

Browne, A., & Bassuk, S. S. (1997). Intimate violence in the lives of homeless and poor housed women: Prevalence and patterns in an ethnically diverse sample. *American Journal of Orthopsychiatry, 67*, 261–278.

Burns, C., & Ross, P. (2011). *Gay and transgender discrimination outside the workplace: Why we need protections in housing, health care, and public accommodations*. Washington, DC: Center for American Progress.

Capps, R. (2001). *Hardship among children of immigrants: Findings from the 1999 National Survey of American Families*. Retrieved from http://www.urban.org/UploadedPDF/anf_b29.pdf

Capps, R., Fix, M., Ost, J., Reardon-Anderson, J., & Passel, J. S. (2004). *The health and well-being of young children of immigrants*. Retrieved from http://www.urban.org/UploadedPDF/311139_ Childrenimmigrants.pdf

Center for the Study of Social Policy. (2011). *The protective factors framework.* Retrieved from http://www.cssp.org/reform/strengthening-families/the-basics/protective-factors

Chiu, S., Redelmeier, D. A., Tolomiczenko, G., Kiss, A., & Hwang, S. W. (2009). The health of homeless immigrants. *Journal of Epidemiology and Community Health, 63,* 943–948.

Clark, W. A. V. (2003). *Immigrants and the American dream: Remaking the middle class.* New York, NY: Guilford Press.

Clervil, R., Grandin, M., & Greendlinger, R. (2010). *Understanding the experience of war fighters: Military literature and resource review.* Needham, MA: The National Center on Family Homelessness.

Cohen, R. (2011). *The impacts of affordable housing on health: A research summary.* Washington, DC: Center for Housing Policy and Enterprise Community Partners.

Culhane, J. F., Webb, D., Grimm, S., Metraux, S., & Culhane, D. P. (2003). Prevalence of child welfare services involvement among homeless and low-income mothers: A five-year birth cohort study. *Journal of Sociology and Social Welfare, 30*(3), 79–95.

DeCandia, C. J. (2012). *Meeting the needs of young families experiencing homelessness: A guide for service providers and program administrators.* Needham, MA: The National Center on Family Homelessness.

Fair Housing Center of Metropolitan Detroit, Fair Housing Center of Southeastern Michigan, Fair Housing Center of Southwest Michigan, & Fair Housing Center of West Michigan. (2007). *Sexual orientation and housing discrimination in Michigan: A report of Michigan's fair housing centers.* Retrieved from http://www.fhcmichigan.org/images/Arcus_web1.pdf

Fairweather, A. (2006). *Risk and protective factors for homelessness among OIF/OEF veterans.* San Francisco, CA: Swords to Ploughshares.

Fontana, A., Rosenheck, R., & Desai, R. (2010). Female veterans of Iraq and Afghanistan seeking care from VA specialized PTSD programs: Comparison with male veterans and female war zone veterans of previous eras. *Journal of Women's Health, 19,* 751–757.

Foster, R. P. (2001). When immigration is trauma: Guidelines for the individual and family clinician. *American Journal of Orthopsychiatry, 71,* 153–170.

Foster, L., & Vince, S. (2009). *California's women veterans: The challenges and needs of those who serve.* Retrieved from California Research Bureau, California State Library. Retrieved from www.library.ca.gov/crb/10/Womenveteransbrieflystated.pdf

Gates, G. J. (2011, November 9). Can homophobia reduce your home equity. *The Huffington Post.* Retrieved from http://www.huffingtonpost.com/gary-j-gates/can-homophobia reduce-you_b_1082729.html

Gates, G. J., & Cooke, A. M. (2010). *United States census snapshot: 2010.* Retrieved from http://williamsinstitute.law.ucla.edu/wp-content/uploads/Census2010Snapshot-US-v2.pdf

Grant, J. M., Mottet, L. A., Tanis, J., Harrison, J., Herman, J. L., & Keisling, M. (2011). *Injustice at every turn: A report of the National Transgender Discrimination Survey.* Washington, DC: National Center for Transgender Equality and National Gay and Lesbian Task Force.

Grant, B. F., Stinson, F. S., Hasin, D. S., Dawson, D. A., Chou, S. P., & Anderson, K. (2004). Immigration and lifetime prevalence of DSM-IV psychiatric disorders among Mexican Americans and non-Hispanic whites in the United States: Results from the national epidemiologic survey on alcohol and related conditions. *Archives of General Psychiatry, 61,* 1226–1233.

Guarino, K., & Bassuk, E. (2010). Working with families experiencing homelessness: Understanding trauma and its impact. *Zero to Three, 30*(3), 11–20.

Guarino, K., Rubin, L., & Bassuk, E. (2007). Trauma in the lives of homeless families. In E. Carll (Ed.), *Trauma psychology: Issues in violence, disaster, health, and illness* (pp. 231–258). Westport, CT: Praeger.

Guarino, K., Soares, P., Konnath, K., Clervil, R., & Bassuk, E. (2009). *Trauma-Informed Organizational Toolkit.* Rockville, MD: Center for Mental Health Services, Substance Abuse and Mental Health Services Administration, and the Daniels Fund, the National Child Traumatic Stress Network, and the W.K. Kellogg Foundation.

Haan, M. (2011). Does immigrant residential crowding reflect hidden homelessness? *Canadian Studies in Population, 38*(1–2), 43–59.

Hankin, C. S., Skinner, K. M., Sullivan, L. M., Miller, D. R., Frayne, S., & Tripp, T. J. (1999). Prevalence of depressive and alcohol abuse symptoms among women VA outpatients who report experiencing sexual assault while in the military. *Journal of Traumatic Stress, 12*, 601–612.

Herbert, M. S. (1994). Feminism, militarism, and attitudes toward the role of women in the military. *Feminist Issues, 14*(2), 25–48.

Hernandez, D. J., Denton, N. A., & Macartney, S. E. (2007). *Children in immigrant families—The U.S. and 50 states: National origins, language and early education.* Retrieved from http://www.childtrends.org/Files/Child_Trends-2007_04_01_RB_ChildrenInImmigrantFamilies.pdf

Hoge, C. W., Castro, C. A., Messer, S. C., McGurk, D., Cotting, D. I., & Koffman, R. L. (2004). Combat duty in Iraq and Afghanistan, mental health problems, and barriers to care. *The New England Journal of Medicine, 351*(1), 13–22.

Joint Economic Committee. (2007). *Helping military moms balance family and longer deployments.* Washington, DC: Author.

Joint Center for Housing Studies of Harvard University. (2010). *The State of the Nation's Housing.* Cambridge, MA.

Kenney, R. R., Fisher, S. K., Grandin, M. E., Hanson, J. B., & Winn, L. P. (2012). Addressing the needs of LGBT youth who are homeless. In S. Fisher, J. Piorier, & G. Blau (Eds.), *Improving emotional & behavioral outcomes for LGBT youth: A guide for professionals* (pp. 207–221). Baltimore, MD: Paul H. Brookes Publishing Co.

Kniskern, M. K., & Segal, D. R. (2010). *Mean wage differences between civilian and military wives.* College Park, MD: RAND Corporation.

LaBash, H. A. J., Vogt, D. S., King, L. A., & King, D. W. (2009). Deployment stressors of the Iraqi war: Insights from the mainstream media. *Journal of Interpersonal Violence, 24*, 231–258.

Lubell, J., Crain, R., & Cohen, R. (2007). *The positive impacts of affordable housing on health: A research summary.* Washington, DC: Center for Housing Policy and Enterprise Community Partners.

MacGregor, C., Hamilton, A. B., Oishi, S. B., & Yano, E. M. (2011). Descriptive, development, and philosophies of mental health service delivery for female veterans in the VA: A qualitative study. *Women's Health Issues, 21*, S138–S144.

Mancini, D. L., & Archambault, C. (2000). *What recent research tells us about military families and communities.* Arlington, VA: Military Family Resource Center.

Marshall, A. D., Panuzio, J., & Taft, C. T. (2005). Intimate partner violence among military veterans and active duty servicemen. *Clinical Psychology Review, 25*, 862–876.

Martin, M. (2009). *Helping new immigrants to access housing resources: What providers should know.* Retrieved from http://homeless.samhsa.gov/Resource/Helping-New-Immigrants-to-Access-Housing-Resources-What-Providers-Should-Know-47254.aspx

Matthews, H. & Jang, D. (2007). *The Challenges of change: Learning from the child care and early education experiences of immigrant families.* Retrieved from http://www.clasp.org/admin/site/publications/files/0356.pdf

Movement Advancement Project, Family Equality Council, & Center for American Progress. (2011). *All children matter: How legal and social inequalities hurt LGBT families.* Denver, CO: Authors.

Murdie, R., Preston, V., Ghosh, S., & Chevalier, M. (2006). *Immigrants and housing: A review of the Canadian literature from 1990 to 2005.* Retrieved from http://www.homelesshub.ca/ResourceFiles/Immigrants&HousingAReview_of_Canadian_Literature_from.pdf

National Association for the Education of Homeless Children and Youth. (NAEHCY). (2006). *Immigrant and homeless: Information for school district title III programs and community agencies.* Retrieved from http://center.serve.org/nche/downloads/briefs/imm_gen.pdf

National Association for the Education of Homeless Children and Youth. (NAEHCY) (2007). *Immigrants, refugees, and homelessness.* Retrieved from http://www.naehcy.org/sites/default/files/images/dl/beam/spr_07.pdf

National Center for Mental Health Promotion and Youth Violence Prevention. (2010). *Military families: Impact on children's and families' mental health.* Waltham, MA: Author.

Perez-Foster, R. (2001). When immigration is trauma: Guidelines for the individual and family clinician. *American Journal of Orthopsychiatry, 71*, 153–170.

Prescott, L., Soares, P., Konnath, K., & Bassuk, E. (2008). *A long journey home: A guide for creating trauma-informed services for mothers and children experiencing homelessness.* Rockville, MD: Center for Mental Health Services, Substance Abuse and Mental Health Services Administration; and the Daniels Fund; National Child Traumatic Stress Network; and the W.K. Kellogg Foundation.

Preston, V., Murdie, R., D'Addario, S., Sibanda, P., Murnaghan, A., Logan, J., & Ahn, M. H. (2011). *Precarious housing and hidden homelessness among refugees, asylum seekers, and immigrants in the Toronto metropolitan area.* CERIS working paper No. 87. Toronto, ON.

Quintana, N. S., Rosenthal, J., & Krehely, J. (2010). *On the streets: The federal response to gay and transgender homeless youth.* Washington, DC: Center for American Progress.

Rentz, E. D., Marshall, S. W., Loomis, D., Casteel, C., Martin, S. L., & Gibbs, D. A. (2007). Effect of deployment on the occurrence of child maltreatment in military and nonmilitary families. *American Journal of Epidemiology, 165*, 1199–1206.

Rosenheck, R., Bassuk, E., & Salomon, A (1999). *Special populations of homeless Americans. Substance Abuse and Mental Health Administration Homelessness Resource Center.* Retrieved from http://www.urbancentre.utoronto.ca/pdfs/elibrary/1998_Special-Pop-HL.pdf

Sadler, A. G., Booth, B. M., Mengeling, M. A., & Doebbeling, B. N. (2004). Life span and repeated violence against women during military service: Effects on health status and outpatient utilization. *Journal of Women's Health, 13*, 799–811.

Sadler, A. G., Booth, B. M., Nielson, D., & Doebbeling, B. N. (2000). Health-related consequences of physical and sexual violence: Women in the military. *Obstetrics and Gynecology, 96*, 473–480.

Sayers, S. L., Farrow, V. A., Ross, J., & Oslin, D. W. (2009). Family problems among recently returned military veterans referred for a mental health evaluation. *Journal of Clinical Psychiatry, 70*(2), 163–170.

Sears, B. & Badgett, L. (2012). *Beyond stereotypes: Poverty in the LGBT community.* Retrieved from http://momentum.tides.org/beyond-the-stereotypes-poverty-in-the lgbt-community/

Shinn, M., & Bassuk, E. L. (2004). Families. In S. Barrow et al. (Eds.), *Encyclopedia of homelessness* (pp. 149–156). Great Barrington, MA: Berkshire Publishing.

Sikich, K. W. (2008). Global female homelessness: A multifaceted problem. *Gender Issues, 25*, 147–156.

Sogomonyan, F., & Cooper, J. L. (2010). *Trauma faced by children of military families.* New York, NY: National Center for Children in Poverty.

Street, A. E., Vogt, D., & Dutra, L. (2009). A new generation of women veterans: Stressors faced by women deployed to Iraq and Afghanistan. *Clinical Psychology Review, 29*, 685–694.

Substance Abuse and Mental Health Services Administration. (2011). *Current statistics on the prevalence and characteristics of people experiencing homelessness in the United States.* Washington, DC: Author.

Tanasescu, A., Classens, M., Turner, D., Richter-Salmons, S., Pruegger, V., & Smart, A. (2009). Hidden in plain sight: Housing challenges of newcomers in Calgary. *United Way of Calgary.*

Tanasescu, A. I., Classens, M., Turner, D., Ritcher-Salmons, S., Pruegger, V., & Smart, A. (2011). *Hidden in plain sight: Housing challenges of newcomers in Calgary.* Calgary: Calgary Homeless Foundation and United Way of Calgary and Area.

Tanielian, T., & Jaycox, L. H. (2008). *Invisible wounds of war: Psychological and cognitive injuries, their consequences, and services to assist recovery.* Santa Monica, CA: The RAND Corporation.

The National Center for Homeless Education. (2006). *Immigrant and homeless: Information for School District Title III Programs and Community Agencies.* Retrieved from http://center.serve.org/nche/downloads/briefs/imm_gen.pdf

The National Center on Family Homelessness. (2011a). *America's youngest outcasts.* Needham, MA: Author.

The National Center on Family Homelessness. (2011b). *The characteristics and needs of families experiencing homelessness*. Retrieved from http://www.familyhomelessness.org/media/306.pdf

The United States Conference of Mayors & Sodexho, Inc. (2006). *Hunger and homelessness survey: A status report on hunger and homelessness in America's cities*. Washington, DC & Gaithersburg, MD: Authors.

Tsai, J., Rosenheck, R. A., & McGuire, J. F. (2012). Comparison of outcomes of homeless female and male veterans in transitional housing. *Community Mental Health Journal* [epub ahead of print]. DOI: 10.1007/s10597-012-9482-5.

U.S. Census Bureau. (2011). *State and county QuickFacts*. Retrieved from http://quickfacts.census.gov/qfd/states/00000.html

U.S. Department of Housing and Urban Development. (2012a). *Equal access to housing in HUD programs regardless of sexual orientation or gender identity* (Federal Register 5359–F–02). Washington, DC: Author.

U.S. Department of Housing and Urban Development. (2012b). *The 2011 annual homeless assessment report to Congress*. Washington, DC: Author.

U.S. Department of Housing and Urban Development. (2012c). *The 2012 point in time estimates of homelessness*. Washington, DC: Office of Community Planning and Development.

United Nations High Commissioner for Refugees (UNHCR). (2006). *The state of The world's refugees 2006: Human displacement in the new millennium*. http://www.unhcr.org/4a4dc1a89.html

United Nations High Commissioner for Refugees (UNHCR). (2011). *Get up and go: Refugee resettlement and secondary migration in the USA*. Retrieved from http://www.unhcr.org/4e5f9a079.html

United Nations High Commissioner for Refugees (UNHCR). (2013). *Refugees*. http://www.unhcr.org/pages/49c3646c2.html

United States Bureau of Labor Statistics. (2012). *Employment situation of veterans—2011*. Retrieved from www.bls.gov/news.release/pdf/vet.pdf

United States Department of Labor, Women's Bureau. (2011). *Trauma informed care for women veterans experiencing homelessness*. Washington, DC: Author.

United States Department of Veterans Affairs. (2004). *Veterans Health Initiative (VHI) study guide*. Washington, DC: Author.

United States Department of Veterans Affairs. (2006). *Strategic plan FY 2006–2011*. Washington, DC: Office of the Secretary.

United States Department of Veterans Affairs. (2012). *Strategies for serving our women veterans*. Washington, DC: Women Veterans Task Force.

United States Department of Veterans Affairs. (2013). Chapter 9: Special groups of veterans, homeless veterans. In *Federal benefits for veterans, dependents and survivors*. Washington, DC: Author Retrieved from http://www.va.gov/opa/publications/benefits_book/benefits_chap09.asp

Wardrip, K. E., Pelletiere, D., & Crowley, S. (2009). *Out of reach 2009*. Washington, DC: National Low Income Housing Coalition.

Weber Castaneda, L., & Harrell, M. C. (2008). Military spouse employment: A grounded theory approach to experiences and perceptions. *Armed Forces & Society, 34*, 389–412.

Yakushko, O., Watson, M., & Thompson, S. (2008). Stress and coping in the lives of recent immigrants and refugees: Considerations for counseling. *International Journal for the Advancement of Counseling, 30*, 167–178.

Part II
Frameworks for Service Delivery and Intervention for Families

Chapter 6
Collaborations Across and Within Systems That Provide Services to Families without Homes

James H. Bray and Andrea Link

Abstract Coordinated intervention from multiple service agencies is a necessity because of the complex set of issues facing families without homes. Barriers to interagency collaboration exist, but are not insurmountable. This chapter presents ten evidence-based principles that can guide successful collaborations that are based on the Federal Strategic Plan to End Homelessness. These principles are illustrated using real-life examples taken from several programs that help people without homes.

> No one should experience homelessness—no one should be without a safe, stable place to call home. (United States Interagency Council on Homelessness, 2010)

Most families without homes need an array of social services in order to establish or regain stable housing and productive lives. Because many homeless persons and families are marginalized by society, they are likely to feel disconnected from or be unaware of social services that can assist them. In addition, many people experiencing homelessness can feel powerless and lack a sense of agency in order to find needed services (Holleman, Bray, Davis, & Holleman, 2004). From the service side, many agencies that provide services are not coordinated and may even compete with each other for funding (USICH, 2010). This situation presents a unique challenge for a person and his/her family to know where to turn for assistance and for agencies to help people get the services they need.

Families without homes include people of all ages, races, ethnicities, cultural backgrounds, sexual orientation, and immigration status (APA, 2010; USICH, 2010). Further, some of these individuals may suffer from mental health, substance abuse and/or other disabilities and problems that complicate their lives. While the majority of people who are homeless are not substance abusers or mentally ill, people with these problems face additional barriers in exiting homelessness and require

Project Total Recovery was supported by grant H79 TI13909 from the Substance Abuse and Mental Health Services Administration, Warren Holleman, project director.

J.H. Bray, Ph.D. (✉) • A. Link, M.D.
Baylor College of Medicine, Houston, TX 77030, USA
e-mail: jbray@bcm.edu

M.E. Haskett et al. (eds.), *Supporting Families Experiencing Homelessness: Current Practices and Future Directions*, DOI 10.1007/978-1-4614-8718-0_6,
© Springer Science+Business Media New York 2014

different services than those without these problems. Further, professionals working with individuals and families need to be aware of cultural diversity and values and also recognize the strengths of families who experience homelessness. To be successful in helping the homeless, collaborations are needed among and within service systems that address family needs as well as those specific to adults and children (Holleman et al., 2004; Rogers et al., 2012). At a systemic level, collaborations should occur among professionals within public health agencies, child welfare agencies, educational and job training programs, and schools, as well as housing programs (APA, 2010; USICH, 2010).

The Federal Response: Federal Strategic Plan to Prevent and End Homelessness

The Obama Administration made ending homelessness a top priority during the first presidential term (USICH, 2010). President Obama stated, "Since the founding of our country, "home" has been the center of the American dream. Stable housing is the foundation upon which everything else in a family's or individual's life is built—without a safe, affordable place to live, it is much tougher to maintain good health, get a good education or reach your full potential (preface, USICH, 2010)." There is also a federal Congressional mandate from the Homeless Emergency Assistance and Rapid Transition to Housing (HEARTH) Act of 2009 and bi-partisan support for moving forward with this priority (US Congress, 2009).

Due in part to the economic recession of 2008–2009, the USA experienced a great expansion of people without homes; the expansion included not only people living in poverty, but also middle class people who found themselves overwhelmed with debt and without a job. In addition, due to the long-standing wars in the Middle East, there were unprecedented numbers of veterans without homes, some of whom could not find jobs after leaving the military and some who suffered from physical and mental health problems due to serving in the military. President Obama recognized the importance of addressing these problems and created the United States Interagency Council on Homelessness that brought together 20 federal agencies, ranging from the Department of Housing and Urban Development to Department of Veterans Affairs to develop a comprehensive strategic plan to end in homelessness in America (USICH, 2010). The Plan focused on four key goals:

"(1) Finish the job of ending chronic homelessness in five years; (2) Prevent and end homelessness among Veterans in five years; (3) Prevent and end homelessness for families, youth, and children in ten years; and (4) Set a path to ending all types of homelessness" (USICH, 2010, p. 4).

The collaboration between and coordination of services among the 20 federal agencies is a model to understand and address problems at state and local levels. The Plan developed a set of strategies for the federal government to partner with state and local governments and the private sector to use comprehensive and cost effective methods to end homelessness (USICH, 2010). President Obama plans to continue this work in his second term and implement the Federal Strategic Plan.

Simultaneously and independently, the first author, while President of the American Psychological Association, created the Presidential Task Force on Psychology's Contributions to Ending Homelessness (APA, 2010). The task force, made up of psychologists who are national leaders, researchers, and clinicians, was charged with reviewing the published literature on people without homes and making recommendations for research, practice, training and public service to end homelessness. The work of the Task Force was incorporated into the Federal Strategic Plan through consultation with the USICH and during a Congressional briefing.

Guiding Principles for Collaboration Across Systems

The Federal Strategic Plan identified a number of key principles for collaborating agencies to follow to meet the needs of people without homes. The Plan provides guidance for interagency collaboration that aligns housing, health, education, and human services to both prevent homelessness and help those without homes regain a productive life (USICH, 2010). Some of these principles will be discussed in the remainder of the chapter and illustrated through examples from our work in several settings that help people without homes. Other principles of collaboration that we found useful in our work are also discussed and illustrated with examples.

Develop a Common Mission

A shared vision and a strong commitment to that vision is a critical first step in any collaboration. In addition to articulating a vision, it is also important to emphasize the need for improved services through collaboration (Carnochan & Austin, 2002; Jacobs, Newman, & Burns, 2001; Jones, Crook, & Webb, 2008; Packard, Patti, Daly, & Tucker-Tatlow, 2012; Rogers et al., 2012). Agencies contemplating a joint endeavor can have different overall missions yet agree on a specific and common goal regarding helping people without homes. In order to have common goals, each group must see some benefit to their own agency's mission.

Chances of success are increased if agencies strongly commit not only to common goals but to a partnership as well (Mizrahi & Rosenthal, 2001). Although there can be differences in the degree to which institutions value a particular mission, the more closely aligned they are, the more likely it will be a successful collaboration. In this chapter, two examples from our work with adults, children, and families experiencing homelessness will be used to illustrate the principles of collaboration across systems.

Project Total Recovery, a joint project between the Baylor College of Medicine Department of Family and Community Medicine (BFM) and the Star of Hope Mission (SoH), a Christian ministry serving Houston's homeless since 1907 (Holleman et al., 2004), was developed to provide comprehensive services to homeless and near-homeless women, children, and families. One of their facilities, the

Transitional Living Center (TLC), is a residential treatment program serving women, children, and families. People accepted into the TLC program were required to participate in an array of activities, such as a 12-step substance abuse recovery program, a personal development program, and a career development program. Following the structured programs, the adults were expected to seek employment or enter an educational program to enhance their job skills.

As part of Project Total Recovery, the Baylor-Star of Hope Center for Counseling began providing individual, family, and group therapy to all TLC clients. Most staff were part-time and included family psychologists and therapists, family physicians, family practice resident physicians, social workers, and trainees from mental health programs. The Center adopted a collaborative, primary care approach to treatment (Frank, McDaniel, Bray, & Heldring, 2004). A more detailed description of our program is found in Holleman et al. (2004). Although the primary mission of the SoH was to help women and children who were homeless and near-homeless find permanent housing and develop productive lives, the primary goal of the Counseling Center was to provide mental and behavioral health and medical services for the women and children at the TLC. Further, the Center provided an important training site for family physician residents, psychology trainees and family therapy trainees. Our work on behavioral and medical health issues was in support of the ultimate goal of the SoH to help end homeless for these women and children.

To create Project Total Recovery, we had to demonstrate to the SoH that our mission of training and service supported their mission of helping families who were experiencing homelessness develop productive lives. Prior to this project, many services were outsourced and required multiple trips to different agencies. Recognizing the splintered nature of services provided to women and children without homes and the stress of locating and obtaining the services at many different locations, we developed a common mission of bringing the care providers to the SoH to unify fractionalized care, break down barriers, and develop creative solutions to better support these women and children.

Another example of successful collaboration is the Jail Outreach Project, a partnership between Healthcare for the Homeless—Houston (HHH), the Harris County Sherriff's Office, and the Mental Health and Mental Retardation Authority of Harris County (MHMRA). This project is a prime example of aligning missions to better serve a population that is often marginalized (Buck, Brown, & Hickey, 2011; Held, Brown, Frost, Hickey, & Buck, 2012). HHH was established in 2001 with a specific focus on integrated primary and mental health care for homeless people in Houston, Texas. The Jail Inreach Program was initiated in 2006 as a response to the increasing number of homeless and mentally ill individuals who were cycling through Harris County, Texas jail system. The Harris County Jail is the largest provider of mental health services in the state of Texas, and the second largest in the country, with an average of 2,400 inmates receiving mental health services on any given day (Buck et al., 2011). Due to the challenges in trying to link released inmates with behavioral health and social services, abrupt termination of care at the time of release was the norm. This resulted in many individuals diagnosed with mental illness and no home cycling between the streets, hospital emergency centers, and jail cells.

A primary goal of the Jail Inreach Project was to improve the health status and support the social reintegration of these individuals through health care based intensive case management (Buck et al., 2011). Key to this project was the involvement of the Harris County Sheriff's Office since the Sheriff controlled access to the inmates prior to release, and a central feature of the program was the case manager's engagement of the inmate *prior to release*.

HHH approached the Sheriff's Office knowing the Office had a strong interest in decreasing recidivism, given the serious issue of jail overcrowding and the expense of housing inmates trapped in the revolving door of incarceration. A successful collaboration was initiated with the Sheriff's Office that gave HHH case managers access to the secure side of the jail. The Sheriff's Office also assisted HHH in establishing "direct releases" whereby inmates were held until morning, at which time an HHH case manager could pick up the client and escort them to the clinic. This is a prime example of successful collaboration between two agencies that might have had different overall missions but had the shared goals of reducing recidivism and increasing linkage to medical care and social services.

All Stakeholders are Represented

To create successful collaborations across agencies and systems, all potential stakeholders need to be identified and included in a meaningful manner for planning and implementation (White & Wehlage, 1995). It is also vital to include as diverse and representative an array of stakeholders as is possible (Foster-Fishman, Berkowitz, Lounsbury, Jacobson, & Allen, 2001). This may include management, consumers, representatives from other agencies and staff at all levels. Enabling staff at all levels to participate in planning as well as implementation of the collaboration can produce more innovative ideas, enhance problem solving and build consensus (Patti et al., 2003). Consensus is valuable because collaboration among agencies will always have positives and negatives, and any kind of change may be met with resistance and concern. By discussing advantages and disadvantages openly and early in the process, the chance of "buy-in" from stakeholders is increased. By keeping partnership negotiations as transparent as possible, staff reservations can be minimized.

Another issue for middle management and frontline staff is the concern that changes in the programs will result in added duties and responsibilities (Packard et al., 2012). Tension is created by change, which can lead to increased levels of stress on personnel (Carnochan & Austin, 2002). However, if management communicates a sympathetic understanding of the increased stress, and encourages honest and open two-way communication, the strain of change will be mitigated (Packard et al., 2012).

The formation of workgroups made up of frontline staff, as well as middle and top management, is another technique to involve staff in a meaningful way (Packard et al., 2012). Frontline staff members are a particularly important group of stakeholders to involve in all levels of planning, as they can be the eyes and ears of the collaborative process given their street-level understanding of the problems. Frontline staff are often perfectly positioned to identify problems and suggest remedies (White & Wehlage, 1995).

This is certainly true of frontline staff serving families who are homeless, as those staff are familiar with the barriers encountered by individuals seeking assistance. Formerly homeless individuals are another helpful resource in planning any collaboration or program, as they bring a unique and usually unheard perspective. At HHH, the "Change Committee" is made up exclusively of individuals who have previous or current experience with homelessness, and they report directly to the Board of Directors (Buck, Rochon, Davidson, & McCurdy, 2004). To further increase their voice in decisions, one member of the Change Committee serves on the HHH Board of Directors.

The Jail Inreach Project also endeavors to involve all stakeholders, and input on the program has been solicited from a wide range of community and government groups. Case managers are empowered to suggest changes to service protocols and there is an "open door" policy all the way to the Chief Executive Officer. Frequent communication between HHH, MHMRA, the Sheriff's Office and other partnering agencies continues to be the norm that includes all levels of the organizational hierarchy.

About 80 % of the women at the Star of Hope Transition Living Center entered the program with substance abuse problems. The TLC has a traditional, 12-step based substance abuse recovery program for the women, called New Hope Recovery. Women stayed in the program until the leaders felt they were ready to graduate and move into the other TLC programs. The decisions to graduate from the New Hope Program were made exclusively by the Licensed Chemical Dependency Counselor leaders of the program. After a year of our collaborative program, it became apparent from working with the women that most of them had experienced physical and sexual abuse as well as trauma. Many also had dual-diagnoses (Anxiety Disorder, Major Depression, and other mental illnesses) in addition to the substance abuse and untreated medical conditions. After leaving the substance abuse program about 20 % had a substance use relapse and were terminated from the TLC. Staff at the SoH expressed frustration in dealing with these kinds of problems as these women had problems complying with the TLC's rules and standards, had angry outbursts due to substance withdrawal and abuse histories, and had difficulty participating in other programs due to mental health problems. For example, women who were depressed were late to class because of sleep problems or unable to complete assignments because of lack of concentration and low energy.

Because of our academic background and funding from the Substance Abuse and Mental Health Services Administration (SAMHSA), we were aware of the research and evidence-based practices that could address these issues. We set up meetings with administrators to address the concerns voiced by staff and the women residents. At first the administration was reluctant to consider our suggestions for implementing changes. However, we decided to ask the frontline staff to attend the next meeting and describe the problems they experienced, and we presented data from our counseling clinic sessions to document the issues. After hearing from the frontline staff and seeing our data, the administration was more open to considering changes in the various programs to address the mental and physical health problems of the women residing in the program. For example, we educated the SoH administration about the high relapse rate for people with substance abuse problems, even after treatment. In response, the administration agreed to change the "zero tolerance" stance about relapse to one in which women found to be using again were given the opportunity to reenter the substance abuse treatment program and also receive individual counseling. The input of the frontline staff was critical to making these types of changes and this resulted in more of the women successfully completing the TLC programs.

Use Evidence-Based and Solution-Driven Approaches

Collaborating agencies may historically have approached the same problem in differing ways, which can potentially lead to discord. However, when interventions are based on evidence-based approaches, the potential for disagreement is diminished. The Federal Strategic Plan found that there are several programs that have strong evidence for their success (USICH, 2010). In addition, as part of implementation of the plan, several federal agencies such as Housing and Urban Development, are now spending substantial funds on evaluating the success or failure of their programs.

Because many agencies that serve individuals and families experiencing homelessness are run by community or faith-based organizations, formal program evaluations or implementation of evidence-based methods and interventions is not necessarily the norm. Many of these agencies do not have access to the knowledge or expertise to implement evidence-based programs. Thus, one of the important roles of outside professionals is to bring this expertise to the various organizations that serve people without homes.

In Project Total Recovery, the Baylor-Star of Hope collaboration brought this type of perspective to our work. Through our prior work in medical settings and with other homeless agencies, we were familiar with the research and evidence-based interventions to help homeless women with substance abuse problems, mental health problems, and trauma. As previously noted, the SoH substance abuse program, New Hope Recovery Program, was a traditional 12-step program run by Licensed Chemical Dependency Counselors (LCDC). In the process of working together we established good relationships that enabled us to share new research on these problems and alternative treatment strategies. To help them implement these, we used funds from our federal grant to hire experts in Motivational Interviewing (Miller & Rollnick, 2002) who treated women who had experienced trauma to provide skills-based workshops. SoH staff members were invited to attend these workshops, which furthered our collaboration and improved our development of a common language and understanding for change. The SoH LCDC staff incorporated aspects of MI into their 12-step program, and they also recognized how trauma and other mental health problems impacted the women's substance abuse. Thus, they were willing to allow these women to simultaneously attend their program and receive counseling in our program. We found that implementation of these changes improved program completion rates (Holleman et al., 2004).

Evidence based models also have informed the Jail Inreach Project since its inception. In formulating this collaborative effort, an exhaustive literature search was performed in addition to soliciting the advice of numerous professionals in the field. The resultant plan not only addressed the needs of homeless ex-offenders identified from the growing body of research, but it also used evidence-based models to formulate protocols for addressing the unique challenges faced by jail releases. One protocol will be discussed later in the chapter.

Develop Agreed-Upon Outcomes and How to Measure Them

Methods for measuring outcomes and endpoints need to be discussed and agreed upon at the beginning of project planning (Hayes, Mann, Morgan, Kelly, & Weightman, 2012). This is always a critical aspect of program development, but it is even more important when definitions of success may differ from one organization to another. It is also beneficial if all members of the partnership develop an outcomes orientation where both short and long-term goals are developed and any successes are celebrated (Foster-Fishman et al., 2001). Realistic expectations, which are distinct from shared goals, need to be developed. When collaborators have short-term objectives that are out of sync, progress is impeded (Liedtka & Whitten, 1998). It is also important to have continuous evaluation of the collaboration itself, with periodic assessments of the coalition mission, objectives, and strategy (Foster-Fishman et al., 2001).

Participating members must identify the types of measures that will be used to gauge success and commit to collecting the data needed to assess the outcome (USICH, 2010). While this can be time-intensive and divert resources away from direct client services, it can help project participants to establish common ground and provide justification for the disruption in services and increase in costs that can be associated with collaboration (Yessian, 1995). Developing a collaborative data collection system can be an especially challenging issue when dealing with multiple agencies, but a mutual database can pay off tremendously when it is time to evaluate and report on a program's effectiveness. It is particularly important to focus on client-outcome measures instead of the standard approach of assessing the number of clients served or the number of linkages established. Documentation of actual changes in client functioning over time is a better measure of the difference the collaboration is making (Yessian, 1995).

HHH, MHMRA, and the Sheriff's Office all agreed that the primary measurable endpoint for the Jail Inreach Project was the reduction in arrest rates of program participants. By using arrest data from Harris County and client data being recorded by HHH, recidivism was monitored and evaluated. To this end, before even the first client was referred to the Jail Inreach Project, an online database was created to track demographics, diagnoses, number of clients linked to services after release, and other pertinent client information. The database tracked client information in a way that was accessible for both research and evaluation (Held et al., 2012). In 2009 and again in 2011, HHH worked with MHMRA, the Harris County Budget Office and the Sheriff's Office to conduct evaluations of the Jail Inreach Project. Data from Harris County was used along with records from the Jail Inreach database to evaluate if the program was impacting recidivism. Data analysis showed that there was a

57 % reduction in recidivism after one year, which demonstrated the tremendous impact of the program (Held et al., 2012).

Various programming features were also assessed for their efficacy in reducing rearrest rates. One area of collaboration turned out to be particularly significant. When clients participated in "direct release" (see earlier explanation) they were much less likely to be rearrested (Held et al., 2012). Knowing the impact of this one programming feature—which was solely possible because of the collaborative effort—solidified relations between the two agencies and helped guide future policy in the jail project.

Develop a Common Language and Similar Definitions

A common language is a necessary step toward helping families without homes negotiate a system that can be fractured (USICH, 2010). Agreeing upon basic definitions is helpful; however, even if agreement is not possible, it is still useful to understand each organization's terms and be aware of conflicting definitions. Different agencies that work with those without a home often have different definitions of homelessness. This can potentially cause conflict when differing intake criteria makes a family eligible for services under one agency's definition but ineligible under the other's. Harris Health System, the county-funded health system, and HHH, for example, have different eligibility criteria for entry into homeless-oriented programs. Cooperation between these two health care entities was critical because many specialty medical services could not be provided at the HHH clinic, but required referral to the county system. To qualify for the county discounted health care plan designed for homeless individuals ("The Homeless Gold Card"), a person had to reside in an emergency shelter or on the street. A different kind of Gold Card was available for those who were considered housed and still indigent, but there was a different intake process for that program. In contrast, to qualify for HHH's services, a client could live on the streets, in a shelter, in a treatment program, be doubled up with family members, or even just be at risk for homelessness. By clearly delineating these differences in definitions, inappropriate linkages were decreased and clients were referred to the program that best fit their needs.

Establish Clear Policies and Procedures

Institutionalizing changes by making formal modifications in policies and procedures is essential for long-term success (Jones et al., 2008; Packard et al., 2012). When ground rules are clearly delineated and agreed upon, the potential for later conflict is diminished. The goal is to make the change permanent and sustainable, yet allow changes in policy to be made as the partnership develops. Project Total Recovery was funded by a grant from the Substance Abuse and Mental Health Services Administration (SAMHSA). Submitting a federal grant required the delineation of formal agreements to implement the project. To develop the grant proposal we needed to create a legal agreement between Baylor College of Medicine and the Star of Hope Mission. The agreement specified the duties and responsibilities of each group and how funds would be allocated. In addition, the grant required written policies and procedures for the services provided. The program services were developed through a series of meetings between BFM staff leaders and SoH staff and administration. Policies and procedures were proposed that would meet the needs of both groups. Agreed-upon outcomes were developed and our project evaluator created measurable outcomes to assess project success.

This process required that the SoH formalize some of its policies and procedures and how BFM staff would interact with their established procedures. Issues around confidentiality, sharing of information across programs, and professional responsibilities had to be delineated. This process set the stage for a successful start to our program. However, as is often the case, this initial set of agreements and plans needed continual process improvement as we implemented the project. Some of these issues are discussed in later sections.

A useful tool to formalize a partnership is creation of a Memorandum of Understanding (MOU). An MOU can formalize the partnership and can also describe the range of services that will be provided. An MOU can allow for sharing of client information, which in turn can improve service delivery. HHH entered into MOU agreements with both MHMRA and the Harris County Sheriff's Office and Harris Health System early in the process of collaboration, which allowed for sharing of patient medical information and also formalized policies and procedures. The MOU allowed case managers to access the Harris County Jail electronic health records, giving HHH medical providers an accurate and up to date record of each client's health issues. This improved the continuity of care for our vulnerable clients. The MOU with MHMRA established the referral process and created a system for the sharing of client records, which in turn improved continuity of care as well as facilitated research and evaluation efforts (Buck et al., 2011).

The Jail Inreach Project also has a comprehensive set of written guidelines that is followed by all project staff. It describes the referral process, the arrangement and agenda of inmate visits, how jail records are to be accessed, and the procedure for direct release and how post-release follow-up should be handled. It also explains how client information and case manager plans should be documented, both in the electronic health record as well as in the research database.

While the Federal Strategic Plan (USICH, 2010) did not explicitly recommend the following guiding principles, we have found the following principles to be supported in the literature and useful in our various projects for the homeless.

Keep Lines of Communication Open

Ongoing, regular, two-way communication is critical for successful collaborations (Packard et al., 2012). Communication can be enhanced by deliberate planning of contact, such as regularly scheduled meetings and updates to stakeholders using a variety of medium, such as emails, newsletters and video conferencing. Face-to-face meetings are essential to develop relationships and enhance communication (Patti et al., 2003). In addition, co-location of staff, as well as cross-disciplinary training, can facilitate better communication (Haas, Bauer-Leffler, & Turley, 2011; Patti et al., 2003).

The collaboration between HHH and MHMRA resulted in placement of a licensed MHMRA clinician within the HHH clinics, marking the first time MHMRA had done this within a Federally Qualified Health Center (FQHC) in Harris County. This had the effect of Jail Inreach staff developing a much clearer idea of MHMRA eligibility criteria as well as MHMRA personnel having a better understanding of the HHH service model. This co-location also helped to develop professional relationships between staff from both agencies. Key HHH staff also underwent training alongside MHMRA personnel, which gave both sides the opportunity to work together in the same physical location, thereby enhancing trust between team members.

Ensure Strong and Consistent Leadership

Competent and visionary leadership is consistently identified as one of the most critical predictors of success in collaborations (Jones et al., 2008; Mizrahi & Rosenthal, 2001; Packard et al., 2012; Yessian, 1995). Leaders of the different agencies need to be committed to the project and be willing to expend personal energy and professional capital to ensure success (Packard et al., 2012). The most effective coalition leaders are visionaries who are credible, trustworthy, articulate, organized, and have good facilitation and political skills (Mizrahi & Rosenthal, 2001). Successful coalition leaders also excel at administration, conflict resolution and resource development (Foster-Fishman et al., 2001).

The Jail Inreach Project benefited tremendously from strong and reliable leadership from all agencies involved. Although the initial idea of this program came from HHH leadership, the sustained commitment from leaders at MHMRA and the Sheriff's Office made the project a reality. The leaders at HHH (the President and the Chief Executive Officer) are well respected in the community with a proven track record of innovating successful programs, so proposals coming from HHH have had immediate credibility.

Respect and Understand Cultures of Different Agencies and Social Systems

It is important to be aware of collaborating agencies' unique cultures and values. Although divergent agency cultures do not preclude a successful collaboration, awareness of areas of difference is key. An agency that prides itself on being fluid and organic may face challenges collaborating with one that is more hierarchical and rigid. Awareness of these differences can decrease the potential for misunderstandings in future interactions. Stereotypes and mistrust can be remedied by joint planning, co-location of staff, cross training, and team building exercises (Patti et al., 2003).

The Star of Hope Mission is a conservative faith-based Christian organization that requires its residents to abide by certain rules that are consistent with its Christian values, such as attending chapel services and abiding by clear rules, regardless of the resident's own belief systems or faith. The SoH was clear that it did not condone or support issues such as homosexual behavior or abortion. These were in direct conflict with their values. On the other hand, Baylor College of Medicine is a traditional medical school with scientific and medical values and ethics. Differences in values set the stage for several conflicts. This came to the forefront after several clients came for counseling with our physicians and behavioral health providers regarding reproductive health issues and their sexual orientation. When the SoH staff learned that we were discussing these issues with the women, they initially gave us an ultimatum to immediately stop addressing these issues or terminate the project. We realized that we had to come to a consensus on how to address these issues in order to continue our work at the SoH.

We used this opportunity to better understand SoH's values and perspectives and reinforce that we respected their perspective and integrity around these issues. Second, we used this as an opportunity to educate them about our code of ethics and inform them that physicians and mental health professionals had varying views on these issues. For example, some physicians are willing to discuss and perform abortions, while others are not. It is up to the individual physician to make that decision. Further, we informed them that if they insisted on telling a physician how to practice, then they would in essence be practicing medicine without a license and this stance would violate federal regulations concerning these issues. The SoH relied heavily on federal housing funding and the funding was important to maintain. Through these discussions, we made several agreements that enabled us to continue to work together in a meaningful way and that respected our differing values. This process resolved the conflict and as a result we were able to forge a stronger partnership in other areas.

Create and Nurture One-to-One Relationships Across Agencies

While trust and relationship building between organizations is critically important, so is the building of one-to-one relationships between staff (Jones et al., 2008; Mizrahi & Rosenthal, 2001). Collaboration between agencies is often only as strong as the personal relationships developed between agency members. As a result, agencies need to allow staff time to build trust with each other and cultivate their professional relationships (Frank et al., 2004; Rogers et al., 2012). Building trust within teams and between hierarchical levels of staff is important, as is building trust between top management (Packard et al., 2012). As mentioned above, joint trainings and co-location of staff can assist with this issue.

When the Jail Inreach Project was first proposed, the established relationship between executive management at HHH and MHMRA was an enormous advantage in implementing the new program. Trust between these individuals and belief in their shared vision was a significant contributor to the early success of the program. Upper management continues to allow time for staff in the Jail Project to nurture collaborative relationships. When case managers are newly hired to work on the project, time is set aside for site visits to many of the agencies with whom they will be working. During these tours, staff not only learn firsthand about services that may benefit their client, but important relationships are formed. When case managers are putting together a service plan for a client, having the ability to connect with a known partner at another agency is a priceless resource. Whether this is a housing manager at a transitional living facility or intake coordinator at a substance abuse treatment program, having a personal connection with a staff person at a collaborating agency can make the difference for the client. The Jail Inreach Project manager also makes a point to meet with key new hires at partnering agencies. Each new employee is invited to tour the clinic and have lunch with Jail Inreach staff. This relatively small investment in time and money pays off repeatedly when Inreach staff tries to help a client access services at another agency, especially if those services are in particularly high demand.

Protocol Example for Collaboration Across Systems

Having a protocol that delineates how client needs should be evaluated and service plans formulated can be very helpful, especially when dealing with the complex needs of the homeless.

The client evaluation and service provision protocol established in the Jail Inreach Project takes into account the anticipated needs of the client population as well as the resources available.

Once referred into the Jail Inreach Program, a case manager is assigned to the client. The majority of the female inmates are assigned to the one female case manager, since many female inmates feel more comfortable working with women. The case manager meets with the inmate approximately 2–3 weeks prior to their release date so that a comprehensive service plan can be formulated. This much lead-time is also needed so that trust can be built between the case manager and client. The HHH service model places a high premium on goal-negotiated care, and this occurs most naturally when there is an established, trusting relationship.

The case manager evaluates client need in several vital areas. The most crucial of these are housing and medical care, so these are generally assessed and attended to first. Based on what the client articulates as his or her goals, appropriate housing options are offered. These can include residential substance abuse treatment programs, transitional living facilities, emergency shelters, or the homes of willing family members or friends. The cultivation of staff relationships and on-the-ground knowledge of partnering programs' intake criteria is critical to this process. Clients are given a range of options that fit their stated goals, and then work begins on securing the housing option they have selected.

Because HHH is primarily a medical clinic, securing healthcare for the client is a straightforward process. A medical appointment is made near to the release date so continuity of care is maintained. Jail medical records are obtained and placed in the patient's chart so that when the client sees the provider, medical care is seamless. Due to the collaboration with MHMRA and their aim for continuity of psychiatric care, clients are referred into their intake program even prior to release.

Next, attention is turned to other medical needs, such as substance abuse treatment and dental care. Through partnerships with numerous residential and outpatient substance abuse treatment programs, clients are offered various options for treatment and arrangements are made for intake, often before the client is even released from jail. Dental care is offered through HHH, and at the first visit, the case manager facilitates referral to the dental clinic.

Identification is the next critical issue to be discussed, as many in this population no longer have government-issued ID and some have never had one. Through an arrangement with the Sheriff's Office, a paper ID can be requested which has the client's booking photo as well as other identifying data. While this rudimentary ID cannot be used as an official government-issued identification, it can be used to establish identity with social service agencies, which often will not serve a client who has no identifying documents. Referral is also made to agencies that help obtain official government-issued ID such as a birth certificate or state photo ID.

Basic necessities such as food, clothing, and transportation are handled next. Food and clothing referral lists are given and free transportation is offered through the Project Access Bus that is run by HHH and travels around the downtown area, stopping at locations known to be useful to people without homes. Information about employment and government aid programs is offered. If interested in employment, clients are directed specifically toward nonprofit employment counseling programs that focus on ex-offenders.

Concomitant to this process, the procedure of direct release is described to the client, and if the client consents, release is arranged with the Sheriff's Office. If agreed to, the client is picked up at jail on the day of release and escorted to the closest HHH clinic, where he/she is linked immediately with medical and psychiatric care. The service plan is reviewed again and any appointment cards, maps, or other useful information is given to the client. Follow-up appointments are made with the case manager and the medical provider, in a timeframe based on client need. Every attempt is made to coordinate these visits, as transportation is always an issue.

At subsequent visits, the service plan is reviewed and linkages to partner agencies are discussed with the client and noted in the chart. An identified need will stay on the client's problem list until successful linkage is made or the need is met in another way. If the original housing plan was either temporary or no longer meets the client's needs, more permanent options are discussed and arranged. Because of the scarcity of permanent housing, this can be a challenging step, but again, through established collaborations, this can be an achievable goal. Medical care continues to be offered, but linkage with the county health system is also pursued. While the commitment to the client is open-ended, contact usually diminishes as the client's situation stabilizes.

By offering primary care with embedded behavioral health care, in addition to intensive case management, clients in the Jail Inreach Project can be shepherded through this period of crisis and return to a more stable life. By pursuing partnerships on an agency and individual level, barriers to coordinated care can be eliminated. Working with trusted partners allows staff to offer clients integrated services that best serve their multifaceted needs.

Summary and Conclusions

It is critical that the various systems that have contact with and serve people and families without homes collaborate and work together to address the multitude of problems experienced by homeless individuals and families (APA, 2010; USICH, 2010). Multiple studies and the experiences of successful programs demonstrate that splintered and fragmented services do not adequately address the needs of these people and that more effective programs require agencies and systems of care to collaborate and coordinate services to end homelessness (APA, 2010; USICH, 2010). The Federal Strategic Plan, supported by the Congressional HEARTH Act of 2009, provides a clear model and set of principles for these types of collaborative services. As Shaun Donovan, Secretary of the Housing and Urban Development Department and chair of the USICH, stated, "By developing the "technology" of combining permanent housing and a pipeline of support services, we've reduced the number of individuals who are chronically ill and experiencing long-term homelessness by one-third in the last five years" (preface, USICH, 2010). It is clear from this work that finding permanent housing is the ultimate goal, but doing this requires that social, psychological, and medical factors, such as substance abuse, mental health problems, and employment, also be addressed through appropriate services (APA, 2010). Without services to address all of these problems, success is not guaranteed. Further, state and local governments, nongovernmental agencies and the private sector need to cooperate and collaborate to reach the ultimate goal of ending homelessness for all Americans.

References

American Psychological Association, Presidential Task Force on Psychology's Contribution to End Homelessness. (2010). *Helping people without homes: The role of psychologists and recommendations to advance training, research, practice and policy.* Washington, DC: Author. Retrieved from http://www.apa.org/pi/ses/resources/publications/endhomelessness.aspx.
Buck, D. S., Brown, C. A., & Hickey, J. S. (2011). Best Practices: The Jail Inreach Project: Linking homeless inmates who have mental illness with community health services. *Psychiatric Services, 62,* 120–122.

Buck, D. S., Rochon, D., Davidson, H., & McCurdy, S. (2004). Involving homeless persons in the leadership of a health care organization. *Qualitative Health Research, 14*, 513–525.

Carnochan, S., & Austin, M. J. (2002). Implementing welfare reform and guiding organizational change. *Administration in Social Work, 26*, 61–77.

Foster-Fishman, P. G., Berkowitz, S. L., Lounsbury, D. W., Jacobson, S., & Allen, N. A. (2001). Building collaborative capacity in community coalitions: A review and integrative framework. *American Journal of Community Psychology, 29*, 241–261.

Frank, R. G., McDaniel, S. H., Bray, J. H., & Heldring, M. (Eds.). (2004). *Primary Care Psychology*. Washington, DC: APA Books.

Haas, S. M., Bauer-Leffler, S., & Turley, E. (2011). Evaluation of cross-disciplinary training on the co-occurrence of domestic violence and child victimization: Overcoming barriers to collaboration. *Journal of Health and Human Services Administration, 34*, 352–386.

Hayes, S. L., Mann, M. K., Morgan, F. M., Kelly, M. J., & Weightman, A. L. (2012). *Collaboration between local health and local government agencies for health improvement status and date: New search for studies and content updated (no change to conclusions), The Cochrane Library, Issue 10*. NY: Wiley.

Held, M. L., Brown, C. A., Frost, L. E., Hickey, J. S., & Buck, D. S. (2012). Integrated primary and behavioral health care in patient-centered medical homes for jail releases with mental illness. *Criminal Justice and Behavior, 34*, 533–551.

Holleman, W. L., Bray, J. H., Davis, L., & Holleman, M. C. (2004). Innovative ways to address the mental health and medical needs of marginalized patients: Collaborations between family physicians, family therapists and family psychologists. *American Journal of Orthopsychiatry, 74*, 242–252.

Jacobs, U., Newman, G. H., & Burns, J. C. (2001). The homeless assessment program: A service-training model for providing disability evaluations for homeless, mentally ill individuals. *Professional Psychology: Research and Practice, 32*, 319–323. doi:10.1037/0735-7028.32.3.319.

Jones, J. M., Crook, W. P., & Webb, J. R. (2008). Collaboration for the provision of services: A review of the literature. *Journal of Community Practice, 15*, 41–71.

Liedtka, J. M., & Whitten, E. (1998). Enhancing care delivery through cross-disciplinary collaboration: A case study. *Journal of Healthcare Management, 43*, 185–205.

Miller, W. R., & Rollnick, S. (2002). *Motivational interviewing: Preparing people for change* (2nd ed.). New York: Guilford Press.

Mizrahi, T., & Rosenthal, B. B. (2001). Complexities of coalition building: Leaders' successes, struggles, strategies and solutions. *Social Work, 46*, 63–78.

Packard, T., Patti, R., Daly, D., & Tucker-Tatlow, J. (2012). Organizational change for services integration in public human service organizations: Experiences in seven counties. *Journal of Health and Human Services Administration, 34*, 471–525.

Patti, R., Packard, T., Daly, D., Tucker-Tatlow, J., Prosek, K., Potter, A., & Gibson, C. (2003). *Seeking better performance through interagency collaboration: Prospects and challenges*. A Report Commissioned by The Southern Area Consortium of Human Services, San Diego State University: Network for Excellence in the Human Services. Retrieved from http://theacademy.sdsu.edu/programs/SACHS/reports/SACHS%20Intergrated%20Services%20Research%20Report%20FINAL%202-16-03.pdf.

Rogers, E. B., et al. (2012). Helping people without homes: Simple steps for psychologists seeking to change lives. *Professional Psychology: Research and Practice, 43*, 86–93.

United States Congress. (2009). *The Homeless Emergency Assistance and Rapid Transition to Housing (HEARTH) Act of 2009*. Washington, DC: Author.

United States Interagency Council on Homelessness (USICH). (2010). *Opening doors: Federal strategic plan to prevent and end homeless*. Washington, DC: Author.

White, J. A., & Wehlage, G. (1995). Community collaboration: If it is such a good idea, why is it so hard to do? *Educational Evaluation and Policy Analysis, 17*, 23–38.

Yessian, M. R. (1995). Learning from experience: Integrating human services. *Public Welfare, 53*, 34–42.

Chapter 7
Trauma-Informed Care for Families Experiencing Homelessness

Kathleen M. Guarino

Abstract Homelessness is a devastating experience that can significantly impact the health and well-being of adults and children. Often these families have experienced ongoing trauma in the form of childhood abuse and neglect, domestic violence, and community violence, in addition to the trauma associated with the loss of home. Traumatic experiences impact how children and adults think, feel, behave, and relate to others, and trauma that goes unrecognized and unaddressed can have potentially devastating implications for development across the life span. Within social service settings, a lack of awareness of trauma increases the risk of causing additional harm. In recognition of this significant public health issue, there is a call to adopt trauma-informed care as a best practice for meeting the needs of trauma survivors across service systems. Trauma-informed care is an organization-wide approach that is grounded in an awareness, understanding, and responsiveness to the impact of trauma, and emphasizes the need to create environments that ensure safety, choice, control, and empowerment for survivors. Often this means changing the policies, practices, and culture of an organization. Key components of trauma-informed care for families experiencing homelessness include: Supporting Staff Development; Creating a Safe and Supportive Environment; Assessing and Planning Services; Providing Services and Trauma-Specific Interventions; Involving Families; and Adapting Policies. This chapter explores the need for a trauma-informed approach to serving families who are homeless, how trauma-informed care is operationalized in homeless service settings, and steps to sustain trauma-informed practice.

The prevalence of traumatic stress in the lives of families experiencing homelessness is extraordinarily high (Caton et al., 2005; Guarino, Rubin, & Bassuk, 2007; Koegel, Melamide, & Burnam, 1995). Often families who experience homelessness

K.M. Guarino, L.M.H.C. (✉)
National Center on Family Homelessness, 200 Reservoir Road, Needham, MA 02494, USA
e-mail: Kathleen.Guarino@familyhomelessness.org

M.E. Haskett et al. (eds.), *Supporting Families Experiencing Homelessness:*
Current Practices and Future Directions, DOI 10.1007/978-1-4614-8718-0_7,
© Springer Science+Business Media New York 2014

have had multiple and ongoing traumatic exposures throughout their lives in the form of childhood abuse and neglect; domestic and community violence; and the significant stress associated with poverty and the loss of home, safety, and sense of security. Exposure to trauma can have a profound effect on how people view themselves and others and move through the world (Herman, 1992; van der Kolk, McFarlane, & Weisaeth, 1996). As traumatic experiences accumulate, the physiological and psychological impact becomes more significant and challenges to daily functioning more intense (Felitti et al., 1998). Losing stable housing and its attendant upheaval can also be profoundly destabilizing. In response to high rates of violence and trauma in the lives of families who are homeless, "trauma-informed care" has emerged as a best practice in homeless service settings (United States Interagency Council on Homelessness, 2010). Providing trauma-informed care requires an organizational commitment to build the knowledge, awareness, and skills needed to support recovery and healing for trauma survivors (Guarino, Soares, Konnath, Clervil, & Bassuk, 2009). Often this means changing the practices, policies, and culture of an entire organization to respond to the needs of traumatized adults and children. Given the high rates of exposure to traumatic stress among families who are homeless, a trauma-informed approach is an essential component of quality care. This chapter will address the need for a trauma-informed approach to serving families without homes, the shift from traditional to trauma-informed care in social service settings, details of core principles and key components of trauma-informed care, and steps to adopt and sustain a trauma-informed service model for families experiencing homelessness.

The Need for Trauma-Informed Services and Systems

Trauma in the Lives of Families Who Are Homeless

Traumatic events occur outside the realm of usual and expected experience; threaten one's physical or emotional integrity; and invoke intense feelings of helplessness, terror, and lack of control (American Psychiatric Association, 2000). These events "overwhelm the ordinary systems of care that give people a sense of control, connection, and meaning" (Herman, 1992, p. 34). The experience of trauma violates one's fundamental sense of safety and security, disrupts long-held belief systems, constricts one's life, and interferes with relationships.

Most families experience multiple traumatic events prior to becoming homeless (Hopper, Bassuk, & Olivet, 2010). Traumatic experiences include childhood abuse and neglect, family separations, violent relationships, and witnessing domestic violence (Bassuk et al., 1996; Bassuk, Dawson, Perloff, & Weinreb, 2001; Browne, 1993; Browne & Bassuk, 1997; Caton et al., 2005; D'Ercole & Struening, 1990; Goodman, 1991; Wood, Valdez, Hayashi, & Shen, 1990). Over 90 % of mothers who are homeless have experienced some form of physical or sexual assault over the course of their lives, mostly in familial or intimate relationships (Bassuk et al., 1996). During childhood, 43 % of women who are homeless report being sexually molested, usually by multiple perpetrators, and violence continues into adulthood with 63 % reporting severe physical assault by an intimate male partner (Bassuk et al., 1996; Browne & Bassuk, 1997). Women who enter adulthood without the skills necessary to manage stress are considerably more vulnerable to the destructive impact of violence, poverty, subsequent experiences of homelessness, and other traumatic stressors (Bassuk et al., 2001).

Children who are homeless often live in chaotic and unsafe environments where there are dramatic and unpredictable life changes. Within a single year, 97 % of children experiencing homelessness move up to three times, 40 % attend two different schools, and 28 % attend three or more different schools (The National Center on Family Homelessness, 1999). By age 12, 83 % of children who are homeless have been exposed to at least one serious violent event, including experiences of abuse and witnessing acts of interpersonal violence within their families and communities (Annoshian, 2005; Bassuk et al., 1996; Bassuk et al., 1997; Buckner, Beardslee, & Bassuk, 2004).

For adults and children who are homeless, the adverse emotional consequences of violence are compounded by severe stress caused by housing instability and living in a chaotic shelter milieu (Fantuzzo & Lindquist, 1989; Goodman, Saxe, & Harvey, 1991; Tischler, Rademeyer, & Vostanis, 2007). Children are negatively impacted by the loss of possessions and familiar surroundings, intrusions upon family autonomy, dislocation from friends and neighborhood supports, and in some cases, interrupted school attendance (Bassuk & Friedman, 2005; Cowan, 2007).

Impact of Trauma

Experiences of trauma in adults and children are first registered at a physiological level and have a profound impact on the brain and body (Perry, 2001; Perry & Pollard, 1998; Saxe, Ellis, & Kaplow, 2006; van der Kolk et al., 1996). The stress response system consists of complex series of neural circuits and connections that span all levels of the brain. The limbic system, known as the brain's emotional control center, is critical to the body's stress response. Within the limbic system, the amygdala plays a key role in identification of incoming sensory experience as threatening (Cohen, Perel, DeBellis, Friedman, & Putnam, 2002; Perry, 2001; Saxe et al., 2006; Shinn, Rauch, & Pitman, 2006; van der Kolk, 2003). Higher, more complex regions of the brain (i.e., the prefrontal cortex) contextualize and evaluate incoming information to determine whether a situation is unsafe and the initial fear response is warranted (Cohen et al., 2002; van der Kolk, 2003). In the face of confirmed threat, structures in the limbic system—particularly the amygdala and hypothalamus—activate the body's survival responses: fight, flight, or freeze (Cohen et al., 2002; Perry, 2001; Perry, Pollard, Blakeley, Baker, & Vigiliante, 1996; Saxe et al., 2006). Neurohormones, including adrenaline and cortisol, prepare the body for action and support a return to a physiological state of balance after the threat has passed (Perry et al., 1996; Perry & Pollard, 1998).

Not all stress is experienced as "traumatic." An event becomes traumatic when it overwhelms the stress response system and leaves people feeling helpless, vulnerable, out of control, and overly sensitive to reminders of the event (Brewin & Holmes, 2003; Herman, 1992; Macy, Behar, Paulson, Delman, & Schmid, 2004). Acute symptoms following a traumatic experience may include nightmares or flashbacks; increased agitation, irritability, and anxiety; hypervigilance; trouble concentrating; and feeling numb or disconnected (American Psychiatric Association, 2000). Younger children may struggle with increased fear and anxiety, difficulty leaving caregivers, regression to an earlier developmental stage (e.g., losing speech and toileting skills), and sleep and eating disturbances (Bassuk, Konnath, & Volk, 2006; National Child Traumatic Stress Network). Older children may experience sleep and eating disruptions, nightmares, difficulties concentrating and learning at school, and physical complaints such as stomach aches or headaches (Bassuk et al., 2006; National Child Traumatic Stress Network).

From a physiological perspective, a "trigger" is a reminder of a previous traumatic experience. Triggers include sights, sounds, smells, or feelings that are associated with a prior traumatic event (Kinniburgh & Blaustein, 2010). When exposed to a trigger (e.g., hearing a siren, seeing someone who looks like a former abuser), the brain perceives this as a danger signal based on past experiences, and automatically activates the body's emergency response (Kinniburgh & Blaustein, 2010; van der Kolk, 1994). At a physiological level, the body is responding to the trigger as if the person is directly experiencing a previous traumatic event, even if there is no current external threat.

Although most people are able to recover relatively quickly from traumatic events, others experience more severe, debilitating, and long-term health and mental health consequences. Whether a person continues to struggle following a traumatic exposure depends on many mediating factors that include the severity of the event, exposures to other traumatic experiences either past or current, biological traits, individual coping styles and skills, family history, attachment to caregiver, and level of social support (Brewin, Andrews, & Valentine, 2000; Pat-Horenczyk, Rabinowitz, Rice, & Tucker-Levin, 2009; van der Kolk et al., 1996). Each of these factors impact whether an individual is able to recover from trauma without developing more significant challenges, including Post-Traumatic Stress Disorder (PTSD).

The hallmark symptoms of PTSD that impact daily functioning are (a) reexperiencing the traumatic event (e.g., nightmares or flashbacks), (b) hyperarousal (e.g., difficulty falling or staying asleep, angry outbursts, difficulty concentrating, hypervigilance), (c) avoiding reminders of the event along with constricted behavior and numbing (e.g., diminished interest or participation in significant activities, feeling detached or estranged from others), and (d) dissociation in which behaviors, feelings, physical sensations, and thoughts associated with the traumatic event are fragmented and walled off from other memories (American Psychiatric Association, 2000; Yehuda, 2002). In children, symptoms associated with PTSD may include fear, worry, sadness, low self-worth, and repeatedly acting out the traumatic event through play. In teens, PTSD may manifest as aggressive or impulsive behaviors, out of place sexual behavior, self-harm, and drug and alcohol abuse (United States Department of Veterans Affairs, 2012).

High rates of PTSD among homeless and extremely poor women are well-documented (Bassuk et al., 1996, 2001; Bassuk, Buckner, Perloff, & Bassuk, 1998; Bassuk, Melnick, & Browne, 1998; Browne, 1993; North & Smith, 1992). More than one-third to one-half of mothers who are homeless have experienced PTSD—a rate three or more times greater than among women in the general population (Bassuk, Buckner et al., 1998; Weinreb, Buckner, Williams, & Nicholson, 2006). In addition to PTSD, 85 % of homeless mothers report a history of major depression (Weinreb et al., 2006).

Mental health issues such as depression and PTSD can significantly impede a parent's ability to bond with her child. The quality of the parent–child relationship has a profound impact on a child's awareness of self and others, social and emotional development, and school adjustment (National Scientific Council on the Developing Child, 2004). Family violence and disruption threatens the quality of parent–child attachments. Parents who have been traumatized often have greater difficulty being responsive and sensitive to their children's needs (Osofsky, 1999). The impact of stress and disruption on homeless families can be seen in the high rates of emotional and behavioral challenges among children. As described in Chaps. 2 and 3 of this volume, many children who are homeless struggle with anxiety, depression, sleep problems, shyness, withdrawal, and aggression (Bassuk & Rosenberg, 1990; The National Center on Family Homelessness, 1999). Overall, homeless children have three times the rate of emotional and behavioral problems compared to non-homeless children (The National Center on Family Homelessness, 1999).

As traumatic experiences accumulate, the physiological and psychological impact becomes more significant and challenges to daily functioning more profound (Cook et al., 2005; Felitti et al., 1998; National Scientific Council on the Developing Child, 2005; van der Kolk, Roth, Pelcovitz, Sunday, & Spinazzola, 2005). The term "complex trauma" describes prolonged, persistent traumatic stress that often originates within the caregiving system during critical developmental stages and leads to both immediate and long-term difficulties in many areas of functioning (Cook et al., 2005). Given the prevalence of chronic interpersonal violence and family disruption, the experiences of families who are homeless often fall within the category of complex trauma.

The Adverse Childhood Experiences (ACE) Study, a groundbreaking study of 17,000 adults, points to the high rates of trauma in the general population and the significant connection between childhood exposure to trauma and negative impact in adulthood. In adults, multiple adverse childhood experiences (e.g., physical, emotional or sexual abuse, witnessing domestic violence, and an incarcerated household member) are associated with long-term challenges that include social, emotional, and cognitive impairment; adoption of high risk behaviors as coping mechanisms (eating disorders, smoking, substance abuse, self-harm); severe and persistent behavioral health, health and social problems; and greater risk of early death (Felitti et al., 1998).

In young children, exposure to traumatic stress can significantly alter the brain and subsequent developmental trajectories (Cohen et al., 2002; National Scientific Council on the Developing Child, 2005; Perry, 2001; Perry et al., 1996; Putnam, 2006; Saxe et al., 2006). According to the National Scientific Council on the

Developing Child (2005) chronic exposure to trauma early in development can lead to changes to brain architecture; alterations in the functioning of neural pathways including those associated with learning, memory, and ability to self-regulate and cope; and heightened baseline state of physiological arousal and increased sensitivity to internal and external triggers. Trauma that continues through childhood and adolescence has a profound impact on affect regulation, behavior, cognition, relationships, and self-concept (Cook et al., 2005; D'Andrea, Ford, Stolbach, Spinazzola, & van der Kolk, 2012; Nader, 2011; Perry et al., 1996; Putnam, 2006; Saxe et al., 2006). Youth may struggle with learning difficulties and challenges planning and anticipating during the course of the day. Behavioral challenges may include self-destructive or self-injurious behaviors, difficulty managing rules and limits, oppositional behaviors, problems with boundaries, and difficulties with peers. The impact of trauma on identity formation can result in low self-esteem and deeply held feelings of shame and guilt.

Post-Trauma Responses in Homeless Service Settings

Adults and children exposed to chronic trauma live at a heightened baseline state of physiological arousal and increased sensitivity to internal and external triggers (i.e., reminders of past trauma) (Perry & Pollard, 1998; Shinn et al., 2006; van der Kolk et al., 1996). Common stressors in service settings (e.g., completing paperwork, participating in multiple assessments, experiencing strict rules and demands from shelter staff, and living with others) may be triggering and lead to heightened or seemingly extreme responses that may be misunderstood by providers as purposefully offensive, rude, or aggressive (Hodas, 2006; Hopper et al., 2010). Post-trauma responses that parents might exhibit include difficulty following through on commitments, avoiding meetings and engaging in other isolating behaviors, engaging in interpersonal conflicts within the shelter, becoming easily agitated and/or belligerent, demonstrating a lack of trust and/or feel targeted by others, continued involvement in abusive relationships, and active substance abuse (Hopper et al., 2010). Traumatized children may be difficult to redirect, seem emotionally out of control, avoid taking responsibility, appear oppositional and disruptive, or withdraw from others (Hodas, 2006). These behaviors can best be understood as adaptive responses to manage overwhelming stress. However, without understanding the connection between trauma and current behaviors, providers may label a parent as "manipulative," "oppositional," "lazy," or "unmotivated," when these behaviors are better understood as survival responses (Prescott, Soares, Konnath, & Bassuk, 2008). Children may be labeled as "hyperactive," "oppositional," "shy," or "spacey," when these behaviors might in fact be fight, flight or freeze responses to ongoing stress (Guarino & Bassuk, 2010).

In addition to being perceived negatively by others, trauma survivors also run the risk of being formally misdiagnosed. To adapt to prolonged traumatic experiences, trauma survivors may develop symptoms that mimic disorders such as anxiety disorders, bipolar disorder, or borderline personality disorder (Luxenberg, Spinazzola, & van der Kolk, 2001). Diagnoses that have been misapplied to traumatized children include ADHD, bipolar disorder, oppositional defiant disorder, depression, and reactive attachment disorder (Cook et al., 2005; D'Andrea et al., 2012). When trauma survivors are diagnosed *solely* on the basis of presenting symptoms, mental health and other providers are likely to miss the underlying traumatic experiences that may be the source of the emotions and/or behaviors and the necessary focus of treatment, which impacts recovery (Cook et al., 2005; D'Andrea et al., 2012).

Impact of Trauma on Help-Seeking and Relationship-Building

People who have experienced ongoing trauma are more likely to view the world and other people as unsafe. Those who have been repeatedly hurt by others may come to believe that people cannot be trusted. Lack of trust and a constant need to be on alert for danger makes it difficult for families without homes to ask for help, trust providers, and form relationships with appropriate boundaries. Family members may interpret providers' efforts to help as controlling. When that help does not yield results, providers' inability to "fix" housing needs and other stressors may be seen by families as purposeful and punishing. Shelter rules and regulations may be perceived as disrespectful and belittling, and not dissimilar to prior acts of victimization. Survivors who are further traumatized within service systems by unrealistic demands and harsh responses by staff become increasingly wary of and triggered by *all* people's efforts to help and may drop out of services altogether (Harris & Fallot, 2001; Prescott et al., 2008).

Vicarious Trauma

Providers working in social service settings face a number of challenges that lead to high rates of burnout and turnover. Working with trauma survivors brings another layer of challenge and stress. Specifically, service providers who work with trauma survivors are at risk of experiencing post-traumatic responses that parallel those of the families being served (Figley, 2002; Saakvitne, Gamble, Pearlman, & Lev, 2001). This phenomenon, known as secondary traumatic stress, vicaious trauma, or compassion fatigue is defined as "a state of tension and preoccupation with the individual or cumulative trauma of clients" (Figley, 2002) that can result in "the transformation or change in the helper's inner experience..." (Saakvitne et al., 2001). Providers who are traumatized by their work may experience diminished ability to trust others and maintain intimate relationships outside of work, increased concerned about their own safety, and intrusive thoughts and images related to the traumatic stories of others (Saakvitne et al., 2001). Vicarious trauma may manifest on the job as increased difficulty leaving work at work, poor interpersonal boundaries, irritability with coworkers and families, and doubts about professional capabilities and impact (Saakvitne et al., 2001). These challenges impact job performance and by extension, the experiences of the families being served.

From Traditional to Trauma-Informed Practice: A Paradigm Shift

Service systems and organizations play a pivotal role in a family's recovery from trauma based on their capacity to offer safe, predictable, compassionate, and informed services that buffer the impact of the traumatic experiences and support resilience. The shift from a traditional to a trauma-informed approach reflects a move away from a reactive, punitive, provider-driven service model, and towards a family-centered, recovery-oriented framework that takes into consideration the impact of trauma on families and those who serve them. This evolution represents a change in service delivery models and reflects a heightened awareness of the role providers play in hindering or fostering recovery for trauma survivors (Harris & Fallot, 2001; Jennings, 2008).

Traditional Approach

Historically, the homeless services system has served individuals and families who have experienced trauma without understanding its impact and the need for tailored responses (Harris & Fallot, 2001). In traditional service systems, the impact of trauma is not well understood by providers and family problems or symptoms are viewed as discrete, separate, and often unrelated to past experiences of trauma. Families are seen as broken, vulnerable, and unable to make decisions for themselves (Prescott et al., 2008). Moreover, in traditional service systems, providers are viewed as experts who know what is best for families; compliance by individuals and families is expected and force or coercion may sometimes occur. In traditional service-delivery approaches, treatment is diagnostically driven and symptom-focused, staff–consumer relationships are based on hierarchies, and power sharing is limited (Bloom, 2000; Jennings, 2008; Prescott et al., 2008).

Trauma-Informed Care

As knowledge and awareness of the prevalence and impact of trauma in the lives of vulnerable individuals and families has increased, there has been a corresponding shift in the way services are designed and delivered across service systems. This evolution represents a movement away from a traditional approach and towards trauma-informed practice. Trauma-informed care is defined as a "strengths-based framework that is grounded in an understanding of and responsiveness to the impact of trauma, that emphasizes physical, psychological, and emotional safety for both providers and survivors, and that creates opportunities for survivors to rebuild a sense of control and empowerment" (Hopper et al., 2010). Trauma-informed organizations "…endeavor to do no harm – to avoid retraumatizing or blaming [clients] for their efforts to manage their traumatic reactions" (Moses, Reed, Mazelis, & D'Ambrosio, 2003). Adopting a trauma-informed approach to serving families who experience homelessness means viewing families through a "trauma lens." This perspective provides a way to better understand family members' behaviors, responses, attitudes, and emotions as a collection of survival skills developed in response to traumatic experiences and respond in ways that support recovery (Bloom, 2000; Guarino et al., 2009; Harris & Fallot, 2001). In the absence of a trauma informed view point, the impact of trauma gets lost amid other mental health, substance use, health, employment, and housing issues in the lives of homeless families (Guarino et al., 2009; Harris & Fallot, 2001; Moses et al., 2003).

Trauma-informed care is driven by a set of core beliefs or principles that inform all aspects of the work between providers and families (Elliott, Bjelajc, Fallot, Markoff, & Reed, 2005; Guarino et al., 2009; Hopper et al., 2010). These core principles include: (1) Understanding Trauma and its Impact; (2) Promoting Safety; (3) Supporting Consumer Control, Choice, and Autonomy; (4) Sharing Power and Governance; (5) Ensuring Cultural Competence; and (6) Integrating Care (Guarino et al., 2009). The chart below sets out the components of these core principles.

Principles of Trauma-Informed Care (Guarino et al., 2009)

Understanding trauma and its impact	Understanding traumatic stress and recognizing that many current behaviors and responses are ways of adapting to and coping with past traumatic experiences
Promoting safety	Establishing a safe physical and emotional environment where basic needs are met, safety measures are in place, and provider responses are consistent, predictable, and respectful
Supporting consumer control, choice, and autonomy	Helping people regain a sense of control over their daily lives. Keeping people well informed about all aspects of the system and allowing them to drive goal-planning and decision-making
Sharing power and governance	Sharing power and decision-making across all levels and roles within an organization, whether related to daily decisions or in the review and creation of policies and procedures
Ensuring cultural competence	Considering the relationship between culture, trauma, and recovery, implementing interventions specific to cultural groups, respecting diversity within the program, providing opportunities for consumers to engage in and share cultural rituals
Integrating care	Maintaining a holistic view of consumers that understands the interrelated nature of emotional, physical, relational, and spiritual health and facilitating communication within and among service providers and systems
Healing happens in relationships	Believing that establishing safe, authentic and positive relationships can be corrective and restorative to survivors of trauma
Recovery is possible	Understanding that recovery is possible for everyone regardless of how vulnerable they may appear, instilling hope by providing opportunities for consumer involvement at all levels of the system, and establishing future oriented goals

Regardless of the services an agency provides, organizations can adopt these trauma-informed principles to assist people in reaching goals and achieving success. Preliminary outcomes of trauma-informed care include improvement in functioning and a decrease in psychiatric symptoms among adults and enhanced self-identity and safety among children. Systems-level changes following adoption of trauma-informed practices include increased housing stability and a decrease in crisis-based service use and greater collaboration among service providers. (Cocozza, Jackson, & Hennigan, 2005; Community Connections, 2002; Finkelstein, Rechberger, & Russell, 2005; Morrissey, Ellis, & Gatz, 2005; Noether, Brown, & Finkelstein, 2007; Rog, Holupka, & McCombs-Thornton, 1995).

Key Components of Trauma-Informed Care for Families

Providing trauma-informed care to families experiencing homelessness requires an organization-wide commitment to translating the principles described above into concrete practices in daily programming. This means taking a proactive approach towards reducing potentially triggering or re-traumatizing experiences while at the same time supporting families as they learn to manage responses and build skills that foster recovery and resilience. Principles of choice, safety, control, shared power, and cultural competence are applied to interactions between providers and families and among staff in all roles within an organization. To sustain trauma-informed practice, organizations must create a culture of respect and empowerment for families and staff.

The following are key components of trauma-informed care for families experiencing homelessness: (1) Supporting Staff Development; (2) Creating a Safe and Supportive Environment; (3) Assessing and Planning Services; (4) Providing Services and Trauma-Specific Interventions; (5) Involving Families; and (6) Adapting Policies. The organizational strategies outlined within these categories are further developed in the *Trauma-Informed Organizational Toolkit*, developed by The National Center on Family Homelessness (Guarino et al., 2009). The *Toolkit* provides organizations with a roadmap for becoming trauma-informed and includes an *Organizational Self-Assessment* tool that consists of trauma-informed practices that can be integrated into daily programming within homeless service settings.

Supporting Staff Development

Organizations serving vulnerable families are often over-taxed, under-resourced, and focused on survival, not unlike the families served. Homeless service settings face significant workforce issues that impact their ability to provide effective care. Staff members are often paraprofessionals who are overworked, underpaid, have few opportunities for training or career development, and lack specific expertise in mental health (Mullen & Leginski, 2010; Olivet, McGraw, Grandin, & Bassuk, 2009). Volk, Guarino, Grandin and Clervil (2008) identified multiple challenges among staff that can lead to high rates of burnout and job turnover. These challenges include heavy workloads with little time to complete tasks, inconsistent supervision, minimal professional development opportunities, and lack of attention to self-care. Staff often struggle with confusion about roles and responsibilities and have minimal input into programming. In addition to these challenges, staff is at high risk of vicarious trauma exposure and post-trauma responses related to intensive work with trauma survivors.

Under stress, organizations, like individuals, can become disorganized, crisis-driven, and reactive, which increases the likelihood of adopting rigid and punitive practices in attempts to structure and control the environment (Bloom, 2006). Staff training, supervision, and ongoing support allow providers to regulate their own reactions to the work and respond in thoughtful, purposeful, and proactive ways. Adequate support for staff ensures that trauma-informed practices will be implemented and reduces the risk for burnout and the use of more traditionally based and potentially ineffective responses.

Building knowledge and skills of the homelessness workforce is the cornerstone of trauma-informed change. Training *all* personnel—administrators, direct care staff, case managers, support staff, etc.—about trauma and trauma-related topics ensures that all staff members have a similar understanding about what families need and respond in similar and appropriate ways. To provide trauma-informed care to families experiencing homelessness, organizations must ensure that all staff receives training and education on a variety of topics that include: (1) education on the homeless service system, resources, families' experiences living in shelters, and the medical and mental health needs of this population; (2) successive stages of human development; (3) caregiver–child attachment processes, including types of attachment and the relationship between attachment and the development of coping skills, identity, and future relationships; (4) the impact of traumatic stress across the life span, including the ways that early trauma impacts the developing brain, early attachments, and child and adult health and functioning; (5) the relationship between trauma and mental health, substance use, and homelessness; (6) culture-specific exposure and responses to trauma; and (7) vicarious trauma.

To fully integrate trauma-informed practices it is essential to create formal structures to support staff over time. Large group trainings are helpful forums for initial staff education about trauma, but these trainings alone are insufficient. Supervision and team meetings offer smaller settings in which to convey and clarify information. Smaller meetings are a forum for open communication, peer support, and additional training and education. Individual supervision by someone who is trained in understanding trauma is an essential follow-up strategy to general trauma training. One-on-one supervision allows the program to meet the individualized needs of each staff member by enabling them to learn how to apply general trauma concepts to real life work situations, discuss and practice specific ways of responding to and supporting families, understand their own responses to families, and monitor job frustration or burnout. Additional strategies for creating healthy work environments and a culture of self-care include: offering necessary training and education about burn-out, vicarious trauma, and self-care; providing adequate supervisory relationships that are grounded in the trauma-informed principles (e.g., safety, control, choice, and shared power); encouraging employee control and input; fostering effective communication; and creating a safe working environment (Volk et al., 2008)

Creating a Safe and Supportive Environment

Traumatic experiences challenge one's belief that the world is a safe and predictable place, and can leave people feeling insecure and distrustful of others. The loss of home can lead to an additional loss of safety, security and control. To begin to heal, families must feel safe. Establishing physical and emotional safety is critical—especially in the immediate aftermath of a traumatic event. Emotional safety involves feeling protected, comforted, in control, heard, and reassured. For children, their primary caregivers often meet this need. However, when the whole family has been affected by traumatic stress, children *and* their caregivers need service providers to help them feel physically and emotionally safe. Service providers must examine their physical space and overall culture to establish and maintain a commitment to safety for all.

Creating Safe Physical Spaces

Creating a safe and welcoming physical space ensures that families will feel secure from the moment they enter an organization. For programs serving families who have experienced trauma, particular attention to physical safety is required. Specific areas within the building, such as bathrooms and bedrooms, can be particularly triggering for those who have abuse histories. Poor lighting or security and a lack of control over personal space and belongings can also trigger feelings of fear and helplessness. Key safety features include providing adequate lighting inside and outside of the program space, having a working security system, maintaining the overall environment to appropriate standards (e.g., fixing things when they are broken, keeping things clean), and ensuring consumers can lock bathroom doors and have locked spaces for their belongings. A safe physical space for children includes having child-friendly areas, decorations, and developmentally appropriate play materials.

Developing Safe and Supportive Relationships

Interpersonal trauma often includes egregious boundary violations that significantly alter a person's ability to trust others and maintain relationships. Trauma survivors often enter service settings with past experiences that include being mistreated, ignored, and silenced. Service providers are faced with the challenge of encouraging honest communication with families and demonstrating an ability to listen to and accept the range of thoughts and feelings that members may share. How families are welcomed and how staff responds to their individual needs sets the stage for future success or difficulty.

Prescott and colleagues (2008) outline numerous strategies for building safe relationships to support recovery from trauma. From the beginning, families should be provided with detailed information about program rules, expectations, and schedules; however, people also should have choices in everything from the types of services they receive and the goals they set, to how staff enters their space or conduct meetings. Establishing and maintaining clear roles and boundaries in relationships with families is considered critical. To create an environment of respect and individuality, it is important to utilize "people-first language" such as "people experiencing homelessness" rather than "homeless people" and avoid negative and derogatory labels that foster disrespect (e.g., referring to the family member as "manipulative" or "lazy"). Agencies should also uphold an awareness of cultural attitudes and beliefs among providers and families and incorporate knowledge of culture into all aspects of programming (physical space, interactions, assessments, interventions, and policies). Finally, establishing regular meetings, keeping and being on time for appointments, following up on parents' requests or concerns, and maintaining empathic responses to parents and children in the face of both successes and setbacks can be helpful in building safe relationships to support recovery from trauma.

Recognizing and Reducing Triggers and Re-traumatizing Practices

To establish and maintain a safe environment, agencies should engage in an ongoing examination of potentially triggering or re-traumatizing practices and strategize about how to minimize and eliminate these experiences. Potential triggers for children include: loud noises; hand or body gestures; confusion or chaos; transitions; change in routine; feelings of anger, sadness or fear that trigger similar feelings connected to past trauma; physical touch; emergency vehicles and police and fire personnel; and separation from caregivers. Potential triggers for parents include: feelings of embarrassment and shame about challenges such as lack of housing; mental health or substance use issues; violence in the home; authority figures; and not having choices or decision-making power. By keeping in mind potential triggers for trauma survivors, organizations can work to eliminate daily practices, policies, and ways of responding to families that compromise safety and diminish control.

Assessing and Planning Services

As noted above, trauma survivors may present with symptoms that could be mislabeled or misinterpreted if experiences of trauma are not addressed. Conducting comprehensive assessments that include questions about trauma is critical to connecting families with the most targeted and beneficial services. For adults in the family, the assessment process includes gathering information about experiences of trauma (e.g., neglect, loss, community violence, and abuse), current level of danger from other people, and injuries resulting from violence, particularly head injuries. Other key domains for caregiver assessments include mental health, substance use, education, employment, housing, and parenting. Assessments should include questions about cultural backgrounds, routines, and rituals as well as family and individual strengths and supports. Given the significant impact of trauma on child development, conducting child-specific assessments is critical to address and mitigate the impact of stressful events on children. Child-specific assessments should be conducted for each child in a family and should include trauma history, achievement of developmental tasks, relationship with caregiver, education, mental health, substance use, and strengths and skills.

Often, the assessment process involves having families meet with a new person and share intimate details about their lives, which can be painful and intense and may trigger difficult emotions for families. It is important for providers to be aware of these challenges throughout the intake and assessment process. Strategies for conducting assessments in a trauma-informed manner include: having private spaces for conversations; offering families options about where to sit, who is in the room with them, and what to expect; asking families how they are doing throughout the assessment; offering water and rest breaks; being aware of body language that may indicate that an individual is feeling overwhelmed; and considering cultural norms and expectations when greeting, engaging, and questioning individuals and families. Using a strengths-based approach also sets a tone of respect for the individual or family and enhances relationship-building.

Developing goals and plans for obtaining housing, employment and other types of services based on assessment results may seem intimidating and overwhelming for people who have experienced trauma. In these situations, it is easy for families to "freeze" and for providers to take over. This pattern leaves families feeling helpless and powerless. Trauma-informed goal planning is individualized and addresses the needs of both parents and children. Encouraging and helping families to create their own goals allows them to take control of their lives and futures. Goals and plans should be reviewed on a regular basis, and updated as needed. Prior to leaving the program, families should work with staff to develop aftercare plans that take into consideration safety and service needs that should be addressed prior to and after discharge. Planning ahead provides a sense of comfort, confidence, and security that is essential to recovery. Anticipating future difficulties before they happen and making a plan to address the potential problem can reduce the likelihood that families will return to a shelter.

Providing Services and Trauma-Specific Interventions

Organizations serving families experiencing homelessness can play a critical role in educating families on trauma and its impact, building coping skills, and supporting caregiver–child attachment. Trauma-related services for children and families include the following:

Nonverbal Interventions

It can be extremely difficult for trauma survivors to verbalize thoughts, feelings, and memories related past traumatic experiences. People who have experienced trauma sometimes disconnect from emotions and physical sensations in an attempt to cope. Body-oriented, nonverbal activities serve as a way for trauma survivors to reconnect to their bodies, manage their feelings, and communicate in nontraditional ways. It is helpful for programs to provide opportunities for parents and children to express themselves using these types of modalities (e.g., art, theater, dance, movement, and music). For younger children, who have fewer words to express how they feel, the use of play and body-based activities help children to manage stress and strengthen coping skills.

Attachment-Focused Interventions

As discussed earlier, the impact of trauma on mothers who are homeless is significant. Challenges that include depression, anxiety, and PTSD can severely compromise a woman's ability to connect with her children and be responsive to their needs. Disrupted parent–child relationships can impact all aspects of a child's functioning, beginning at the most fundamental, neurobiological level. Research suggests that "relationships children have with their caregivers play critical roles in regulating stress hormone production during the early years of life" (National Scientific Council on the Developing Child, 2005). Strategies for fostering parent–child attachment and parent skill-building include providing parent education about child development, attachment, and the impact of stress on children. Staff can model healthy interactions with parents and their children (e.g., tone of voice, eye contact, asking permission around personal space, asking them about their needs).Agencies can strengthen parent–child relationships through activities such as family nights and joint parent–child groups. See Chap. 9 of this volume for specific parenting interventions that have been used with this population.

Trauma-Specific Mental Health Services

While trauma-informed care refers to an organization-wide approach to acknowledging and responding to trauma, "trauma-specific" services are interventions or treatments designed to address trauma symptoms and the impact of trauma on mental health (Hopper et al., 2010). Offering trauma-specific interventions to families who require more intensive mental health services is an important component of trauma-informed care. Within the field of homelessness, there is a need for increased access to mental health services such as witness to violence services, mental health professionals who provide services in shelter and housing programs, and connections with community agencies that can provide these types of trauma-related services. Trauma-specific services for children and families may include individual and family therapy and interventions that focus on helping children and adults to manage traumatic stress and strengthen connections. Organizations can learn about a range of evidence-based and promising approaches to meeting the mental health needs of children and families exposed to trauma through a variety of initiatives, including the National Child Traumatic Stress Network (www.nctsn.org).

Integrated services

Programs serving families may not be able to provide all of the necessary services in house. Therefore, organizations often refer families to services in the community, including legal and educational advocacy, employment services, and mental health and substance abuse treatment. When families are referred to mainstream settings, many of these services are provided separately, in isolation from each other. A trauma-informed organization makes it a priority to facilitate communication among different service providers, as integration of services is a key principle of trauma-informed care. This reduces the risk of treating each symptom or challenge individually and overlooking the impact of trauma and the roots of many of these difficulties. See Chap. 6 for a full discussion of methods to insure collaboration across agencies that can enhance integration of services.

Involving Families

Recovery and success for trauma survivors is based largely on their ability to regain control of their lives. Organizations support control and choice by giving families a voice in what happens in the program on a daily basis. Ways to involve families include running a "resident voice" meeting and putting residents in charge of developing the agenda and facilitating the discussion; providing families with choices about their services, and if there is a minimum requirement of mandatory services, making more services available to offer choices; giving families opportunities to evaluate the program and offer their suggestions for improvement in anonymous and/or confidential ways (e.g., suggestion boxes, regular satisfaction surveys, meetings focused on necessary improvements, etc.); involving families in developing program activities; and including families on the organization's board. This level of input enhances the quality of the services provided and affirms the belief that families are the experts in what works best for them.

People who have experienced homelessness in the past have a unique and invaluable perspective. They know first-hand what was helpful and what was not along their road to housing stability. To capitalize on this first-hand expertise, programs can make a commitment to hire former "consumers" at all levels of the organization, from the board of directors and administrative staff to direct care staff. It is also important to involve former consumers directly in program development and service provision (e.g., peer-run support, educational, and therapeutic groups). Whether they are on staff, visiting the program to share their stories, or volunteering, the presence of former consumers can reinforce the message that homelessness is not a permanent condition.

Adapting Policies

Trauma-informed organizations craft policies based on an understanding of the impact of trauma on families, with the goal of reducing triggering or re-traumatizing situations. Policies are strengths-based, accompanied by explanations of why they are needed, and available in multiple formats and in different languages. Policies that are particularly important in trauma-informed agencies include a commitment to providing trauma-informed and culturally competent care and to hiring former consumers. Procedures for addressing issues of safety and crisis, emergency procedures, and professional conduct for staff should be clearly defined.

As the needs of consumers evolve and an organization learns more about trauma, policies that were once effective may no longer be as helpful or relevant. Continual review of policies is strongly suggested. When reviewing individual policies and procedures, organizations may begin by asking the following questions: (1) Is this policy or rule necessary? (2) What purpose does it serve? (3) Who does it help? (4) Who does it hurt? (5) Does the policy facilitate/hinder family inclusion and control? (6) Were families included in its development? (7) Could this policy or rule re-traumatize families (e.g., limit consumer control and power and lead to fear and confusion)? Asking and answering these questions can allow organizations to determine whether existing policies should be changed or eliminated and if new policies should be included. Review of policies should be done with both staff and consumer input.

Trauma-Informed Practices in Homelessness Service Settings (Guarino et al., 2009)

Supporting staff development	Training staff in trauma, trauma-informed care, and vicarious trauma. Discussing trauma-related concepts in supervision and team meetings. Incorporating ongoing, trauma-related consultation. Making an organizational commitment to supporting staff self-care
Creating a safe and supportive environment	Creating a clean, well-maintained, accessible physical space. Creating a welcoming and respectful environment that includes: asking families about the least intrusive ways for staff to check on them and their spaces; providing private spaces for staff and families to discuss personal issues; respecting cultural/spiritual rituals and practices
Assessing and planning services	Including questions about trauma in assessment protocol. Conducting child assessments for each child that include questions about violence and trauma. Providing or referring children and families to trauma-specific mental health services when needed
Involving consumers	Providing opportunities for families to have input into program rules, policies, practices, and service offerings. Including formerly homeless families in critical positions (e.g., as staff, on the board)
Adapting policies	Policies include a commitment to trauma-informed care. Policies are examined for their risk of triggering or re-traumatizing families. Policies are reviewed on a regular basis for extent to which they support family control, empowerment, and recovery from trauma

Becoming Trauma-Informed: Next Steps for Organizations Serving Families

Creating a trauma-informed organization requires system-wide transformation. This type of change is not found just at the direct care level or only in the administrative arena. Becoming trauma-informed requires a commitment to adapt the practices, policies, and culture of an entire organization. For those leaders who are interested in championing this type of organizational change, programs can follow the steps outlined here.

Step one: *Building knowledge and gaining buy-in*. Becoming trauma-informed is an ongoing process that begins by providing agency staff with education on trauma and its impact, the relationship between homelessness and trauma, and the principles of trauma-informed care. Training should include all staff in an agency, from the executive director to administrative assistants and maintenance employees. This type of agency-wide education ensures that everyone is using the same language and working from a similar level of understanding. Introductory training is also helpful for ensuring buy-in among staff to make additional changes.

Step two: *Evaluating your organization*. Once agency staff receives training on trauma and there is consensus that people are interested in adopting a trauma-informed approach, organizations can evaluate current programming and the extent to which they incorporate trauma-informed practices. Methods for gathering this information may include surveys, focus groups with staff and consumers, and discussions in staff meetings. For organizations that are interested in engaging in a more formal assessment process, there are tools that are easily accessible via the Web and can be used for this purpose (e.g., the *Trauma-Informed Organizational Toolkit* developed by The National Center on Family Homelessness, www.family-homelessness.org). After agencies evaluate their current programming, they can begin to develop goals for integrating trauma-informed practices associated with the key components of trauma-informed care discussed above.

Step three: *Establishing structures to support change*. After agency leaders and staff members identify goals for incorporating trauma-informed practices, it is helpful to put structures in place to monitor progress towards goals and keep the commitment to being trauma-informed in the forefront. One way that an organization can do this is by creating a multidisciplinary "trauma workgroup" consisting of a core group of staff representing all roles in the agency. This group makes a commitment to: (1) ensure short-term and long-term goals are met; (2) generate new ideas about additional changes that may be necessary as the process continues; and (3) seek out additional training opportunities for the program at large. It is critical that consumers be involved in both the initial evaluation of programming and any strategic action planning based on assessment results. The trauma workgroup should maintain ongoing contact with residents as one key method of assessing whether they are making progress on identified goals. This can be done via surveys, one-on-one interviews, focus groups, and having current and/or former residents as members of the workgroup. The *Trauma-Informed Organizational Toolkit* discussed earlier includes a consumer version of an organizational self-assessment that can be used to gather concrete consumer feedback about organizational practices.

Step four: Sustaining a trauma-informed approach. Sustaining agency-wide changes can be challenging. Staff turnover, diminishing resources, and competing demands for an agency's time and attention can threaten any change process. To ensure an organizational commitment to incorporate trauma-informed practices and uphold trauma-informed principles, agencies may consider the following strategies: (1) Maintaining the trauma workgroup; (2) Engaging in ongoing self-assessment and reviewing progress towards goals; (3) Providing continuous trauma training (e.g., trauma training as part of the new hire process, offering refresher trainings on trauma-related topics); (4) Establishing connections with experts who can provide ongoing support and consultation; (5) Developing and/or participating in a community of practice with other organizations who are incorporating a trauma-informed service model; and (6) Bringing trauma-informed concepts to the broader system (e.g., educating other service systems and providers working with families about the need for trauma-informed care).

Concluding Remarks

Families who are homeless face multiple challenges as they attempt to stay together, obtain permanent housing, and access necessary supports and resources. Experiences of trauma have a significant impact on the health and well-being of children and adults. Given the prevalence of trauma in the lives of families who are homeless, it is imperative that service providers adopt a trauma-informed approach. Trauma-informed practices include educating staff, creating safe environments, conducting thorough assessments, examining policies, giving families a voice, and helping parents and children build on strengths and learn new skills. Families who are homeless come into contact with service providers in a variety of settings (e.g., shelters, mental health agencies, child welfare departments, schools, and child care centers). Becoming trauma-informed involves creating an integrated web of trauma-informed service systems that are united in the goal of open communication, cross-system education, and joint service planning to best assist families in their transition from homelessness.

References

American Psychiatric Association. (2000). *Diagnostic and statistical manual of mental disorders* (4th ed., text rev.). Washington, DC: Author.
Annoshian, J. L. (2005). Violence and aggression in the lives of homeless children. *Journal of Family Violence, 20,* 373–387.

Bassuk, E. L., Buckner, J. C., Perloff, J. N., & Bassuk, S. S. (1998). Prevalence of mental health and substance abuse disorders among homeless and low-income housed mothers. *The American Journal of Psychiatry, 155*(1), 1561–1564.

Bassuk, E. L., Buckner, J. C., Weinreb, L. F., Browne, A., Bassuk, S. S., Dawson, R., et al. (1997). Homelessness in female-headed families: Childhood and adult risk and protective factors. *American Journal of Public Health, 87*(2), 241–248.

Bassuk, E. L., Dawson, R., Perloff, J., & Weinreb, L. (2001). Post-traumatic stress disorder in extremely poor women: Implications for health care clinicians. *Journal of the American Medical Women's Association, 56*(2), 79–85.

Bassuk, E., & Friedman, S. (2005) Facts on trauma and homeless children. *National Child Traumatic Stress Network Homelessness and Extreme Poverty Working Group.* Retrieved from http://nctsn.org/nctsn_assets/pdfs/promising_practices/Facts_on_Trauma_and_Homeless.

Bassuk, E., Konnath, K., & Volk, K. (2006). *Understanding traumatic stress in children.* Newton, MA: National Center on Family Homelessness. Retrieved from www.familyhomelessness.org.

Bassuk, E. L., Melnick, S., & Browne, A. (1998). Responding to the needs of low-income and homeless women who are survivors of family violence. *Journal of the American Medical Women's Association, 53*(2), 57–64.

Bassuk, E. L., & Rosenberg, L. (1990). Psychosocial characteristics of homeless children and children with homes. *Pediatrics, 85*(3), 257–261.

Bassuk, E. L., Weinreb, L. F., Buckner, J. C., Browne, A., Salomon, A., & Bassuk, S. S. (1996). The characteristics and needs of sheltered homeless and low-income housed mothers. *The Journal of the American Medical Association, 276*(8), 640–646.

Bloom, S. (2000). Creating sanctuary: Healing from systemic abuses of power. *Therapeutic Communities: The International Journal for Therapeutic and Supportive Organizations, 21*(2), 67–91.

Bloom, S. L. (2006). *Organizational stress as a barrier to trauma-sensitive change and system transformation.* White Paper for the National Technical Assistance Center for State Mental Health Planning (NTAC), National Association of State Mental Health Program Directors. Retrieved from http://www.nasmhpd.org/publications.cfm.

Brewin, C. T., Andrews, B., & Valentine, J. D. (2000). Meta-analysis of risk factors for posttraumatic stress disorder in trauma-exposed adults. *Journal of Consulting Clinical Psychology, 68*(5), 748–766.

Brewin, C. R., & Holmes, E. A. (2003). Psychological theories of posttraumatic stress disorder. *Clinical Psychology Review, 23*, 339–376.

Browne, A. (1993). Family violence and homelessness: The relevance of trauma histories in the lives of homeless women. *American Journal of Orthopsychiatry, 63*(3), 370–383.

Browne, A., & Bassuk, S. S. (1997). Intimate violence in the lives of homeless and poor housed women: Prevalence and patterns in an ethnically diverse sample. *American Journal of Orthopsychiatry, 72*, 261–277.

Buckner, J. C., Beardslee, W. R., & Bassuk, E. L. (2004). Exposure to violence and low-income children's mental health: Direct, moderated, and medicated relations. *American Journal of Orthopsychiatry, 74*, 413–423.

Caton, C., Boarnerges, D., Schaner, B., Hasin, D., Schrout, P., Fexlix, A., et al. (2005). Risk factors for long term homelessness: Findings from a longitudinal study of first time homeless single adults. *American Journal of Public Health, 95*(10), 1753–1759.

Cocozza, J. J., Jackson, E. W., & Hennigan, K. (2005). Outcomes for women with co-occurring disorders and trauma: Program-level effects. *Journal of Substance Abuse Treatment, 28*, 109–119.

Cohen, J., Perel, J., DeBellis, M., Friedman, M., & Putnam, F. (2002). Treating traumatized children: Clinical implications of the psychobiology of posttraumatic stress disorder. *Trauma, Violence & Abuse, 3*(2), 91–108.

Community Connections (2002). *Trauma and abuse in the loves of homeless men and women.* Online PowerPoint presentation. Washington, DC. Retrieved from www.pathprogram.samhsa.gov/ppt/Trauma_and_Homelessness.ppt.

Cook, A., Spinazzola, J., Ford, J., Lanktree, C., Blaustein, M., Cloitre, M., et al. (2005). Complex trauma in children and adolescents. *Psychiatric Annals, 35*, 390–398.

Cowan, B. A. (2007). Trauma exposure and behavioral outcomes in sheltered homeless children: The moderating role of perceived social support. *Psychology Dissertations*. Paper 39. Retrieved from http://digitalarchive.gsu.edu/psych_diss/39.

D'Andrea, W., Ford, J., Stolbach, B., Spinazzola, J., & van der Kolk, B. (2012). Understanding interpersonal trauma in children: Why we need a developmentally appropriate trauma diagnosis. *American Journal of Orthopsychiatry, 82*(2), 187–200.

D'Ercole, A., & Struening, E. (1990). Victimization among homeless women: Implications for service delivery. *Journal of Community Psychology, 18*, 141–151.

Elliott, D. E., Bjelajc, P., Fallot, R. D., Markoff, L. S., & Reed, B. G. (2005). Trauma-informed or trauma-denied: Principles and implementation of trauma-informed services for women. *Journal of Community Psychology, 33*(4), 461–477.

Fantuzzo, J. W., & Lindquist, C. U. (1989). The effects of observing conjugal violence on children: A review and analysis of research methodology. *Journal of Family Violence, 4*, 77–94.

Felitti, V. J., Anda, R. F., Nordenberg, D., Williamson, D. F., Spitz, A. M., Edwards, V., et al. (1998). Relationship of childhood abuse and household dysfunction to many of the leading causes of death in adults. The Adverse Childhood Experiences (ACE) Study. *American Journal of Preventive Medicine, 14*(4), 245–258.

Figley, C. H. (2002). *Treating compassion fatigue*. New York: Routledge.

Finkelstein, N., Rechberger, E., & Russell, L. A. (2005). Building resilience in children of mothers who have co-occurring disorders and histories of violence: Intervention model and implementation issues. *Journal of Behavioral Health Services and Research, 32*, 141–154.

Goodman, L. A. (1991). The prevalence of abuse among homeless and housed poor mothers: A comparison study. *American Orthopsychiatric Association, 61*(4), 489–500.

Goodman, L., Saxe, L., & Harvey, M. (1991). Homelessness as psychological trauma. *American Psychologist, 46*(11), 1219–1225.

Guarino, K., & Bassuk, E. (2010). Working with families experiencing homelessness: Understanding trauma and its impact. *Zero to Three, 30*(3), 11–20.

Guarino, K., Rubin, L., & Bassuk, E. (2007). Trauma in the lives of homeless families. In E. Carll (Ed.), *Trauma psychology: Issues in violence, disaster, health, and illness* (pp. 231–258). Westport: Praeger.

Guarino, K., Soares, P., Konnath, K., Clervil, R., & Bassuk, E. (2009). *Trauma-informed organizational toolkit*. Rockville, MD: Center for Mental Health Services, Substance Abuse and Mental Health Services Administration, and the Daniels Fund, the National Child Traumatic Stress Network, and the W.K. Kellogg Foundation. Retrieved from www.homeless.samhsa.gov and www.familyhomelessness.org.

Harris, M., & Fallot, R. (Eds.). (2001). *New directions for mental health services: Using trauma theory to design service systems*. San Francisco: Jossey-Bass.

Herman, J. (1992). *Trauma and recovery*. New York: Basic Books.

Hodas, G. R. (2006). *Responding to childhood trauma: The promise and practice of trauma informed care*. Pennsylvania Office of Mental Health and Substance Abuse Services. Retrieved from http://www.nasmhpd.org/docs/publications/docs/2006/Responding%20to%20Childhood%20Trauma%20-%20Hodas.pdf.

Hopper, E., Bassuk, E., & Olivet, J. (2010). Shelter from the storm: Trauma-informed care in homelessness service settings. *The Open Health Services and Policy Journal, 3*, 80–100.

Jennings, A. (2008). *Models for developing trauma-informed behavioral health systems and trauma-specific services*. Alexandria, VA: National Association of State Mental Health Program Directors, National Technical Assistance Center for State Mental Health Planning. Retrieved from http://www.annafoundation.org/MDT.pdf.

Kinniburgh, K., & Blaustein, M. (2010). *Treating traumatic stress in children and adolescents: How to foster resilience through attachment, self-regulation, and competency*. New York: The Guilford Press.

Koegel, P., Melamide, E., & Burnam, A. (1995). Childhood risk factors for homelessness among homeless adults. *American Journal of Public Health, 85*, 1642–1649.

Luxenberg, T., Spinazzola, J., & van der Kolk, B. (2001). Complex trauma and disorders of extreme stress (DESNOS) diagnosis, Part one: assessment. *Directions in Psychiatry, 21*(25), 373–392.

Macy, R. D., Behar, L. B., Paulson, R., Delman, J., & Schmid, L. (2004). Community based acute post-traumatic stress management: A description and evaluation of a psychosocial intervention continuum. *Harvard Rev Psychiatry, 12*(4), 217–228.

Morrissey, J. P., Ellis, A. R., & Gatz, M. (2005). Outcomes for women with co-occurring disorders and trauma: Program and person-level effects. *Journal of Substance Abuse Treatment, 28*, 121–133.

Moses D. J., Reed B. G., Mazelis R., & D'Ambrosio, B. (2003). *Creating trauma services for women with co-occurring disorders: Experiences from the SAMHSA women with alcohol, drug abuse, and mental health disorders who have histories of violence study*. Delmar, NY: Policy Research Associates. Retrieved from http://www.prainc.com/wcdvs/pdfs/CreatingTraumaServices.pdf.

Mullen, J., & Leginski, W. (2010). Building the capacity of the homeless service workforce. *The Open Health Services and Policy Journal, 3*, 101–110.

Nader, K. (2011). Trauma in children and adolescents: Issues related to age and complex trauma reactions. *Journal of Child and Adolescent Trauma, 4*, 161–180.

National Child Traumatic Stress Network. *Symptoms and behaviors associated with exposure to trauma*. Retrieved from http://www.nctsn.org/trauma-types/early-childhood-trauma/Symptoms-and-Behaviors-Associated-with-Exposure-to-Trauma.

National Scientific Council on the Developing Child (2004). *Young children develop in an environment of relationships: Working Paper No. 1*. Retrieved from www.developingchild.harvard.edu.

National Scientific Council on the Developing Child (2005). *Excessive stress disrupts the architecture of the developing brain: Working Paper No. 3*. Retrieved from www.developingchild.harvard.edu.

Noether, C. D., Brown, V., & Finkelstein, N. (2007). Promoting resiliency in children of mothers with co-occurring disorders and histories of trauma: Impact of a skills-based intervention program on child outcomes. *Journal of Community Psychology, 35*, 823–843.

North, C. S., & Smith, E. M. (1992). Posttraumatic stress disorder among homeless men and women. *Hospital and Community Psychiatry, 43*(10), 1010–1016.

Olivet, J., McGraw, S., Grandin, M., & Bassuk, E. (2009). *Staffing challenges and strategies for organizations serving individuals who have experiences chronic homelessness*. Rockville, MD: Center for Mental Health Services, Substance Abuse and Mental Health Services Administration.

Osofsky, J. D. (1999). The impact of violence on children. *The Future of Children, 9*(3), 33–49.

Pat-Horenczyk, R., Rabinowitz, R. G., Rice, A., & Tucker-Levin, A. (2009). The search for risk and protective factors in childhood PTSD. In D. Brom, R. Pat-Horenczyk, & J. D. Ford (Eds.), *Treating traumatized children risk, resilience and recovery* (pp. 51–71). New York: Routledge.

Perry, B. D. (2001). The neurodevelopmental impact of violence in childhood. In D. Schetkey & E. Benedek (Eds.), *Textbook of child and adolescent forensic psychiatry* (pp. 221–238). Washington, DC: American Psychiatric Press, Inc.

Perry, B. D., & Pollard, R. (1998). Homeostasis, stress, trauma, and adaptation: A neurodevelopmental view of childhood trauma. *Child and Adolescent Psychiatric Clinics of North America, 7*(1), 33–51.

Perry, B. D., Pollard, R., Blakeley, T., Baker, W., & Vigiliante, D. (1996). Childhood trauma, the neurobiology of adaptation and use-dependent development of the brain: How 'states' becomes 'traits. *Infant Mental Health Journal, 16*(4), 271–291.

Prescott, L., Soares, P., Konnath, K., & Bassuk, E. (2008). *A long journey home: A guide for creating trauma-informed services for mothers and children experiencing homelessness*. Rockville, MD: Center for Mental Health Services, Substance Abuse and Mental Health Services Administration; and the Daniels Fund; National Child Traumatic Stress Network; and the W.K. Kellogg Foundation. Retrieved from www.homeless.samhsa.gov.

Putnam, F. W. (2006). The impact of trauma on child development. *Juvenile and Family Court Journal, 1–11.*

Rog, D. J., Holupka, C. S., & McCombs-Thornton, K. L. (1995). Implementation of the homeless families program: Service models and preliminary outcomes. *American Journal of Orthopsychiatry, 65*, 502–513.

Saakvitne, K. W., Gamble, S., Pearlman, L. A., & Lev, B. T. (2001). *Risking connection: A training curriculum for working with survivors of childhood abuse.* Baltimore: Sidran Institute.

Saxe, G. N., Ellis, B. H., & Kaplow, J. B. (2006). *Collaborative treatment of traumatized children and teens: The trauma systems therapy approach.* New York: Guilford Press.

Shinn, L. M., Rauch, S. L., & Pitman, R. K. (2006). Amygdala, medial prefrontal cortex, and hippocampal function in PTSD. *Annals New York Academy of Sciences, 1071*, 67–79.

The National Center on Family Homelessness. (1999). *Homeless children: America's new outcasts.* Newton, MA: Better Homes Fund.

Tischler, V., Rademeyer, A., & Vostanis, P. (2007). Mothers experiencing homelessness: Mental health, support and social care needs. *Health & Social Care in the Community, 15*(3), 253–256.

United States Department of Veterans Affairs, National Center on PTSD (2012). *PTSD in children and adolescents.* Retrieved from http://www.ptsd.va.gov/professional/pages/ptsd_in_children_and_adolescents_overview_for_professionals.asp.

United States Interagency Council on Homelessness (2010). *Opening doors: Federal strategic plan to prevent and end homelessness.* Retrieved from http://www.usich.gov/PDF/OpeningDoors_2010_FSPPreventEndHomeless.pdf.

van der Kolk, B. (1994). The body keeps the score: Memory and the evolving psychobiology of post traumatic stress. *Harvard Review of Psychiatry, 1*(5), 253–265.

van der Kolk, B. A. (2003). The neurobiology of childhood trauma and abuse. *Child and Adolescent Psychiatric Clinics, 12*, 293–317.

van der Kolk, B., McFarlane, A. C., & Weisaeth, L. (Eds.). (1996). *Traumatic stress.* New York: Guilford Press.

van der Kolk, B. A., Roth, S., Pelcovitz, D., Sunday, S., & Spinazzola, J. (2005). Disorders of extreme stress: The empirical foundation of a complex adaptation to trauma. *Journal of Traumatic Stress, 18*(5), 389–399.

Volk, K., Guarino, K., Grandin, M., & Clervil, R. (2008). *What about you? A workbook for those who work with others.* Needham, MA: The National Center on Family Homelessness. Retrieved from http://www.familyhomelessness.org/resources.php?p=sm.

Weinreb, L., Buckner, J. C., Williams, V., & Nicholson, J. (2006). A comparison of the health and mental health status of homeless mothers in Worcester, Mass: 1993 and 2003. *American Journal of Public Health, 96*, 1444–1448.

Wood, D., Valdez, R. B., Hayashi, T., & Shen, A. (1990). Homeless and housed families in Los Angeles: A study comparing demographic, economic, and family function characteristics. *American Journal of Public Health, 80*(9), 1049–1052.

Yehuda, R. (2002). Postraumatic stress disorder. *New England Journal of Medicine, 346*(2), 108–114.

Chapter 8
Cultural Competence and Individualized Care in Service Provision

BraVada Garrett-Akinsanya

Abstract The population of Americans without homes, especially those with children, is becoming increasing diverse. As their diversity increases, so should provider efforts to accommodate those families by facilitating their transitions in more culturally appropriate ways. Thus, three objectives are met through this chapter. First, this chapter focuses on the disproportional representation of historically marginalized families among those who experience homelessness. Through the use of case examples, it explores the notions of culture and cultural competence as they relate to providing cultural adaptations in services to homeless families. Second, this chapter addresses both the personal and systemic barriers (including the development of Oppression Reaction Syndromes) that families face in their attempts to access adequate housing resources. Barriers ranging from economic disparities, parental wellness, distrust of health/mental health systems, historical trauma, exposure to violence, and adverse childhood experiences are discussed. Finally, this chapter reviews promising programs for parents experiencing homelessness. Case examples are provided to illustrate how systems can overcome barriers by offering culturally competent services that include fathers, provide holistic support (such as childcare, meals, transportation access, and financial stipends), address the needs of adolescents, parental anger/stress, community violence, trauma, as well as cultural affirmation and community engagement strategies. In conclusion, it is surmised that culturally competent service delivery systems for families who experience homelessness must be *family-directed*, *family-centered*, *culturally affirming*, and *trauma-informed*.

B. Garrett-Akinsanya, Ph.D., LP (✉)
Brakins Consulting & Psychological Services, LLC, African American Child Wellness
Institute, Inc., Minneapolis, MN, USA
e-mail: bravadaakinsanya@hotmail.com

M.E. Haskett et al. (eds.), *Supporting Families Experiencing Homelessness:*
Current Practices and Future Directions, DOI 10.1007/978-1-4614-8718-0_8,
© Springer Science+Business Media New York 2014

"She who can not dance, will say the Drum is Bad."

(Ancient Yoruba proverb)

It can be said that cultural competence is the ability to "dance to the rhythm of the cultures one serves;" yet, cultural competence in service provision has posed a challenge for many providers—as clearly no one individual or agency can master the full knowledge of an ever-evolving phenomenon as complex as "culture." Nonetheless, the need to provide culturally competent services exists, especially in the area of serving homeless populations.

It is no secret that historically marginalized minority populations are overrepresented among those families that experience homelessness, and that families with children are the fastest growing group of Americans who are without homes. According to the "point-in-time" estimates produced by the US Department of Housing and Urban Development's 2012 Annual Homeless Assessment Report to Congress, on a given night in January 2011, 78.9 % of homeless people in families (186,482 people) were in shelters or transitional housing programs, and 49,699 people in families (21 % of all homeless persons) were in unsheltered locations or on the streets. While ethnic and racial minority groups currently represent approximately 45 % of all US families, among the sheltered families with children, they represented 71.9 % of the sheltered family population in 2011. African Americans comprised 43.6 % of the sheltered people in families, while 28.1 % of the sheltered family population was white, non-Hispanic/non-Latino. The remaining population was Latino (20.6 %), Asian (0.6 %), American Indian or Alaska Native (4.8 %), Native Hawaiian or Pacific Islander (0.9 %), or several races (12.6 %). Notably, these findings are not surprising as minorities were also overrepresented among the families living in poverty in 2011 such that 34.3 % were Hispanic/Latino, 24.1 % were African American, 20.3 % were another single race or of multiple race, and 34.8 % were white, non-Hispanic/non-Latino.

Some researchers (Friedman, Meschede, & Hayes, 2003) contend that the data on homeless families suggests that they are often headed by young, poorly educated single mothers who are either unemployed or underemployed, with a large proportion of the population raising children under the age of 5. Also of concern are the needs of adolescents, who may (or may not) be accompanied by adults. This is critically important as research suggests that homeless adolescents of color are at greater risks for incarceration (Metraux & Culhane, 2006); school failure (Kurtz, Jarvis, & Kurtz, 1991); substance abuse (Greene et al., 1997; Kipke, Montgomery, & Mackenzie, 1993); exposure to violence; and chronic physical, emotional, and sexual abuse (Powers et al., 1990; Rotheram-Borus, 1991). It is also possible that the description of homeless families may be inaccurate as some shelter regulations restrict family size, the inclusion of fathers, or children over a certain age.

Hanson (1992) estimated that by the year 2030, in the USA there will be 5.5 million more Latino children, 2.6 million more African-American children, 1.5 million more children of other races, and 6.2 million fewer white, non-Hispanic children born. Consequently, if these trends in population growth continue, it will become more imperative that those who work with diverse communities become increasingly skilled at culturally competent strategies to meet their multiple service needs in areas such as employment, health, and housing.

In fact, the US Surgeon General David Satcher released a ground-breaking publication in 2001 entitled *Mental Health: Culture, Race, and Ethnicity*. The document was a supplement to a previously released study on mental health, and reviewed multiple studies on racial/ethnic disparities and the negative health trajectories for people of color (James, 1994; Koegel et al., 1995). Since the release of the document, the patterns of negative health outcomes for people of color have persisted (Lekan, 2009). Finally, studies have revealed that the psychological stress affiliated with the subjective experiences of racism and discrimination has been linked to health status (Ahmed, Mohammed, & Williams, 2007; Steffen, McNeilly, Anderson, & Sherwood, 2003).

According to the Surgeon General's document, when compared to their white counterparts, minority populations are less likely to use services. Furthermore, when they do receive services, these groups experience a poorer quality of care. Consequently, a higher proportion of minority group members have unmet mental health needs. This problem is further compounded by the fact that minority populations are overrepresented among the homeless and incarcerated subpopulations that have higher rates of mental disorders than do people living in the general population (Burt et al., 1999; Koegel et al., 1995; Metraux & Culhane, 2006).

Finally, one of the largest barriers faced by culturally diverse communities who experience homelessness is the exposure to adversity in multiple forms. Researchers (Anda, Butchart, Felitti, & Brown, 2010) have described the deleterious and long-term effects of adverse childhood experiences on the trajectory of later life well-being. In fact, some researches (Felitti et.al., 1998) contend that childhood abuse and household dysfunction are linked to many of the leading causes of death in adults. Women, in particular African-American women, bear enormous burdens of both daily and historical stress (Garrett-Akinsanya, 2003; Hall, Garrett-Akinsanya, & Hucles, 2008). For instance, routine trauma and exposure to violence among African-American children and adults have resulted in up to a 33 % prevalence of Posttraumatic Stress Disorder (Alim, 2006) being diagnosed among this population.

According to the Surgeon General's report, when compared to whites, racial and ethnic minorities also experience a higher disability burden due to unmet mental health needs. While these groups face barriers such as stigmatization, high costs, and poorly coordinated services, they also face barriers of provider ignorance and ias—which results in limited access to linguistically or culturally appropriate care. Finally, many ethnic and minority clients experience fears and mistrust of treatment that are rooted in both historical and ongoing experiences of racism and discrimination. Systems that endorse trauma-informed care (Guarino, Soares, Konnath, Clervil, & Bassuk, 2009) support the Surgeon General's notion that "culture counts" in virtually every aspect of institutional and interpersonal processes. Further, the document stipulated that the negative impact of cultural biases contributes to a downward trajectory of families from cultural and ethnic communities. The negative trajectory was described by Bowen (1978) as a transgenerationally transmitted set of processes, an inherited status so to speak, that disproportionally impacts those in poverty. For example, a study conducted by the Insight Center for Community Economic Development in California (2011) found that children of color, in comparison to their white peers, were four times more likely to be born into poverty and experience life-long consequences of poverty, starting from diminished academic advancement to higher rates of financial insecurity. Unfortunately, according to a Kaiser Foundation report (2011), because ethnic minority groups (especially African Americans) are more likely to continue to experience poverty, it comes to reason that those who experience homelessness are more likely to come from ethnic minority populations (SAMSHA, 2011). Poverty among families has also been associated with higher rates of housing instability, exposure to environmental hazards, unsafe neighborhoods and family violence (including abuse), untreated medical and emotional conditions, and higher incidences of substance and alcohol abuse (Bassuk et al., 1998; Garbarino, 2001; Graham-Bermann, Coupet, Egler, Mattis, & Banyard, 1996).

In order to understand the prevalence of cultural disparities and why multicultural groups in the United States continue to face universal challenges with access to housing around issues of poverty, one needs to look no further than to the recent racial history of this country. For example, the Jim Crow laws of this country were enacted in 1876 and lasted until 1965. The Jim Crow laws were state and local laws that *mandated segregation* in all public facilities in the formerly confederate Southern states. The laws resulted in the development of the practice of "separate but equal" status for people of African descent. The separatist laws, however, resulted in the establishment of conditions for African Americans that tended to be inferior when compared to those enjoyed by white Americans. Additionally, while Jim Crow was based on *"de jure"* laws that primarily applied to Southern states, Northern segregation practices were generally de facto in nature and produced patterns of segregation in housing that have been maintained for decades by the implementations of covenants, bank lending practices, and job discrimination. While the *legal* access to fair housing has been granted to African Americans for only 48 years, the period of sociocultural access to housing continues to be a challenge.

It is well-understood that wide systemic and individual differences exist in the adjustments made by parents and children who are homeless. The diversity within this population points to the importance of addressing individual and collective needs inclusive of respect for cultural norms in approaches to strengthening these families (see also Chap. 5, DeCandia et al., this volume, for a discussion of needs of special populations without homes). Consequently, this chapter addresses ways in which programs that support families can maximize effectiveness via the use of culturally competent approaches to service delivery. Further, this chapter defines components of cultural competence, elements of service delivery that promote cultural competence, and addresses some innovative models for overcoming systemic barriers to change.

What Is Cultural Competence?

Mario Orlandi (1991) describes cultural competence as "a set of academic and interpersonal skills that allow individuals to increase their understanding and appreciation of cultural differences and similarities within, among, and between groups." Orlandi (1991) further proposes that cultural competency requires a willingness and ability to draw on community-based values, traditions, and customs. Additionally, it requires a willingness to work with *knowledgeable persons of and from the community* in developing focused interventions, communications, and other supports. Finally, cultural competency requires a *self-awareness and self-acceptance of one's own cultural biases and identity development.*

Darrell Wing Sue and his colleagues (Sue & Sue, 2003; Sue & Torino, 2005) purport that cultural competence must be comprised of three basic elements: (1) knowledge of the population being served; (2) an awareness of how one's own biases, values, attitudes, and beliefs impact the intervention process; and (3) skills to translate those elements into practice through culturally relevant adaptations. Thus, the core components of the vehicle that drives cultural competence with populations who experience homelessness must be inclusive of cognitive, affective, and skill dimensions in the dance between providers and the communities being served.

Orlandi (1991) consolidates the constructs of cultural competence within the context of a Cultural Sophistication Model. His model describes the developmental stages (and overall impact) of institutions or individuals as being *culturally incompetent (destructive)*, *culturally sensitive (neutral)*, or *culturally competent (constructive)* as assessed along cognitive, affective, and skills dimensions. On the other hand, a more explicit developmental model of cultural competence is proposed by Terry Cross (1988) and his colleagues (Cross, Bazron, Dennis, & Isaacs, 1989). Terry Cross (1988) describes cultural competence as occurring on a six-stage continuum of development, ranging from culturally destructive to culturally proficient. According to his model, when it comes to cultural competence, individuals or institutions may experience the following stages: (1) Cultural Destructiveness, (2) Cultural Incapacity, (3) Cultural Blindness, (4) Cultural Pre-Competence, (5) Basic Cultural Competence, and (6) Cultural Proficiency/Advanced Cultural Competence. From his perspective, institutions and individuals can be at different stages of development *concurrently.* For example, an institution or an individual may function at the Basic Culturally Competent stage in terms of dealing with the issue of sexual orientation, but may be at the Cultural Incapacity stage with regard to dealing with issues pertaining to race. Furthermore, Cross contends that in order to offer minimally competent services to diverse groups, a provider must (1) have acceptance and respect for differences, (2) expand his or her own cultural knowledge, (3) be aware of the dynamics that difference creates, (4) adapt service models and skills, (5) seek consultation from the cultural community of the client, and (6) engage in continuous self-assessment during the engagement process. In addition, providers are expected to hold culture and differences in high esteem, and engage in continuous efforts to expand knowledge and continued advocacy for cultural competence at all service levels.

Thus, individuals or institutions working with families that experience homelessness are considered to be "Culturally Destructive" when they develop policies and practices that decimate the cultural infrastructure of families. Individuals who are culturally destructive tend to assess their own cultural values and ways of being to be superior to those of others. On an institutional level, culturally destructive organizations engage in activities that eradicate "lesser" cultures. One of the most egregious examples of a "Culturally Destructive" policy in housing is the historical practice of developing boarding schools for Native American youths. For American Indian tribes during the late nineteenth and early twentieth centuries, the Bureau of Indian Affairs created boarding schools in an attempt to "assimilate" Native American children into European American culture by changing their appearance with haircuts and clothing. The traditional names given to Native American children were replaced by new Anglo-American names. Likewise, the children were forbidden to speak their native language, practice their native religions or participate in cultural rituals. Historical accounts (Adams, 1995) suggest that the children were ripped from their parents and exposed to boarding school conditions that were often harsh and plagued with exposure to sexual, physical, and mental abuse. The number of boarding schools reached their apex in the 1970s enrolling over 60,000 Native American youth. Today, shelters and supportive housing complexes that are designed for single women and their children, but exclude the presence of fathers, continue to replicate the process of breaking up the family units.

Within Cross' model, an individual or institution that functions at the *Cultural Incapacity* stage is characterized by a lack of cultural awareness and skills, and generally adhere to a belief in the racial superiority of the dominant group, and maintain a paternalistic view toward ethnic minority populations. Individuals or organizations that operate within this stage of awareness engage in discriminatory hiring practices, and hold assumptive stereotypical beliefs such as all single parents are inferior parents, or all homeless people are faulty or flawed somehow. The essence of this stage is that those who operate from this context are incapable of serving others in a respectful, equitable manner. *Cultural Blindness* is defined as the stage during which individuals or organizations are so ethnocentric that they view the cultural needs, beliefs, and values of all groups from the vantage point of the majority culture. From this perspective, all people are believed to be exactly alike, consequently culture makes no difference. Because they believe that all people are the same, groups and individuals functioning within the Cultural Blindness phase operate from a "cookie cutter" perspective, "erase" culture as an important variable and implement policies and practices that treat everyone the same way regardless of significant differences in religion, race, etc. According to Cross, only the most assimilated of ethnic or racial groups benefit from programs developed from this perspective.

Cross' model incorporates the *Cultural Pre-Competence* stage as the level of cultural competence during which individuals or institutions recognize cultural differences and attempt to educate themselves concerning these differences. Furthermore, this stage allows for the discovery of shortcomings in interfacing with diverse communities, and is characterized by an attempt to address diversity issues by activities such as offering cultural sensitivity training or hiring/promoting diverse staff. At this stage, there is limited knowledge about what needs to be done to address cultural issues in a competent manner. The next phase of Cross' model is known as the *Basic Cultural Competence* stage. During this stage, organizations and individuals demonstrate an ability to understand and manage the multiple intersections of cultural dynamics. This phase is characterized by the ability to accept, appreciate, and accommodate cultural differences, exhibit respect, value and acceptance of difference, as well as the willingness to explore cross-cultural interactions, promote community inclusion, and develop culturally specific services. The final phase of this model is the *Cultural Proficiency/Advanced Cultural Competence* stage. Institutions and individuals at this stage tend to operate from a higher level by seeking out knowledge about diverse cultures and developing skills in interacting within the context of diverse environments. Members of majority culture groups develop cross-cultural alliances and move beyond simply accommodating cultural differences. They become activists in promoting educational experiences for individuals who are less knowledgeable of, or comfortable with multicultural groups. Finally, at the organizational level, groups operating within the Advanced Cultural Competence stage tend to hire cultural competence specialists, advocate for historically marginalized groups, and conduct research on diversity issues. At this stage, there is a collaborative "joining" process that takes place with the communities being served.

Along that same vein, Tervalon and Murray-Garcia (1998) have introduced the concept of *"Cultural Humility"* that requires providers to explore their own limited cultural perspectives with efforts toward overcoming them through processes of self-awareness and self-reflection. In this model, the failure to provide culturally appropriate care is not the result of a lack of knowledge about any given culture; it is due to the failure on the part of a provider to develop a self-reflective and respectful community engagement process in response to diverse perspectives and individuals.

One core element in the process of self-reflection is the acknowledgement of power differentials between providers and the clients they serve. The Domestic Containment Program in Duluth, Minnesota (Pense and Paymar, 1993) utilizes a Power and Control Wheel that describes eight abuse behaviors associated with domestic violence. Lenore Walker (1994) highlighted the similarities that exist between sociocultural abuse and domestic violence. She suggests that domestic violence researchers and practitioners incorporate the definitions of psychological violence or terrorism endorsed by Amenesty International, as they closely resemble the ways that male batterers control and intimidate their female partners. Thus, in order to capture the sociocultural constructs of psychological violence, Garrett-Akinsanya (2004) introduced the Sociocultural Models of Abused and Shared Power and Control. The model is characterized by eight systemic oppressive elements that develop and maintain power abuses resulting in discrimination and prejudice in American society: (1) *Cultural Isolation*, (2) *Emotional abuse*, (3) *Economic abuse*, (4) *Sexual abuse*, (5) *Using children*, (6) *Using Threats*, (7) *Using Intimation*, (8) *Using white, male and American privilege*. According to this model, systemic corrections can only occur when individuals and organizations share power. Sharing power requires that those who are in power recognize and become perceptive to those who are not. A tenant of this model is that sharing power creates healthy connections, and healthy connections yield healthy individuals, families, and societies.

The Model of Shared Power and Control mandates that power is shared through: (1) Community Inclusion (versus isolation), (2) Respect for Physical Health/ Sexuality (versus Physical/Sexual Abuse), (3) Emotional Affirmation/respect for diversity (versus Emotional Abuse), (4) Honesty and Accountability/restorative justice and restitution (verses Intimidation), (5) Shared Value and Responsibility for all Children (versus Using Children), (6) Equal Opportunity/dismantling privilege through fairness (versus Using White, Male and American Privilege), (7) Non-Threatening Behavior/creating safety for challenge and risks (versus Use of Threats), and (8) Economic Empowerment (versus Economic Abuse).

Why Does Cultural Competence Matter Within the Context of Family Homelessness?

As can be seen, the goal of culturally competent engagement strategies is to yield effective, respectful and affirming processes that capitalize on the cultural strengths of the families served. In order to fully understand the concept of cultural competence as a strategy to integrate cultural strengths, it is critical to more deeply understand the construct of "culture." The anthropologist Muriel Saville-Troike (1985) describes culture as "a set of shared, learned behaviors that are transmitted from one generation to another for purposes of human adjustment, adaptation and growth." It is important to understand that one's indigenous culture influences everything that one knows, thinks, and feels in reference to the world. According to Saville-Troike, culture has both external and internal referents and the degree to which individuals adhere to cultural referents or adopt attitudes, values, behaviors, and beliefs outside the mainstream of their culture may be influenced by other factors such as the individual's stage of ethnic/cultural identity, the situational salience of identity, as well as other acculturation and assimilation processes (Atkinson, Morten, & Sue, 1989; Cross, 1971,1991; Gordon, 1961; Helms, 1990,1992; Sattler, 1995).

Therefore, Saville-Troike (1985) further postulates that the cultural context of families must be considered because culture impacts several life areas. For example, culture dictates the presentation of *familial roles* (e.g., What roles are available and to whom? How are roles acquired?), *interpersonal relationships* (e.g., How do people greet each other? How are respect and/or insults expressed?), as well as *decorum and discipline* (e.g., How do people behave at home and in public? What means of discipline are used?). Surely, in order to be effective, providers in homeless shelters and other supportive housing environments need to be aware of how roles are shared, how to engage respectfully, as well as how decorum and discipline are exhibited across cultures. For example, Harkness and Super (1995, 1996) contend that being culturally competent in parenting requires that one has a basic understanding of the general dimensions of a culture as well as the specific aspects of the backgrounds of children and their families served. They believe that by gaining culturally informed knowledge about the individualized needs of children and their families will reveal how families operate and how a given behavior can serve different cultural goals.

As an example, Silber (1989) demonstrated that white American professionals prefer democratic child-rearing practices as illustrated by lower levels of parental assertion and greater use of explanation, negotiation, and question-answer techniques. On the other hand, others (Philips, 1972; Tafoya, 1982) reported that more visual, low-key verbal styles were apparent among Native American parents. Conversely, McLoyd (1990) found that when low-income African-American families live in unsafe neighborhoods, a more directive, authoritarian parenting style may be warranted—especially when parents also pass on the negative consequences of ignoring strict rules. Additionally, when it came to parental strategies for punishment of misbehavior by children, Kalyanpur and Rao (1991) reported that a traditional belief in corporal punishment is common among African-American, Asian, and Latino families; shaming was a normative disciplinary practice among Asian groups. Finally, Delpit (1988) compared the more explicit expression of authority used by African-American parents to that of middle class Caucasian Americans and concluded that the strength of either relationship resides in the child's recognition that the parent's authority is being exercised in love.

The case example of Laticia provides evidence of this phenomenon. Laticia was a young African-American mother with two children (6 and 4 years of age). Her husband and she had broken up; consequently, her husband moved back to Chicago to be around his family and to find a better-paying job. Laticia worked as a teacher's aid at a local daycare, but was laid off at the end of the summer because the center had lost income when a number of children began to attend public school. Although she was eligible for unemployment, it was not enough money for her to maintain her apartment, consequently, she found herself seeking supportive housing. While staying in the supportive housing unit, she and her children were frequently observed to be involved in activities such as sitting together on a blanket having lunch, playing on the swings, or snuggling on the couch reading books.

Besides her children, Laticia had no family in town, but quickly became friends with several of the women who were also residents in the housing complex. Laticia contends that she and the other African-American women perceived that they were often the last ones to gain the supportive attention of the staff. She related that she felt pressured and angry because she would frequently hear the primarily European-American staff members refer to her or the other African-American women as "welfare moms." She described experiencing pervasive feelings of shame and isolation. One day, she reported that her oldest daughter Kenya took candy from the store and to punish her, Laticia loudly and harshly scolded the child, smacked her bottom, and told her that she would *"Knock the black off of her."* One of the staff members overheard the interaction and reported Laticia to the manager. According to Laticia, the staff member and the woman's supervisor called Laticia to the office and threatened to not only evict her from the housing unit, but to contact Child Protection Services because of her "terrorist threats" to harm her child. Despite her efforts to explain, Laticia related that she felt even more disrespected and unsafe in that environment. Eventually, she left and went back home to Chicago.

Clearly, culture impacts how parents behave within the context of supportive housing environments. The rules of these environments, on the other hand, may not be tailored to meet the individual, cultural "ways of being" that are common among diverse ethnic groups. Instead, more Eurocentric models may be perceived as being "best practices" when it comes to child-rearing and iatrogenic outcomes may result due to identifying culturally adaptive strategies as being culturally maladaptive. Conversely, not knowing what is culturally adaptive may also lead an agency or individual to unknowingly describe a maladaptive behavior as being "cultural" in nature.

It may be obvious to many providers that culture also impacts other life areas such as religion, dress, holidays and food. Nonetheless, in order for agencies to appropriately serve communities of color, they may have to adapt the ways in which their services are provided. As an example, Aatifa was an Ethiopian Muslim woman who came to America as a refugee. She had three children—two daughters (ages 11 and 9) and one son (age 7). Aatifa's husband was among the 123,000 people killed in the Eritrean–Ethiopian war that took place from May 1998 to June 2000. When she came to America, she initially lived with her sister where she learned to speak some English; however, her sister did not have room at her small home for Aatifa to stay permanently. Eventually, Aatifa had to find temporary housing support in a shelter.

While in the shelter, Aatifa rarely slept and had frequent nightmares of her husband dying. She would get up early in the mornings to pray and was told that she needed to go back to her area as she would be "abandoning her children" and "disrupting others" in the shelter. She also found herself being pushed out early in the mornings with her children after a breakfast of fruit, cereal, and milk. She described being afraid to feed the cereal to her children as she was told by her sister as well as other Muslim women that some cereals had animal fat (from pigs) and that she would be committing a grave sin by eating the available meals. She was reluctant to share this information with the shelter manager, but realized that after a few days when they continued to provide the same meals she must respectfully request different food. After she summoned the courage to speak with the shelter manager, Aatifa was sadly disappointed by the manager's reply that because the shelter had limited financial resources she would have to "*find another shelter or eat what* [they] *had to serve.*" By not making individualized cultural accommodations for Aatifa's dietary, religious and mental health needs, the providers of the shelter engaged in culturally destructive practices that resulted in poor service provision.

Cultural adaptations are also necessary in other life areas such as health and hygiene. For example, many cultures—including Black, Native, Latino, and Asian American—routinely perceive symptoms of mental illness as related to spiritual causes. Additionally, because those groups (especially African American and Native Americans) have been historically exploited as experimental subjects in physical health areas, there continues to be a tendency within these communities to avoid medical professionals of all types. One cannot overlook the infamous Tuskegee syphilis experiment, which was a clinical study conducted between 1932 and 1972 by the US Public Health Services. The study was used to explore the natural progression of untreated syphilis among rural black men who thought that they were receiving free health care from the government. Even after a viable treatment (penicillin) was found, the participants were "sacrificed" unknowingly in the service of science. While the vehicle driving the experiments was a predominately white institution, those who delivered the syphilis were African Americans from their communities! Thus, even when African-Americans are the primary health service providers, "intra-group" issues arise as to whether those African Americans are "sell-outs" and have been "co-opted" as coconspirators to the dominate white culture to implement strategies that will lead to the demise of their communities. As a result, today, African Americans exhibit large disparities in mental and physical health outcomes due to discomfort with, and mistrust of, the medical community.

Consequently, instead of seeking medical support, multicultural communities (American Indians, African Americans, and Asian Americans) tend to utilize natural remedies that have been passed down transgenerationally. As an example, according to the Coalition for Asian American Children and Families (Lee & Lee, 2002), many Asian parents may choose to use traditional Asian medicine to treat ailments before seeking treatment from Western clinics or emergency rooms. Some forms of traditional medical treatments, such as "coining" or "spooning" may leave red marks on the child's skin that can be mistaken for evidence of abuse. Therefore, having a lack of knowledge about a culture's traditional healing techniques (or marginalizing it) may lead to misjudgments in serving culturally different populations.

Understanding the importance of history and traditions is also a key element in the process of integrating culture into the work that is done with families that experience homelessness. When exploring one's cultural history, key questions are asked, such as the following: "How are history and tradition passed on to the young? How do cultural understandings of history differ from "scientific" facts or literate history?" For example, historians tell us that the Atlantic Slave Trade took place from the sixteenth to the nineteenth centuries in an effort to address a shortage in the labor market required for European colonists to exploit New World land and resources for capital profits. Initially, Native peoples were utilized as slave labor until a large number of them died due to overwork and exposure to European-borne diseases. Then Africans were used as they were able to physically handle the intensive heat and weather conditions of the south. The first Africans imported to the English colonies came as "indentured servants" or "apprentices for life." By the middle of the seventeenth century, however, they (and their offspring) were legally treated as merchandise or units of labor and were sold at "stock markets" with other goods and services. Soon thereafter, estimates are that well over 12 million African slaves were stolen from Africa and brought to America over the course of the next 300 years. Notably, many millions more died in African wars and in route through the Middle Passage to America. They become "involuntary" immigrants, and were stripped of their cultural ways of life including language, religion, rituals, etc. This process, known as "deracination" continues to leave its legacy and impact on the lives of the offspring of Natives and Africans that experienced what may be referred to as "historical trauma."

Consequently, although Crispus Attucks (a Black man) was the first man shot in the American revolution, for many African Americans celebrating the 4th of July as a day for commemorating freedom is not as meaningful as celebrating "Juneteenth" as a holiday around freedom. The "Juneteenth" holiday is formally celebrated on June 19th throughout the United States (and other parts of the world) as a day to acknowledge emancipation from slavery. As part of America's racial history, many are unaware that while Abraham Lincoln issued the Emancipation Proclamation on September 22, 1862, with an effective date of January 1, 1863, many slaves in the south and parts of the northern states remained in bondage (Foner, 2007). Texas, as a Confederate state, was particularly recalcitrant and doggedly resisted the federal proclamation to free the slaves. It was not until June 19, 1865 (Juneteenth) that Union General Gordon Granger arrived in Galveston, Texas along with 2,000 federal troops to take possession of the state and enforce the emancipation of its slaves. Culturally competent agencies serving African Americans, then, would incorporate this event into their plans for service provision (Franklin, 1963). Furthermore, within the context of culture, programs designed for families experiencing homelessness should also provide trauma-informed environments for care. See Chap. 7 (Guarino) in this volume for a comprehensive discussion of the importance of trauma-informed practices.

Another example of the relevance of cultural history in the delivery of support to homeless populations includes those services provided to Native Americans. Many Americans observe Columbus Day and Thanksgiving Day as primary holidays by commemorating the "bounty and discovery" of America with feasts, parades, school, and office closures as well as official proclamations. Nonetheless, for many Native Americans, Columbus Day is observed as "Native American Day" and Thanksgiving Day is perceived as a National Day of Mourning (Feagin, 2009). Native Americans describe the origins of their mourning as being linked to when Columbus came to America, and when the first pilgrims landed on Plymouth Rock bringing disease and exploitation. In fact, historians and sociologists (Feagin, 2009) write accounts of pilgrims, who during their first years in America, confessed to the opening of Indian graves, pillaging the Indians' wheat and bean supplies, and selling Indians as slaves at a rate of 220 shillings each. Thus, when shelters serving African American or Native American clients hold a lack of perspective in terms of the historical implications of their experiences, there is a broadening of cultural disconnections among program participants and service providers.

Another example of important life areas impacted by culture include cultural perspectives of work and play (i.e., What behaviors are considered "work" and "play"? What kinds of work are prestigious and why?) Due to the legacy of slavery, for instance, many African Americans prefer to work inside of buildings as opposed to outside—even though the wages may be higher for jobs outdoors. This phenomenon is closely related to the social positioning of field slaves as opposed to house slaves. House slaves were frequently the offspring of slave holders and their female slaves. Consequently, they were given better accommodations (e.g., food, clothing, shelter) and social positioning when compared to those slaves who were forced to be in the fields all day. The result of those sexually exploitative conditions—"colorism," (the tendency to display social preference for lighter skin and devalue darker skin) remains a problem among people of color.

Culture also influences a community's perception of time and space (What is considered "on time?" What is the importance of punctuality? How important is speed of performance?). Several writers (Hall, 1983; Helman, 1987, 2001; Jenkins, 2009) describe the cultural variations among groups in terms of how people understand and use time. When it comes to their use of time, cultural groups can be divided into two categories such that they are either monochromic or polychromic. A monochromic culture is one that views time in a linear way so that there is a discrete beginning and ending of the construct. Additionally, the use of time mandates that there is a differentiation between task-oriented activities and relational ones. Cultural examples of the monochromic type of temporal orientation include the USA, Israel, Switzerland, and Germany. On the other hand, some countries (i.e., Africa, the Middle East, and Latin America) have a polychromic orientation and perceive time in a different way. Polychromic groups are more flexible with time and perceive time as an opportunity to integrate both relational and task-oriented activities. Thus "cultural time" is identified as an orientation to time that is fluid, relational, and socially determined. This orientation impacts many multicultural community members and is often in stark contrast to the temporal expectations of employers, housing authorities, or other sociocultural systems that mandate access to support and care.

When clients come for appointments, holding the construct of polychromic time may lead them to be late, slow to "get down to business" and perceived as being "resistant." On the other hand, culturally competent providers will understand and interpret the origins of the use of time among ethnic minority populations and make adaptations to policies and procedures to accommodate the cultural differences. Accommodations may be offered in a variety of ways such as creating procedures that allow more time to connect with clients, identifying "walk-in" hours for clients to access supportive services, or assisting clients in gaining the skills of operating in monochromic systems by providing cultural coaching.

Another key life area impacted by culture is communication (What languages and dialects are spoken? How are conversations opened or closed? How are silence, humor, and interruptions integrated into the conversations?). The case of Marquetta demonstrates how cultural differences in discourse, including the use of slang, can result in confusion. Marquetta was an African-American woman who lived in a supportive housing unit with her two children and her husband Jamar. Jamar had recently been hired at a local building company and was being recognized at the company's monthly luncheon meeting. New employees were asked to bring their families to the meeting. When Marquetta returned to the housing office, she proceeded to praise her husband's efforts and told the assistant housing manager that Jamar was "a hard-working brother." Later that evening, she received a call from the housing manager telling her that the apartments were for parents and their children, and that her "brother" would have to move out. Obviously, the ordinary cultural use of the word "brother" in reference to her partner was outside the cognitive schema of the office staff.

Other life areas influenced by culture include values (What traits and attributes in self, others are important, good or bad? What attributes in the world are important, good or bad?). Of all of the variables impacting cultural work, the role of cultural values is perhaps the most important. Cultural values delineate what is desirable within the individual and society (Gollnick & Chinn, 1990) and contribute to the ways in which people think, feel, and behave in larger society. Theorists (Gilligan, 1982; Gushue & Constantine, 2003; Kambon, 1992; Markus & Kitayama, 1994; Triandis, 1989; Utsey, Adams, & Bolden, 2000) have categorized systems of cultural values as being based on a dichotomy of "individualist" versus "collectivist" orientations.

Although North Americans are often cited for placing an emphasis on individualism, other cultures are described as more "collectivist" in nature (Triandis, Brislin, & Hui, 1988). In fact, some researchers (Kambon, 1992; Utsey et. al, 2000) contend that the mental health of African Americans or other ethnic minority populations traditionally has required that they be more collectivistic in orientation, while others (Gushue & Constantine, 2003) contend that a more bicultural orientation combining both collectivist and individualist worldviews may be necessary for navigating today's dominant culture-driven systems.

Thus, two key cultural transformation processes exist that may change our values and worldviews. First, values change through acculturation, which is the process by which an individual gradually becomes accustomed to another culture and inevitably adopts that culture as her own. The second way in which values may change is through assimilation, which occurs when two distinct cultural groups experience a merging of cultural traits. With that in mind, the cultural transformation processes of assimilation and acculturation create variability in the degree to which one family (or its members) adheres to traditional cultural values or not. Specifically, "Collectivism" is affiliated with an emphasis on interdependence, communal and relational models of engagement among self and others, while "Individualism" is construed as focusing on independence, autonomy, and separatists' models of the self in relation to others. In basic terms, individualism focuses on the individual, while collectivism focuses on the group. The groups most impacted by homelessness tend to be those whose roots are deeply mired in the value of collectivism. For example, African cultures have a concept known as "Ubuntu," which integrates the individual to the whole. Ubuntu reflects a greater commitment to consubstantiation—the belief that among all living creatures there is an "interconnection." Within this vein, the "African self" only exists within the context of a larger group system and consequently Ubuntu is exemplified in the saying: "*I am because we are*," and "*we are*" because "*I am*." Many theorists (Gilligan, 1982; Kambon, 1992; Nobles, 2006) believe that the individualist characteristic of society and the value of looking out only for oneself are contrary to the well-being of marginalized and multicultural communities.

Thus, the tendency of mainstream American providers to gravitate to processes that are "individualized" promotes acculturation while simultaneously creating cultural clashes for many multicultural families. To them, the emphasis on individualism is reflective of a "save yourself" mentality and is especially evident when housing programs are designed solely for women and their children instead of being designed to promote the *whole* family's survival. The individualist mentality is also demonstrated by institutionally driven economic support programs that penalize families for legally being married by withdrawing or limiting access to economic support or medical supplements because (together) the family is not far enough under the poverty level to gain adequate assistance. For this reason, the failure to implement processes, policies, and practices that promote Ubuntu (survival of the individual and the entire family as a group) may be the least culturally responsive way of bringing cultural strengths into service delivery systems.

A good case example of this problem involves an African-American teenage father, James. James was a senior in high school who was sleeping on the couches of friends and family for several months while on the waiting list for a housing unit designed for homeless youth. As a relatively good student, he had continued to go to school and had hoped to go to college as soon as he graduated. Once he got the call that a housing unit would be coming available and prior to being interviewed, James was told that to qualify to live in the housing unit, he could not be a full-time student and could not currently have a place to stay. James reported that he immediately withdrew from school and lied about staying with friends so that he could land a stable place to live. Within a few weeks of living in his apartment, James' pregnant girlfriend Laura (who was living at her sister's house) delivered their baby. Laura's sister was pressuring her to move out. James wanted Laura and the baby to live with him as he now had stable housing; however, he could only allow them to visit for 3 days at a time. So, he would have them stay at 3-day intervals with a day or two between visits. He sought housing for the entire family, but could find no place available that would accept them all. The young couple grappled with the issue of whether it was best to be on the streets together or have individual housing arrangements apart. After sneaking his girlfriend and newborn child into the apartment for a period of more than 3 days in a row, the program manager put James on visitation restriction for breaking the rules. Consequently, he was not allowed to have visitors in his apartment for 2 weeks and the early attachment needs of the newborn were compromised. This dilemma reflects the problem of funding streams that are culturally destructive, staff who do not engage in self-reflective cultural humility practices, and the lack of cultural competence in systems that serve "collectivist" cultures but do not promote collectivism.

What Barriers Do Communities of Color Face in Gaining Access to Culturally Competent Services in Housing Support?

Although many barriers to adequate housing may be due to externally driven systems that impact economic and social instability, some barriers experienced by marginalized communities are the result of oppression including interpersonal, internalized and historical traumas. Garrett-Akinsanya (2004) writes about *"Oppression Reaction Syndromes*, which are dysfunctional interpersonal relationships that are the result of racial oppression. Oppression Reaction Syndromes are often perpetuated through the use of racial micro-aggressions (Sue et al., 2007), which are described as "brief and commonplace daily verbal, behavioral or environmental indignities, whether intentional or unintentional, that communicate hostile, derogatory or negative racial slights and insults toward people of color." According to Garrett-Akinsanya (2004), the act of marginalizing and dehumanizing others is not a natural phenomenon and therefore such practices create cognitive dissonance in both the victim and the perpetrator of oppression. Consequently, for oppressors to incorporate and normalize the process of victimizing others, they must reformulate reality through the use of Oppression Reaction Syndromes. Similarly, the internalization of oppressive beliefs by victims is the way in which victims of oppression "buy into" or participate in the reformulated realities of their oppressors.

Oppression reaction syndromes consist of, but are not limited to, symptoms commonly observed in posttraumatic stress disorder such as lowered self-esteem, decreased sense of self-worth, loss of own self-identity, reduced self-confidence in abilities/decreased sense of competence, restricted sense of possible life options, increased self-doubt, lack of trust in others, hyper-vigilance, feelings of loneliness and social isolation, feelings of helplessness and hopelessness, embarrassment, humiliation, shame, guilt, depression, anxiety, rage, anger, and blocking (or difficulty concentrating or processing information). Additional symptoms include fear of abandonment; fear of serious physical, economic or social harm to oneself, one's children, or other family members; emotional paralysis; as well as poverty of spirit and spiritual depletion. Because many providers who serve families who experience homelessness may not recognize these symptoms, they may misjudge parental behaviors as being indicative of mental illness or character defects rather than being reactions to the trauma of systemic oppression.

Garrett-Akinsanya (2004) has categorized existing theories of bias, prejudice, and discrimination as being Oppression Reaction Syndromes. Thus, constructs such as the White Racial Frame (Feagin, 2009), Fly in the Buttermilk Syndrome (Garrett-Akinsanya, 2004), the Invisibility Syndrome (Franklin, 1993), Stereotype Threat (Steele, 1997), Post Traumatic Slave Syndrome (DeGruy-Leary, 2005), and Aversive Racism (Dovidio & Gaertner, 1991)—just to name a few, represent core examples of this phenomenon.

Sociologist Joe Feagin (2009) describes one Oppression Reaction Syndrome, *White Racial Framing*, as a critical aspect of the societal reality of "systemic racism." He contends that this framing is a deeply held, broad, generic meaning system held by most whites that shape human action and behavior in a myriad of ways that are often automatic or unconscious. According to Feagin, white racial framing has racial images, interpretations, emotions, and action inclinations that are closely tied to racial cognitions that support standards, policies, and practices within systems that endorse white cultural values, while rejecting the cultural practices of marginalized groups as inferior or dysfunctional in nature. Thus, within the context of working with homeless families of color, white providers may identify "family functioning" and wellness within a Eurocentric context without consideration of which factors constitute culturally defined wellness.

Another Oppression Reaction Syndrome is the "Fly in the Buttermilk" Syndrome, which may be observed among ethnic minority families who are isolated and living in shelters when they report that (in comparison to their white counterparts) they perceive as if they are under constant observation and that their differences or mistakes are magnified and their accomplishments or similarities to others are minimized. This process is evidenced by their perceived experiences of being "singled out" as demonstrated through perpetrator generated practices such as racial profiling while driving, shopping, or living in housing facilities.

The Fly in the Buttermilk Syndrome is the opposite of the Invisibility Syndrome. The "*Invisibility Syndrome*," introduced by A. J. Franklin (1993), was originally used to describe the experience of African Americans in reaction to the tendency of the dominant culture to ignore, minimize, or marginalize the existence, contributions and needs of Blacks in America. This syndrome was most notable on a sociocultural level during Hurricane Katrina, when the transportation needs of the poor, mostly ethnic minority, communities were "not seen." Although the community was warned to evacuate the city of New Orleans, nobody considered the fact that a large part of the ethnic minority community used mass transit as their primary means of movement throughout the city. Thus, they had no means with which to evacuate, and unfortunately many of them perished due to the invisibility of their needs. In attempts to meet the housing needs of low-income families, providers may engage in this process by building new low-income housing stock in suburban neighborhoods—without considering the needs of families to have access to mass transit in order to reach jobs, schools, or other community infrastructural support systems such as churches or family members. In order to have a place to live, these families, in essence, have to become isolated and stranded in suburban communities because their unique needs are invisible.

"*Stereotype Threat*" is another Oppression Reaction Syndrome introduced by Dr. Claude Steele (1997). Stereotype Threat occurs in reaction to circumstances in which there exists a negative stereotype or cultural bias about one's group. Individuals with Stereotype Threat internalize those negative biases and, consequently, their resultant behavior is modified because of those biases. They unconsciously engage in "self-fulfilling prophesies." For example, if stereotypes exist that most families are homeless because of substance abuse, then many housing programs will be designed that require participants to go through substance abuse counseling. To get housing, participants may lie or begin to engage in drug or alcohol abuse in order to be housed.

Another excellent example of an Oppression Reaction Syndrome is the construct of *Aversive Racism* (Gaertner & Dovidio, 1986) which surmises that unconscious, implicit biases, and negative attitudes towards minority groups are acquired early in life, resulting from immersion in a society with a long history of racial bias. Yet, because pressures exist against *overt* expression of negative attitudes towards minority group members, dominant-culture members only demonstrate their racist attitudes *covertly* when acting upon their biases can be attributed to other factors besides race. Therefore, individuals who engage in aversive racism tend to profess holding egalitarian beliefs and deny engaging in racially motivated behaviors. Yet, when ambiguous situations arise that require judgment calls relative to members of minority groups, aversive racists unconsciously exhibit behaviors that are incongruent with their professed non-racist beliefs. As an example, Dovidio and his colleagues (Dovidio, Gaertner, Kawakami, & Hodson, 2002; Gaertner & Dovidio, 2000; Pearson, Dovidio, & Gaertner, 2009) experimentally demonstrated that when a white candidate had less job experience than a black candidate (but she had more education) the white candidate would be recommended for hire with the assumption that she could gain on-the-job training. Conversely, when a white candidate had less education than the black candidate, yet she had more experience, the white candidate would still be recommended for hire based on the assumption that she could gain "continuing education."

Families who experience Aversive Racism within the context of homelessness often complain that the rules keep changing or shifting and describe that dominant-culture providers may disproportionately help majority culture families by recommending them sooner for supports or for placements in better facilities. Thus, staff may appear to hide behind policy and their rationale for making decisions on factors such as family size, length of time waiting, past housing experiences, availability of program funds, etc. may appear arbitrary to the ethnic minority family members.

Dr. Joy DeGruy-Leary (2005) describes the *"Post Traumatic Slave Syndrome"* as a set of multigenerational maladaptive behaviors that were developed by African Americans in order to survive hundreds of years of chattel slavery. Gone (2009) eloquently describes a similar impact of historical trauma on Native American communities. Drs. Gone and DeGruy-Leary contend that these behaviors have been perpetuated because parents who experienced trauma continue to indoctrinate their children into exhibiting unhealthy survival-based coping strategies, although many posttrauma circumstances have changed. Similarly both researchers contend that programming for these families must provide opportunities for them to reclaim their heritage, focus on identity, and embrace spirituality as part of their recovery processes.

How Can Systems Overcome Barriers to Parent Success?

For systems to overcome barriers and promote resilience, providers must look at what has been working already. Consequently, this component of the chapter reviews a few promising parenting programs that have occurred within the context of family homelessness by highlighting their cultural strengths in promoting family change. Also see Chap. 9 (Gewirtz et al.) of this volume for a complete review of the literature on parenting programs to support positive parenting.

It is recognized that most shelters and programs for homeless parents are designed to be delivered solely to mothers. Interestingly, Ferguson and Morley (2011) explored a comprehensive supportive housing program created to increase paternal involvement in child rearing among a group comprised primarily of African-American men. In order to qualify for supportive housing, fathers were mandated to participate in weekly individual therapy sessions, peer support group sessions, as well as the Parents As Teachers (PAT) program. According to the researchers, the PAT curriculum was designed to teach fathers how to engage in activities that advance child development and increase their confidence as parents. Problems with this program were that participation was mandatory and not voluntary, sample size of the participant group was small ($n = 7$) and no information was provided about the fidelity to the PAT curriculum. Outcomes reported from a focus group conducted with four of the seven participants revealed that the fathers conveyed that they enjoyed the group, improved their relationships with their children (and the children's mothers), and increased their ability to manage anger. Details about the components of the intervention were limited, which would pose a difficulty in replicating the program. Nonetheless, the fact that the program targeted fathers and provided more holistic strategies (in the form of psychotherapy, housing, and social support) increased its likelihood of being culturally relevant.

Gewirtz and Taylor (2009) designed a study to explore the feasibility of implementing the *Parenting Through Change* curriculum as delivered in a domestic violence shelter for women as part of an extensive collaboration between university and community partners. The curriculum was delivered over 14 weekly group sessions, with homework and weekly check-in phone calls. Results suggested that parents reported feeling more empowered, consistent in their parenting roles and supported by group facilitators. The strength of this program was that it created a collectivist environment for women to grow and learn. It minimized participation barriers by providing childcare, financial incentives, food, individual contact, and social support. These factors, though not culturally specific in nature, created a culturally relevant environment for program participants.

Puterbaugh (2009) evaluated the use of the Adolescent Transitions Program as delivered in 12 individual sessions completed in a long-term shelter over a period of 10 weeks with 13 single mothers with adolescents serving as the program participants (4 Latinos, 5 African Americans, 4 Caucasians). All Latino participants dropped out of the program prematurely. The remaining participants completed self-report pre- and post-intervention measures of child behavior and parental stress. Results suggested that significant reductions in the intensity of some adolescent behavior problems were noted. Concerns with the study included small sample size and the fact that all of the Latino members dropped out of the intervention; however, the strength of the program was in its attempt to address parental stress, especially among parents with adolescents since homeless adolescents of color are at greater risk for multiple life problems (e.g., incarceration, school failure, substance abuse, exposure to violence).

Garrett-Akinsanya (2013) described the Project Murua: Pre-meditated Parenting Boot Camp, a military-style African-centered parenting program that integrates parents living in shelters with general community members to create a sense of community once parents transition from the shelter to the community. Project Murua: Pre-meditated Parenting Boot Camp relies upon an African-Centered Wellness Model and that targets parents raising children of African descent (ages 6–18 years). Parents voluntarily participate in a 10-week program for 3 hours each week, including both didactic lectures and kinesthetic exercises with a Drill Sergeant who teaches cadences and drills that affirm positive parenting strategies. Families are provided with dinner, childcare/homework help, transportation, and a $100 stipend upon graduation. Project Murua is a wellness promotion and violence prevention program designed to improve family functioning and communication; build adult and youth self-esteem; increase social support; and facilitate efforts to combat child abuse, substance abuse, parent-school relationships, juvenile delinquency, gang violence, behavioral problems, and emotional disturbances. Participants develop Family Wellness Plans that are monitored by a Wellness Coach, with weekly phone calls for follow-up on progress. Along with homework and pre-post measures for each module, participants complete measures on knowledge of community resources, basic parenting practices/skills, exposure to violence, and normative beliefs about aggression. After they graduate from the program, Project Murua graduates come back to serve as paid program facilitators, and are "deployed" to community events to provide lectures and support for other parents. The program has trained over 200 parents with approximately 15 parents per Boot Camp class. Project Murua participants have consistently reported positive outcomes in terms of increased knowledge of parenting, increased wellness strategies, and decreased violence. Challenges with the program are related to fact that it is resource intensive, has 30 h of programming, and its longitudinal impact has not been studied. Strengths of the program include its robust use of pre–post measures, large sample size, culturally specific design and engagement of both shelter and community members, voluntary nature of participation, ongoing involvement of participants after the course is completed, and its emphasis on family functioning as well as violence prevention and wellness promotion.

Conclusions and Recommendations for Cultural Competence and Individualized Care in Service Provision

Among sheltered families with children, ethnic minority families are overrepresented in the system. Thus, the need for cultural competence is critical. This chapter has offered a definition of cultural competence as "a set of academic and interpersonal skills that allow individuals to increase their understanding and appreciation of cultural differences and similarities within, among, and between groups." Within that context, groups providing services to culturally diverse families experiencing homelessness must be willing to draw on community-based values, traditions, and customs. They must also engage knowledgeable persons of and from the communities served in developing focused interventions, communications, and other supports. Cultural adaptations to services and intervention programs should integrate culturally meaningful values and practices including religious accommodations, dietary options, holidays celebrated, clothing, games, etc. They will also require that providers do not succumb to the temptation to create interventions that are culturally blind or culture-free, rather, that they make a commitment to adjusting their service delivery models to be consistent with the cultures of those served.

It has been noted that no two families are alike; consequently, adaptations to the unique needs and barriers of individual family-based cultural practices will be required. Likewise, solutions to overcoming the barriers of homelessness and the need to individualize parental support systems will require providers to understand the contextual nature of each family's unique experiences and the cultural history of the groups to whom they belong. Additionally, culturally competent providers will be required to create ongoing policies and practices that foster cultural humility and an increased understanding of how provider biases, values, attitudes, and beliefs impact the intervention process. Therefore, successful, culturally competent services must focus on understanding oppression reaction syndromes, trauma recovery, cultural parenting practices (inclusive of fathers), as well as the development of culturally relevant attachment rituals and values. In fact, this chapter has reviewed diverse promising parenting programs that have targeted fathers, provided holistic support (such as childcare, meals, transportation access, and financial stipends), addressed the needs of at-risk adolescents, parental anger/stress, community violence, trauma, cultural affirmation, and community engagement strategies. From the review, it is clear that providers should be mindful of how individual and sociocultural power is shared or abused. Rather than implementing policies or practices that force families to participate in programs that they do not value (in order to gain housing or other services needed to live), providers should offer a menu of well-planned support systems, with goals co-created by families that meet their needs.

Providers should make efforts to strengthen the capacity of diverse clients to develop a sense of agency and self-empowerment by close attention to institutional practices of sharing power by hiring diverse staff and managers and creating collaborative processes with families that minimize the unconscious messages of white superiority. Finally, the creation of substantive changes in the delivery of services to culturally diverse families experiencing homelessness will also require improved policies on the parts of service organizations and funders that promote family preservation through community-building practices that are *family-directed, family-centered, culturally affirming*, and *trauma-informed*.

References

Adams, D. W. (1995). *Education for extinction: American Indians and the boarding school experience, 1875–1928*. Lawrence, KS: University of Kansas Press.

Ahmed, A. T., Mohammed, S. A., & Williams, D. R. (2007). Racial discrimination & health: Pathways & evidence. *Indian Journal of Medical Research, 126*, 318–327.

Alim, T. N. (2006). An overview of posttraumatic stress disorder in African Americans. *Journal of Clinical Psychology, 62*, 801–813.

Anda, R. F., Butchart, A., Felitti, V. J., & Brown, D. W. (2010). Building a framework for global surveillance of the public health implications of adverse childhood experiences. *American Journal of Preventive Medicine, 39*, 93–98.

Atkinson, D. R., Morten, G., & Sue, D. W. (1989). A minority identity development model. In D. Atkinson, G. Morten, & D. W. Sue (Eds.), *Counseling American minorities* (pp. 35–52). Dubuque, IA: W. C. Brown.

Bassuk, E. L., Buckner, J. C., Perloff, J. N., & Bassuk, S. S. (1998). Prevalence of mental health and substance use disorders among homeless and low-income women. *American Journal of Psychiatry, 155*, 1561–1564.

Bowen, M. (1978). *Family therapy in clinical practice.* New York: Jason Aronson.

Burt, M. R., Aron, L. Y., Douglas, T., Valente, J., Lee, E., & Iwen, B. (1999). *Homelessness: Programs and the people they serve (summary report).* Washington, DC: Urban Institute.

Cross, W. E., Jr. (1971). Toward a psychology of Black liberation: The Negro-to-Black conversion experience. *Black World, 20*, 13–27.

Cross, T. (1988). Services to minority populations: Cultural competence continuum. *Focal Point, 3*, 1–9.

Cross, W. E., Jr. (1991). *Shades of Black: Diversity in African-American identity.* Philadelphia: Temple University Press.

Cross, T., Bazron, B., Dennis, K., & Isaacs, M. (1989). *Towards a culturally competent system of care* (Vol. 1). Washington, DC: Georgetown University Child Development Center, CASSP Technical Assistance Center. In M. Isaacs, & M. Benjamin. (1991). *Towards a culturally competent system of care, volume 2, programs which utilize culturally competent principles.* Washington, DC: Georgetown University Child Development Center, CASSP Technical Assistance Center.

DeGruy-Leary, J. A. (2005). *Post traumatic slave syndrome: America's legacy of enduring injury and healing.* Baltimore, MD: Uptone.

Delpit, L. D. (1988). The silenced dialogue: Power and pedagogy in educating other people's children. *Harvard Educational Review, 58*, 280–299.

Dovidio, J. F., & Gaertner, S. L. (1991). Changes in the expression and assessment of racial prejudice. In H. J. Knopke, R. J. Norrell, & R. W. Rogers (Eds.), *Opening doors: Perspectives on race relations in contemporary America* (pp. 119–148). Tuscaloosa, AL: University of Alabama Press.

Dovidio, J. F., Gaertner, S. L., Kawakami, K., & Hodson, G. (2002). Why can't we just get along? Interpersonal biases and interracial distrust. *Cultural Diversity & Ethnic Minority Psychology, 8*, 88–102.

Feagin, J. R. (2009). *The White racial frame: Centuries of racial framing and counter-framing.* New York, NY: Routledge.

Felitti, V. J., Anda, R. F., Nordenberg, D., Williams, D. F., Spitz, A. M., Edwards, V., et al. (1998). Relationship of childhood abuse and household dysfunction to many of the leading causes of death in adults: The Adverse Childhood Experiences (ACE) Study. *American Journal of Preventive Medicine, 14*(4), 245–258.

Ferguson, S., & Morley, P. (2011). Improving engagement in the role of father for homeless, noncustodial fathers: A Program evaluation. *Journal of Poverty, 15*, 206–225.

Foner, E. (2007). *Nothing but freedom: Emancipation and its legacy.* Baton Rouge, LA: Louisiana State University Press.

Franklin, J. H. (1963). *The emancipation proclamation.* New York: Doubleday.

Franklin, A. J. (1993). The invisibility syndrome. *Networker, 17*(4), 33–39.

Friedman, D. H., Meschede, T., & Hayes, M. (2003). Surviving against the odds: Families' journeys off welfare and out of homelessness. *Cityscape: A Journal of Policy Development and Research, 6*(2), 187–206.

Gaertner, S. L., & Dovidio, J. F. (1986). The aversive form of racism. In J. F. Dovidio & S. L. Gaertner (Eds.), *Prejudice, discrimination and racism: Theory and research* (pp. 61–89). Orlando, FL: Academic.

Gaertner, S. L., & Dovidio, J. F. (2000). *Reducing intergroup bias: The common ingroup identity model.* Philadelphia, PA: Psychology.

Garbarino, J. (2001). An ecological perspective on the effects of violence on children. *Journal of Community Psychology, 29*, 345–361.

Garrett-Akinsanya, B. M. (2003). Stress management for women. In L. Slater, J. Henderson Daniel, & A. Banks (Eds.), *The complete guide to mental health in women.* Boston, MA: Allyn & Bacon.

Garrett-Akinsanya, B. (2004). The sociocultural abuse of power: A model for shared power. In C. Jean Lau (Ed.), *The psychology of prejudice and discrimination: Disability, religion, physique, and other traits. The psychology of prejudice and discrimination (Race and Ethnicity in Psychology)* (Vol. 4). Westport, CT: Preager.

Garrett-Akinsanya, B. M. (2013). *Beyond Trayvon: Exposure to violence and critical treatment issues among African-American youth.* Workshop presented at American Psychological Association, National Multicultural Conference and Summit, Houston, TX

Gewirtz, A. H., & Taylor, T. (2009). Participation of homeless and abused women in a parent training program: Science and practice converge in a battered women's shelter. In F. Columbus (Ed.), *Community participation and empowerment*. Hauppage, NY: Nova.

Gilligan, C. (1982). *In a different voice: Psychological theory and women's development.* Cambridge, MA: Harvard University Press.

Gollnick, D. M., & Chinn, P. C. (1990). *Multicultural education in a pluralistic society*. Columbus, OH: Merrill.

Gone, J. (2009). A community-based treatment for Native American historical trauma: Prospects for evidence-based practice. *Journal of Consulting and Clinical Psychology, 77*, 751–762.

Gordon, M. M. (1961). Assimilation in America: Theory and reality. *Journal of the American Academy of Arts and Sciences., 90*, 263–285.

Graham-Bermann, S. A., Coupet, S., Egler, L., Mattis, J., & Banyard, V. (1996). Interpersonal relationships and adjustment of children in homeless and economically distressed families. *Journal of Clinical Child Psychology, 25*, 250–261.

Greene, J. M., Ennett, S. T., & Ringwalt, C. L. (1997). Substance use among runaway and homeless youth in three national samples. *American Journal of Public Health, 87*, 229–235.

Guarino, K., Soares, P., Konnath, K., Clervil, R., & Bassuk, E. (2009). *Trauma-informed organizational toolkit.* Rockville, MD: Center for Mental Health Services, Substance Abuse and Mental Health Services Administration, and the Daniels Fund, the National Child Traumatic Stress Network, and the W.K. Kellogg Foundation. Retrieved May 7, 2013, from http://www.homeless.samhsa.gov

Gushue, G. V., & Constatine, M. (2003). Examining individualism, collectivism, and self-differentiation in African American college women. *Journal of Mental Health Counseling, 25*(1), 185.

Hall, E. T. (1983). *The dance of life: The other dimension of time.* Garden City, NY, USA: Anchor/Doubleday.

Hall, R. L., Garrett-Akinsanya, B., & Hucles, M. (2008). Voices of Black feminist leaders: Making spaces for ourselves. In J. L. Chin, B. J. K. Lott, J. K. Rice, & J. Sanchez-Hucles (Eds.), *Women and leadership: Transforming visions and diverse voices* (pp. 281–296). Oxford, UK: Blackwell.

Hanson, M. J. (1992). Ethnic, cultural, and language diversity in intervention settings. In E. W. Lynch & M. J. Hanson (Eds.), *Developing cross-cultural competence: A guide for working with young children and their families*. Baltimore, MD: Brookes.

Harkness, S., & Super, C. (1995). Culture and parenting. In M. H. Bornstein (Ed.), *Handbook of parenting* (Biology and ecology of parenting, Vol. 2, pp. 211–234). Hillsdale, NJ: Erlbaum.

Harkness, S., & Super, C. M. (1996). Introduction. In S. Harkness & C. M. Super (Eds.), *Parents' cultural belief systems, their origins, expressions, and consequences* (pp. 1–26). New York: The Guilford.

Helman, C. G. (1987). Heart disease and the cultural construction of time: The type A behaviour pattern as a Western culture-bound syndrome. *Social Science & Medicine, 25*, 969–979.

Helman, C. G. (2001). *Culture, health and illness* (4th ed.). London, UK: Arnold.

Helms, J. E. (1990). Toward a model of white racial identity development. In *Black and white racial identity: Theory, research and practice* (pp. 49–66). New York: Greenwood.

Helms, J. E. (1992). *A race is a nice thing to have: A guide to being a white person or understanding the white persons in your life.* Topeka, KS: Content Communications.

Henry J, Kaiser Family Foundation. (2011). State health facts: Poverty rate by race/ethnicity. Retrieved November 13, 2012, from http://kff.org/other/state-indicator/poverty-rate-by-raceethnicity

Insight Center for Community Economic Development in California. (2011). *Measuring up: Aspirations for economic security in the 21st century*. Retrieved April 18, 2013, from http://www.insightcced.org/

James, S. A. (1994). John Henryism and the Health of African-Americans. *Culture, Medicine and Psychiatry, 18*, 163–182.

Jenkins, O. B. (2009). Time – A cultural concept. Retrieved January 12, 2013, from http://orville-jenkins.com/whatisculture/timecul.html

Kalyanpur, M., & Rao, S. S. (1991). Empowering low-income black families of handicapped children. *American Journal of Orthopsychiatry, 61*, 525–532.

Kambon, K. K. K. (1992). *The African personality in America: An African-centered framework*. Tallahassee, FL: Nubian Nation.

Kipke, M. D., Montgomery, S., & Mackenzie, R. G. (1993). Substance use among youth seen at a community-based health clinic. *Journal of Adolescent Health, 14*, 289–294.

Koegel, P., Melamid, E., & Burnam, M. A. (1995). Childhood risk factors for homelessness among homeless adults. *American Journal of Public Health, 85*, 1642–1649.

Kurtz, P. D., Jarvis, S. V., & Kurtz, G. L. (1991). Problems of homeless youths: Empirical findings and human services issues. *Social Work, 36*, 309–314.

Lee, J., & Lee, L. (2002). *Crossing the divide: Asian American families and the child welfare system, Report for the Coalition for Asian American Children and Families, New York*. Retrieved May 5, 2013, from http://www.cacf.org/documents/Crossing_the_Divide.pdf

Lekan, D. (2009). Soujourner syndrome and health disparities in African American women. *ANS. Advances in Nursing Science, 32*, 307–321.

Markus, H. R., & Kitayama, S. (1994). A collective fear of the collective: Implications for selves and theories of selves. *Personality and Social Psychology Bulletin, 20*, 568–579.

McLoyd, V. C. (1990). The impact of economic hardship on Black families and children: Psychological distress, parenting, and socioemotional development. *Child Development, 61*, 311–346.

Metraux, S., & Culhane, D. P. (2006). Recent incarceration history among a sheltered homeless population. *Crime & Delinquency, 52*, 504–517.

Nobles, W. (2006). *Seeking the Sakhu: Foundational writings for an African psychology*. USA: Third World.

Orlandi, M. A. (1991). Defining cultural competence: An organizing framework. In M. A. Orlandi (Ed.), *Cultural competence for evaluators*. Rockville, MD: U.S. Department of Health and Human Services, Office for Substance Abuse Prevention.

Pearson, A. R., Dovidio, J. F., & Gaertner, A. L. (2009). The nature of contemporary prejudice: Insights from aversive racism. *Social and Personality Psychology Compass, 3*, 1–25.

Pense, E., & Paymar, M. (1993). Education groups for men who batter: The Duluth Model. New York: Springer Publications.

Philips, S. (1972). Participant structures and communicative competence: Warm Springs children in community and classroom. In C. Cazden, D. Hymes, & V. John (Eds.), *Functions of language in the classroom*. New York: Teachers College Press.

Powers, J., Eckenrode, J., & Jaklitsch, B. (1990). Maltreatment among runaway and homeless youth. *Child Abuse & Neglect, 14*, 87–98.

Puterbaugh, F. G. (2009). *The impact of the Adolescent Transition Program's parent management curriculum on risk factors for delinquency and perceived parenting efficacy*. Unpublished Doctoral Dissertation, Alliant International University

Rotheram-Borus, M. J. (1991). Serving runaway and homeless youths. *Family and Community Health, 14*, 23–32.

SAMSHA. (2011). *Current statistics on the prevalence and characteristics of people experiencing homelessness in the United States*. Retrieved August 18, 2012, from http://www.homeless.samhsa.gov/ResourceFiles/hrc_factsheet.pdf

Sattler, J. M. (1995). *Assessment of children (3rd ed. Revised)*. San Diego: Sattler.

Saville-Troike, M. (1985). The place of silence in an integrated theory of communication. In D. Tannem & M. Saville-Troike (Eds.), *Perspectives on silence* (pp. 3–18). Norwood, NJ: Ablex.

Silber, S. (1989). Family influences on early development. *Topics in Early Childhood Special Education., 8*(4), 1–23.

Steele, C. M. (1997). A threat in the air: How stereotypes shape intellectual identity and performance. *American Psychologist, 52,* 613–619.

Steffen, P. R., McNeilly, M., Anderson, N., & Sherwood, A. (2003). Effects of perceived racism and anger inhibition on ambulatory blood pressure in African Americans. *Psychosomatic Medicine: The Journal of Bio-behavioral Medicine., 65,* 746–750.

Sue, D. W., Capodilupo, C. M., Torino, G. C., Bucceri, J. M., Holder, A. M. B., Nadal, K. L., et al. (2007). Racial microaggressions in everyday life: Implications for clinical practice. *American Psychologist, 62*(4), 271–286.

Sue, D. W., & Sue, D. (2003). *Counseling the culturally diverse: Theory and practice* (4th ed.). New York: Wiley.

Sue, D. W., & Torino, G. C. (2005). Racial-cultural competence: Awareness, knowledge, and skills. In R. T. Carter (Ed.), *Handbook of racial-cultural psychology and counseling: Training and practice* (Vol. 2, pp. 3–18). Hoboken, NJ: Wiley.

Tafoya, T. (1982). Coyotes eyes: Native cognition styles. *Journal of American Indian Education, 21*(2), 21–33.

Tervalon, M., & Murray-Garcia, J. (1998). Cultural humility versus cultural competence: a critical discussion in defining physician training outcomes in multicultural education. *Journal of Health Care for the Poor and Underserved, 9*(2), 117–125.

Triandis, H. C. (1989). The self and social behavior in differing cultural contexts. *Psychological Review, 96,* 506–520.

Triandis, H. C., Brislin, R., & Hui, C. H. (1988). Cross-cultural training across the individualism-collectivism divide. *International Journal of Intercultural Relations, 12,* 269–289.

U.S. Department of Health and Human Services. (2001). *Mental health: Culture, race and ethnicity- A supplement to the mental health: A report of the Surgeon General.* Rockville, MD: U.S. Department of Health and Human Services, Public Health Service, Office of the Surgeon General.

U.S. Department of Housing and Urban Development. (2011). *2010 Annual homeless assessment report to Congress.* Retrieved on May 5, 2013, from https://www.onecpd.info/resources/documents/2010HomelessAssessmentReport.pdf

Utsey, S. O., Adams, E. P., & Bolden, M. (2000). Development and initial validation of the Africultural coping systems inventory. *Journal of Black Psychology, 26,* 194–215.

Walker, L. E. A. (1994). *Abused women and survivor therapy: A practical guide for the psychotherapist.* Washington, DC: APA Press.

Part III
Evidence Based and Promising Approaches to Service Provision and Intervention

Chapter 9
Research on Programs Designed to Support Positive Parenting

Abigail Gewirtz, Kimberly Burkhart, Jessica Loehman, and Beth Haukebo

Abstract Supporting parenting in homeless families is particularly important because the nature of homelessness itself may directly affect a parent's capacity to be an effective parent. Shelters and supportive housing sites offer an important portal for service delivery because they often are grassroots agencies, embedded in communities, with strong local ties. In this chapter, a brief overview of evidence-based parenting programs to promote children's healthy adjustment under conditions of adversity is presented. Following that, the very limited research that has been published to date on empirically supported parenting programs delivered and/or tested in shelters or supportive housing settings for families experiencing homelessness is reviewed. The barriers to implementing effective parenting programs in shelters and housing are discussed, followed by recommendations for strategies to address those barriers.

Introduction

Homelessness and associated stressors (e.g., residential instability, hunger, and exposure to violence) present significant threats to children's psychosocial development (Lee et al., 2010; Masten, Miliotis, Graham-Bermann, Ramirez, & Neemann, 1993;

A. Gewirtz, Ph.D., L.P. (✉)
Department of Family Social Science and Institute of Child Development,
University of Minnesota, St. Paul, MN, USA
e-mail: agewirtz@umn.edu

K. Burkhart, Ph.D.
Nationwide Children's Hospital, Columbus, OH, USA

J. Loehman, M.S.
Department of Psychology, North Carolina State University, Raleigh, NC, USA

B. Haukebo, B.S.
Family Supportive Housing Center/Hart-Shegos and Associates, St. Paul, MN, USA

M.E. Haskett et al. (eds.), *Supporting Families Experiencing Homelessness:*
Current Practices and Future Directions, DOI 10.1007/978-1-4614-8718-0_9,
© Springer Science+Business Media New York 2014

Vostanis, Grattan, & Cumella, 1998). Parenting is a crucial mediator of children's psychosocial adjustment. Although relatively few studies have examined parenting in the context of homelessness (e.g., Gewirtz, DeGarmo, Plowman, August, & Realmuto, 2009), multiple studies have demonstrated how stressful family contexts impair parenting and consequently child adjustment. Particularly relevant to the context of homelessness is research on economic hardship and family transitions. These studies demonstrated that disrupted family processes mediated the relationship between family stressors and children's adjustment. For example, Elder and colleagues (e.g. Conger et al., 2002; Elder, Caspi, & Downey, 1986) demonstrated how economic stress functioned to amplify negative family interactions, reducing the quality of parenting and increasing child behavior problems. Among families experiencing homelessness, Bassuk and colleagues (1997) found self-reported parenting practices to be one of several correlates of adjustment among preschoolers. Comparing homeless and low-income housed African–American mothers of young children, Koblinsky, Morgan, and Anderson (1997) reported that homeless mothers were rated as providing a less structured environment, stimulation for learning, and warmth and acceptance, compared to housed mothers. This is not surprising given the literature demonstrating high rates of adverse early experiences among homeless adults. Herman, Susser, Struening, and Link (1997) reported that child abuse and significant separation from primary caregivers is associated with homelessness rates in adulthood that are 26 times the rate in the general population. In addition, significantly more children in foster care have parents who are homeless (Zlotnick, Kronstadt, & Klee, 1998). Homeless adults may therefore lack effective parenting role models. In turn, impaired parenting places children at risk for poor behavioral and emotional outcomes. See Chap. 4 (Perlman et al.), this volume, for a full discussion of parenting in the face of homelessness.

In high-risk environments, effective parenting offers a critical source of protection for children and is a key correlate of resilience (Masten, 2001). Supporting parenting in homeless families is particularly important because the nature of homelessness itself (e.g., lacking a private space in which to parent) may directly affect a parent's capacity to be an effective parent. Shelters and supportive housing sites offer an important portal for service delivery because they often are grassroots agencies, embedded in communities, with strong local ties (Gewirtz & August, 2008). We define shelters as temporary housing for families who are homeless or are fleeing domestic violence. Shelters may house multiple families in a single living space; length of stay varies widely across the United States from several days to 6 months or more.

Supportive housing, formally established with the McKinney Homelessness Act of 1987, combines subsidized housing with support services to families in order to increase the likelihood of housing stability (CSH, 2005). Federal funding through the US Department of Housing and Urban Development (HUD) allocated to permanent supportive housing for families, limits funding to caregivers with disabilities (primarily mental illness, chemical dependence, and HIV/AIDS), or those fleeing domestic violence, who have experienced chronic homelessness. From 2002 to 2007, an estimated 65,000–72,000 units (about half the supply) of supportive housing were created in the United States. About half of the new units added were targeted towards chronically homeless individuals, and one-fifth were for homeless families (US Interagency Council on Homelessness, 2010). A small number of studies focused on families residing in supportive housing have highlighted the significant experiences of child and family risks and adversity, and associated adjustment challenges (Gewirtz, 2007; Gewirtz, Hart-Shegos, & Medhanie, 2008; Lee et al., 2010).

In the next section, we provide a brief overview of evidence-based (also known as empirically supported) parenting programs to promote children's healthy adjustment under conditions of adversity. Following that, we review the very limited research that has been published to date on empirically supported parenting programs that have been delivered and/or tested in shelters or supportive housing settings for families experiencing homelessness. We discuss the barriers to implementing effective parenting programs in shelters, and provide recommendations for strategies to address these barriers.

Empirically Supported Parenting Programs for Families Under Stress: A Brief Overview

In this section we provide a very brief overview of selective- and indicated parenting prevention programs (i.e., those targeting specific families at risk for, or demonstrating, impaired parenting). These programs are relevant for families experiencing homelessness because studies have demonstrated that homeless children have similar levels of risk as housed children who have already been identified with behavior problems (see Chaps. 2 and 3 of this volume). For example, Lee et al. (2010) compared 146 children in housed families participating in a community-based indicated prevention program, with 111 children in homeless families residing in supportive housing. Child emotional and behavioral problems and emotional strengths were similar across both groups. However, compared to housed mothers, mothers in homeless families reported significantly higher levels of mental health problems, less optimal parenting practices, and higher rates of service utilization.

Over 40 years of research has produced a proliferation of parenting programs that have been demonstrated effective at improving parenting practices, reducing maltreatment risk, and demonstrating improvements in a broad range of child outcomes (e.g., Furlong et al., 2012; Lundahl, Risser, & Lovejoy, 2006; Thomas & Zimmer-Gembeck, 2007). In infancy and early childhood, parenting programs generally focus on improving the parent–child relationship (e.g., by targeting caregiver responsiveness, sensitivity, or infant attachment), increasing parental knowledge of children's developmental needs, and supporting parents in managing the behavior of toddlers and preschoolers. As developmental tasks change with the transition to school, parenting programs that focus on middle childhood and beyond generally target behavior management strategies, healthy parent–child communication, and monitoring.

A comprehensive description of effective parenting programs may be found in a variety of federal, state, and local databases. For example, the California Evidence-Based Clearinghouse for Child Welfare (http://www.cebc4cw.org/) lists and rates parenting programs that reduce parents' risk for child maltreatment, and the Substance Abuse and Mental Health Services Administration's National Registry of Evidence-Based Programs and Practices includes effective parenting programs that reduce mental health and substance use problems in children (http://www.nrepp.samhsa.gov/).

Behavioral parent training (BPT) programs form the majority of the model programs listed on federal clearinghouses. Programs including The Incredible Years, Parent Management Training-Oregon Model, and the Triple P program have been widely disseminated nationally and internationally, and have shown improvements in parenting practices and child adjustment in diverse families, including those in socioeconomically fragile families (e.g., Forgatch & Patterson, 2010; Prinz, Sanders, Shapiro, Whitaker, & Lutzker, 2009; Webster-Stratton, Jamila Reid, & Stoolmiller, 2008). BPT programs generally share a common theoretical framework based on a social interactional learning perspective (SIL) (Patterson, 2005), which suggests that children learn antisocial behavior through interactions in the home and later at school. The frequency and intensity of negative, coercive parent–child interactions predicts subsequent disruptive behavior, out of home placement, and police arrests (Dishion & Patterson, 2006; Snyder et al., 2008). Family stressors (including financial stress, divorce, parental bereavement, and parental psychopathology) impair parenting by increasing coercion and subsequently increasing child maladjustment (Calzada, Eyberg, Rich, & Querido, 2004; DeGarmo, Patras, & Eap, 2008; Mistry, Vanderwater, Huston, & McLoyd, 2002). BPT programs reduce coercive parenting by targeting key positive, effective parenting practices. These include teaching through positive reinforcement, effective discipline, communication and problem-solving skills, and monitoring/supervision (e.g., Forgatch & DeGarmo, 1999). BPT programs have demonstrated positive effects on parenting and child behavior in a wide range of populations including families in transition (i.e., divorce and remarriage, Bullard et al., 2010; Forgatch & DeGarmo, 1999; parental bereavement, Sandler et al., 2003; and foster placement, Fisher, Burraston, & Pears, 2005).

While the focus of this chapter is parenting programs, it seems important to note that case management and coordination (sometimes called advocacy) is a key resource used to help homeless families access services (e.g., Anderson, Stuttaford, & Vostanis, 2005). Advocacy or case management is often the central service that is provided in a shelter or supportive housing site. Advocates or case managers might assist families who are homeless to access social service benefits, medical appointments, jobs, education, training services, and school placement (see Chap. 6, Bray & Link, of this volume for a discussion of collaboration across systems that serve homeless families). Case management may also be an integral part of effective parenting programs. For example, the Nurse Family Partnership (Olds, 2002), a parenting program for new mothers, who are pregnant or have children under 2 years of age, includes case management and coordination as an integral element of its program.

Innovative Parenting Programs in Shelters and Supportive Housing: Current State of the Research and Gaps in Knowledge

Empirical research on the impact of parenting programs in shelter settings is at an inchoate stage, and lags far behind the larger literature on parenting interventions. A recent review conducted by the American Psychological Association's Task Force on Promoting Positive Parenting in the Context of Family Homelessness identified only seven published papers on the implementation or outcomes of parenting interventions in shelters (Haskett, Loehman, & Burkhart, in press). The review included *empirical research* in which *qualitative and/or quantitative data* were collected to examine the *process and/or outcome* of parenting programs in shelters (i.e., descriptive papers were not included). Just three of the papers used an empirically supported intervention (Gewirtz & Taylor, 2009; Jouriles et al., 2009; Puterbaugh, 2009); one paper described case management services for homeless families in the UK (Anderson et al., 2005); two papers described newly developed, short-term (three sessions; one weekend) parenting programs (Davey, 2004; Jones, 2003), and one article focused on training shelter staff to implement a parenting program (Kelly, Buehlman, & Caldwell, 2000).

Most of the articles provided some feasibility and acceptability data for the programs studied. Given the early stage of research on parenting programs in supportive housing, it seems important to ascertain whether parenting programs can be delivered in residential locations serving families in transition (i.e., whether participants attend, return for subsequent sessions, and are satisfied with the program; whether staff can be trained to deliver the program and shelters provide the resources necessary to run the program). The studies reviewed suggested that, in general, families in shelters were open to parenting programs and reported enjoying the interventions and gaining information about parenting and family relationships. Retention in parenting programs varied from very poor (Davey, 2004) to excellent (Gewirtz & Taylor, 2009; O'Neil-Pirozzi, 2009). Establishing feasibility and acceptability of parenting programs in shelters is necessary, in part because there is an assumption among some service providers that shelters should simply provide "three hots and a cot"—i.e., that families in crisis may not be able to meaningfully participate in programming when basic needs are in jeopardy (Gewirtz & Taylor, 2009). Of course, feasibility and acceptability, though necessary, are not sufficient elements in establishing whether a parenting program is effective in shelter or housing settings.

Across those studies that analyzed change from pre- to post-test, and that included a control group, findings were mixed and many expected benefits were not found. Lack of a randomized control group prevents concluding whether the few changes that were demonstrated can be attributed to the specific parenting program delivered (compared with changes occurring naturally over time or due to parents simply receiving attention to parenting).

Of the articles reviewed, just one (Jouriles et al., 2009) used a randomized controlled design, the gold standard for establishing program effectiveness. The intervention, Project Support, is a parent training and advocacy program that targets mothers exposed to domestic violence and includes two primary components: (1) teaching child management skills and (2) providing instrumental and emotional support to mothers during their transition from the shelter. Although families were recruited from domestic violence shelters, the intervention was initiated only after families were discharged from the shelter to housing due to limited length of stay (30 days or less) and the need to address urgent issues (i.e., determining living arrangements after families leave the shelter and how families will support themselves).

Women with 4- to 9-year-old children who reported experiencing at least one act of physical intimate partner violence (IPV) from a male partner during the previous 12 months were eligible to participate. Mothers also had to have one child who met criteria for a disruptive behavior disorder who was not in treatment. Families were judged to be ineligible if significant psychiatric or substance use could negatively impact participation. Of the 200 potentially eligible families identified in shelters, 66 were found eligible and consented to participate (families were considered ineligible if, after their stay at the shelter, they could not be located, had moved more than 50 miles away, or the mother's abusive partner lived with the family). Of the 66 families deemed eligible for participation, 32 were randomly assigned to Project Support and 34 were assigned to the comparison condition. All families were provided financial compensation for their participation.

The intervention consisted of an average of 20 home visits over a maximum of 8 months. Skills were taught to mothers through didactic instruction accompanied by written materials, role plays, in vivo practice, corrective feedback, between-session homework assignments, and mastery checklists. Project Support staff attempted to contact families in the comparison condition monthly, either in person or by telephone, to provide support.

Children's conduct problems were measured by parent report on the Child Behavior Checklist and Eyberg Child Behavior Inventory. Harsh parenting was measured by parent reports on the Conflict Tactics Scale-Revised and Parenting Dimensions Inventory. Mothers' expressed negative affect and harsh behavior toward the child was coded from observational data. Observational data consisted of 1-min ratings summed for each day in which the mother was observed (45 min per day) and daily scores were averaged to derive a Mother Expressed Negative Affect and Behavior score. Mothers' psychiatric symptoms and trauma symptoms were measured by self-report on the SCL-90-R and Impact of Events Scale. Measures were administered at baseline, 4, 8, 12, 16, and 20 months. Parental inconsistency was observed during parent–child interaction periods that lasted for 45 min (observations were conducted at baseline, 8, and 16 months).

Growth curve modeling was used to evaluate the effects of treatment on child conduct problems, mothers' parenting, and mothers' psychiatric symptoms. Children in the Project Support condition evidenced a greater reduction in conduct problems in comparison to children in the control condition. Children's conduct problems not only decreased over the course of the intervention period but also continued to decrease throughout the follow-up period. Mothers participating in Project Support also showed greater reductions in inconsistent and harsh parenting over the course of the intervention period and during the follow-up period in comparison to mothers in the control condition. Results also indicated that maternal psychiatric symptoms decreased during the intervention period for participants in the intervention group *and* comparison group.

This is one of the most methodologically sound studies completed on parenting interventions for families experiencing homelessness. Strengths of the study include random assignment to experimental and control groups, use of psychometrically sound tools, observations of parenting, and long-term follow-up assessment. Although the study included a multi-method assessment of child conduct problems, mothers' parenting, and mothers' psychiatric symptoms, it would have been helpful to have an additional respondent (e.g., a teacher) to provide input on child behavior outside the home. Gathering data on changes in child internalizing problems also would have been beneficial. Furthermore, treatment dosage varied widely based on number of sessions delivered. Therefore, future research should consider examining dosage effects.

Availability of a manual enhances the degree to which this intervention could be replicated in shelter settings. However, shelters rarely have the resources to provide such extensive treatment with well-trained and closely supervised therapists. The intervention was delivered after families exited the shelter system and might not be feasible, without modification, in shelter settings. Some families that might have been most challenging to treat were ineligible for the study, so generalizability is somewhat limited.

A very recent study (whose findings went to press after the literature review was completed) examined the effectiveness of a family-based prevention program in 16 shelters and family supportive housing sites in a randomized controlled trial (Gewirtz, DeGarmo, Lee, & August, in preparation). This study evaluated the Early Risers conduct problems prevention program, an empirically supported multicomponent program that included—but was not limited to—a parent training component (Parenting Through Change). Sixteen housing sites (1 shelter, 15 transitional and supportive housing sites) were randomly assigned to participate in the Early Risers program or services-as-usual; all families with 5–12-year-old children within those sites were invited to participate in the study ($N = 136$ families).

The Early Risers/ER intervention targets reduction of conduct problems via a multicomponent approach that builds child and parenting competencies (August, Realmuto, Hektner, & Bloomquist, 2001). The program is of 2 years duration and includes an after school program and summer camp program (using the Promoting Alternative Thinking Skills/PATHS curriculum; Kusche & Greenberg, 1993), as well as a parent training program (Parenting Through Change; Forgatch & DeGarmo, 1999), and a school-based monitoring and mentoring program. Family advocates with prior human service experience received training and regular coaching in the ER program and delivered the intervention. Fidelity was assessed using observations and found to be adequate to high. Multi-method, multi-informant data (including videotaped observations of parenting practices) were gathered from parents, children, and teachers, at baseline, and at the end of each of two subsequent years.

Intent-to-treat longitudinal analyses indicated that parents in the ER condition significantly improved their parenting self-efficacy compared with those in the control condition, and child depression symptoms (parent report) also were significantly improved in the ER condition. Although there were no main effects of the intervention on positive parenting practices, over time, average levels of parenting self-efficacy predicted observed effective parenting practices, and effective parenting practices predicted improvements both in teacher- and parent-reported child behavior problems.

This is the first study to report positive effects on parenting and child outcomes of an empirically supported prevention program conducted within family supportive housing or shelters. However, there are several limitations to this study that also may mitigate its applicability. First, the program was not limited to parenting—program components also included activities targeting children only (i.e., afterschool and summer camp). Thus, improvements in parenting and child outcomes may or may not be directly linked to the parent training component (Parenting Through Change) within ER. Second, the comprehensive nature of this program limits its applicability in housing sites with few resources and staff. The multiple components require resources (e.g., curricula for programming, training, adherence to fidelity requirements) as well as additional staff (one advocate can provide service for up to 20 children).

We know little about the types of programs that are most feasible, efficient, and effective in shelters. Significant barriers to program implementation and data collection in shelter settings have slowed progress in this field. Most of the studies are limited by small sample sizes, lack of experimental control, and failure to use psychometrically sound measures of program impact. Only the two studies described above (Gewirtz et al., in preparation; Jouriles et al., 2009) have followed parents or children to determine whether positive changes are sustained. Most of the interventions are not manualized, so replication would be quite difficult. Further, there is limited theoretical and empirical justification for many program features and components. With few exceptions, fidelity of implementation is not addressed.

Research Recommendations

Larger randomized controlled studies using multi-informant, multi-method measures need to be conducted. Such studies would allow for better understanding of how parenting interventions can help homeless families and would allow investigations of mediators and/or moderators of intervention effects. Given the extent of the challenges for both parents and service providers in shelters and supportive housing, it seems sensible that a research agenda aimed at testing modifications of programs that are known to be effective in other contexts—particularly those contexts serving high-risk families—might be most effective and efficient (e.g., Gewirtz & Taylor, 2009).

Research also is needed to understand further the service needs of sheltered families. Most mental health prevention programs still are provided on a "one size fits all" basis, with few programs tailoring the services to a client's risk status or level of need (see, e.g., Dishion & Kavanagh, 2000). Lee et al.'s (2010) finding that children in shelters and supportive housing showed comparable adjustment to housed children identified with disruptive behavior problems suggests that, overall, sheltered children are at higher risk for mental health difficulties. However, there is clearly diversity in service needs among parents and children residing in shelters, and thus a "menu" of services to support parenting may be useful. See Chap. 10 (Herbers & Cutuli) for a presentation of research on programs to support children experiencing homelessness.

The new field of implementation science may inform the transporting of evidence-based practices into shelter settings (Fixsen, Naoom, Blasé, Friedman, & Wallace, 2005). Implementation research is particularly needed to uncover organizational factors within shelters and housing settings that may impede or facilitate training of practitioners, and sustainability of empirically supported parenting programs, given the unique characteristics of shelters as small, often grassroots organizations, providing services to families in crisis and transition.

Barriers and Strategies for Providing Parenting Programs in Shelters and Supportive Housing

Shelters and transitional and supportive housing sites provide natural opportunities as portals to psychosocial prevention services in general, and parenting programs in particular. Families live on-site, and childcare and case management services often are provided as routine support services. Key staff, typically advocates or case managers, provide many of the services to families and often provide ad hoc parenting services as part of general support.

However, these strengths also represent challenges; many shelters and housing sites are small, with limited financial resources, dependent upon the vagaries of state and local funding. Ironically, shelters often see increasing demand during times of financial hardship or recession—at precisely the time when governments and nonprofits are attempting to contain costs and cut budgets.

Shelter and housing staff providing psychosocial services to families are typically "generalists"—providing services that may include advocacy (legal, housing, benefits, etc.), case management, counseling, and parenting support. Few shelter advocates have advanced education or training, and no professional, state, or national organization licenses or monitors the services provided by shelters or housing sites (unlike for example, daycare centers). Staff members are often highly committed and hardworking but salaries are low, and thus experience and education may be limited. Staff turnover in shelters is typically extremely high—up to 50 % per year (Olivet, Grandin, & Bassuk, 2010), meaning little return on investments in intensive or lengthy staff training.

Despite the challenges, many shelters offer a variety of family-based services including parenting services (Gewirtz & Menakem, 2004). Parenting resources vary widely and may include "home grown" parenting curricula, informal drop-in groups, or simply ad hoc parenting advice. A very small minority of shelters provides evidence-based parenting programs (Gewirtz et al., 2008).

Not surprisingly, given the reasons for needing shelter or housing support, many families who reside in shelters are highly mobile. A recent study of families residing in temporary or permanent supportive housing indicated that families, on average, had moved 1.5 times in the prior 12 months. Most shelters are designed to provide short-term housing for families in crisis; transitional and supportive housing sites offer more stability but, even in permanent supportive housing, families' average length of stay is less than 2 years (U.S. Conference of Mayors, 2008). The high mobility of families provides challenges for both research and practice—parenting programs delivered over weeks or months may not be practical for families in short-term shelters, and following families over even a year or two following their participation in a parenting program may result in extremely high attrition (Gewirtz et al., in preparation). Despite these barriers, the literature reviewed indicates that shelters and housing sites can and do offer effective parenting programs, and moreover, that when families are able to participate in such programs, they enjoy and report benefiting from them.

Program and Policy Recommendations for Implementing Effective Parenting Programs in Shelters and Supportive Housing Sites

Given the small number and methodological limitations of studies conducted to date, there is no *empirical* basis for making recommendations to shelter administrators about programs to consider for their own settings. Reliance on the larger body of literature on effectiveness of parenting programs delivered in non-shelter settings will have to suffice until the base of research on programs in shelter settings builds. The recommendations below are based upon the literature reviewed, as well as the authors' experiences working with shelter and housing settings serving diverse provider and family populations.

1. *Consider carefully the family, staff, and agency attributes of the shelter or housing site before selecting a parenting program or group of programs.* For example, crisis shelters serving families whose average length of stay is just a week or two will require very different kinds of programs than permanent supportive housing sites. Similarly, provider turnover is an important consideration for investment in training in evidence-based parenting programs. In high-turnover sites, short training modules for providers to offer brief psycho-educational programming may be most useful (e.g., Psychological First Aid for families in shelter: http://66.104.246.25/ucla/PFA_Families_homelessness.pdf), combined with individualized, ad hoc parenting advice (e.g., using tip sheets from the Triple P program: http://triplep-america.com/). In low-turnover, longer-term stay housing, multi-week parent training programs (e.g., Parenting Through Change; Forgatch & DeGarmo, 1999) may be implemented successfully. Provision of group parenting programs is optimal in single site, housing; for scattered site transitional or supportive housing, individual programming may be optimal.

2. *Train shelter case managers or advocates to deliver, as well as broker services.* As noted above (Anderson et al., 2005), a family support model—where an individual case manager provides and brokers services for families—is perceived as helpful by families. Training shelter staff to deliver effective parenting programs builds internal shelter capacity to deliver and sustain services and increases self-efficacy

of providers. In addition, service delivery by (familiar) shelter staff may increase the likelihood of participation and engagement by resident families.

3. *Bringing agencies together for training increases cost-efficiencies and peer support.* Although shelters and housing agencies do not typically belong under a single umbrella organization (e.g., professional organization or licensing board), encouraging agencies to collaborate and coordinate joint training can provide much-needed cost-efficiencies. For example, Minnesota's Family Housing Fund convenes a large group of almost 20 shelters, transitional, and supportive housing agencies in a monthly training series focused on psychosocial issues for children and families, including parenting (Gewirtz, 2007). The monthly forum and associated training opportunities offer case managers, advocates, and other shelter staff a chance to convene, share practice experiences, and provide peer support, in addition to receiving training on evidence-based practice and strategies to use with parents and families.

4. *Partner with local mental health professionals or agencies, to colocate parenting programs.* Where resources or related challenges prevent training shelter staff to deliver parenting programs, consider partnerships with local human service agencies to enable parenting programs to be delivered on-site in shelters by trained local professionals. In some cases, mental health providers may be able to bill Medicaid or local government contracts for services provided. For example, San Francisco's Homeless Children's Network provides colocated parenting programs and other child and family mental health services in shelters and housing sites across the city (Gewirtz & Menakem, 2004; http://www.hcnkids.org/our-services.html).

5. *Adapt evidence-based parenting programs to meet contextual needs of shelters without changing core principles or practices.* Where possible, partner with intervention developers or local experts to modify the selected program. Once staff has been trained in the intervention, they may be in the best position to modify the program (rather than addressing modifications prior to being trained in the intervention). For example, after having received training in a parent training intervention (Parenting Through Change), shelter staff suggested ideas for incentive chart rewards that might be good fits for a shelter (free, involving local resources or "goodies" available in the shelter), as well as incentives that would not be relevant or possible (e.g., incentives requiring one's own kitchen or financial cost). Similarly, giving time out in a shelter may require specific modifications (e.g., finding a location that is not too well-trafficked but still can be monitored by a parent).

6. *Collaborate with local university and other researchers and intervention experts to adapt and evaluate parenting programs.* Most shelters and housing sites do not have evaluation resources, but evaluations are often the sine qua non for receipt of grant funding. Similarly, local clinical researchers also may have access to program development expertise (e.g., connections with program developers) that can support local agencies to access county, state, and federal dollars to improve the standard of care for vulnerable children. For example, SAMHSA provides funds (up to $50,000) for meetings that bring together researchers and providers around evidence-based practices.

References

Anderson, L., Stuttaford, M., & Vostanis, P. (2005). A family support service for homeless children and parents: User and staff perspectives. *Child & Family Social Work, 11*, 119–127.

August, G. J., Realmuto, G. M., Hektner, J. M., & Bloomquist, M. L. (2001). An integrated components preventive intervention for aggressive elementary school children: The Early Risers program. *Journal of Consulting and Clinical Psychology, 69*, 614–626.

Bassuk, E. L., Weinreb, L. F., Dawson, R., Perloff, J. N., & Buckner, J. C. (1997). Determinants of behavior in homeless and Low-income housed preschool children. *Pediatrics, 100*, 92–100.

Bullard, L., Wachlarowicz, M., DeLeeuw, J., Snyder, J., Low, S., Forgatch, M., et al. (2010). Effects of the Oregon model of Parent Management Training (PMTO) on marital adjustment in new stepfamilies: A randomized trial. *Journal of Family Psychology, 24*, 485.

Calzada, E. J., Eyberg, S. M., Rich, B., & Querido, J. G. (2004). Parenting disruptive preschoolers: Experiences of mothers and fathers. *Journal of Abnormal Child Psychology, 32*, 203–213.

Conger, R. D., Wallace, L. E., Sun, Y., Simons, R. L., McLoyd, V. C., & Brody, G. H. (2002). Economic pressure in African American families: a replication and extension of the family stress model. *Developmental Psychology, 38*, 179–193.

CSH. (2005). Corporation for supportive housing. Retrieved December 15, 2005.

Davey, T. L. (2004). A multiple-family group intervention for homeless families: The weekend retreat. *Health & Social Work, 29*, 326–329.

DeGarmo, D. S., Patras, J., & Eap, S. (2008). Social support for divorced fathers' parenting: Testing a stress buffering model. *Family Relations, 57*, 35–48.

Dishion, T. J., & Kavanagh, K. (2000). A multilevel approach to family-centered prevention in schools: Process and outcome. *Addictive Behaviors, 25*, 899–911.

Dishion, T. J., & Patterson, G. R. (2006). The development and ecology of antisocial behavior. In D. Cicchetti & D. Cohen (Eds.), *Developmental psychopathology. Vol. 3: Risk, disorder, and adaptation* (Revised ed., pp. 503–541). New York: Wiley.

Elder, G. H. J., Caspi, A., & Downey, G. (1986). Problem behavior and family relationships: Life course and intergenerational themes. In A. B. Sorensen, F. Weinert, & L. R. Sherrod (Eds.), *Human development and the life course: Multidisciplinary perspectives* (pp. 293–340). New York: Lawrence Earlbaum.

Fisher, P. A., Burraston, B., & Pears, K. (2005). The early intervention foster care program: Permanent placement outcomes from a randomized trial. *Child Maltreatment, 10*, 61–71.

Fixsen, D. L., Naoom, S. F., Blasé, K. A., Friedman, R. M., & Wallace, F. (2005). *Implementation research: A synthesis of the literature*. Tampa: University of South Florida, Louis de la Parte Florida Mental Health Institute, the National Implementation Research Network.

Forgatch, M. S., & DeGarmo, D. S. (1999). Parenting through change: An effective prevention program for single mothers. *Journal of Consulting and Clinical Psychology, 67*, 711–724.

Forgatch, M. S., & Patterson, G. R. (2010). Parent Management Training – Oregon Model: An intervention for antisocial behavior in children and adolescents. In J. R. Weisz & A. E. Kazdin (Eds.), *Evidence-based psychotherapies for children and adolescents* (2nd ed., pp. 159–178). New York: Guilford.

Furlong, M., McGilloway, S., Bywater, T., Hutchings, J., Smith, S. M., & Donnelly, M. (2012). Behavioural and cognitive-behavioural group-based parenting programmes for early-onset conduct problems in children aged 3–12 years.

Gewirtz, A. H. (2007). Promoting children's mental health in family supportive housing: A community-university partnership for formerly homeless children and families. *Journal of Primary Prevention, 28*, 359–374.

Gewirtz, A. H., & August, G. J. (2008). Incorporating multifaceted mental health prevention services in community sectors-of-care. *Clinical Child and Family Psychology Review, 11*, 1–11.

Gewirtz, A. H., DeGarmo, D., Lee, S., & August, G. J. (in preparation). *Twenty-four month outcomes from the Early Risers Supportive Housing prevention trial.*

Gewirtz, A. H., DeGarmo, D. S., Plowman, E., August, G. J., & Realmuto, G. (2009). Parenting, parental mental health, and child functioning in families residing in supportive housing. *American Journal of Orthopsychiatry, 79*, 336–347.

Gewirtz, A. H., Hart-Shegos, E., & Medhanie, A. (2008). Psychosocial status of children and youth in supportive housing. *American Behavior Scientist, 51*, 810–823.

Gewirtz, A. H., & Menakem, R. (2004). Working with young children and their families: Recommendations for domestic violence agencies and batterer intervention programs. In S. Schecter (Ed.), *Domestic violence, poverty and young Children*. David and Lucile Packard Foundation. (Reprinted from: http://www.uiowa.edu/~socialwk/publications.html).

Gewirtz, A., & Taylor, T. (2009). Participation of homeless and abused women in a parent training program: Science and practice converge in a battered women's shelter. In M. F. Hindsworth & T. B. Lang (Eds.), *Community participation and empowerment* (pp 97–114). Hauppage, NY: Nova Science Publishers.

Haskett, M. E., Loehman, J., & Burkhart, K. (in press). Parenting interventions in shelter settings: A qualitative systematic review of the literature. *Child and Family Social Work*.

Herman, D. B., Susser, E. S., Struening, E. L., & Link, B. L. (1997). Adverse childhood experiences; Are they risk factors for adult homelessness. *American Journal of Public Health, 87*, 249–255.

Homelessness, U. S. I. C. o. (2010). *Supplemental document to the federal strategic plan to prevent and end homelessness*. Retrieved from http://www.usich.gov/resources/uploads/asset_library/BkgrdPap_ChronicHomelessness.pdf

Jones, S. L. (2003). *Homeless families: A crisis management program for parents*. Dissertation: James Madison University.

Jouriles, E. N., McDonald, R., Rosenfield, D., Stephens, N., Corbitt-Shindler, D., & Miller, P. C. (2009). Reducing conduct problems among children exposed to intimate partner violence: a randomized clinical trial examining effects of project support. *Journal of Consulting and Clinical Psychology, 77*, 705–717.

Kelly, J. F., Buehlman, K., & Caldwell, K. (2000). Training personnel to promote quality parent–child interaction in families who are homeless. *Topics in Early Childhood Special Education, 20*, 174–185.

Koblinsky, S. A., Morgan, K. M., & Anderson, E. A. (1997). African-American homeless and low-income housed mothers: Comparison of parenting practices. *American Journal of Orthopsychiatry, 67*, 37–47.

Kusche, C. A., & Greenberg, M. T. (1993). *The PATHS (Promoting alternative thinking strategies) Curriculum*. Deerfield, MA: Channing-Bete Company.

Lee, S., August, G. J., Gewirtz, A. H., Klimes-Dougan, B., Bloomquist, M. L., & Realmuto, G. M. (2010). Identifying unmet mental health needs in children of formerly homeless mothers living in a supportive housing community sector of care. *Journal of Abnormal Child Psychology, 38*, 421–432.

Lundahl, B., Risser, H. J., & Lovejoy, M. C. (2006). A meta-analysis of parent training: Moderators and follow-up effects. *Clinical Psychology Review, 26*, 86–104.

Masten, A. S. (2001). Ordinary magic: Resilience processes in development. *American Psychologist, 56*, 227–238.

Masten, A. S., Miliotis, D., Graham-Bermann, S. A., Ramirez, M., & Neemann, J. (1993). Children in homeless families: Risks to mental health and development. *Journal of Consulting and Clinical Psychology, 61*, 335–343.

Mayors, U. S. C. o. (2008) Status report on hunger & homelessness.

Mistry, R. S., Vanderwater, E. A., Huston, A. C., & McLoyd, V. C. (2002). Economic well-being and children's social adjustment: The role of family process in an ethnically diverse low-income sample. *Child Development, 73*, 935–951.

Network, H. C. s. Retrieved from http://www.hcnkids.org/our-services.html

O'Neil-Pirozzi, T. M. (2009). Feasibility of and benefit of parent participation in a program emphasizing preschool child language development while homeless. *American Journal of Speech-Language Pathology, 18*, 252–263.

Olds, D. L. (2002). Prenatal and infancy home visiting by nurses: From randomized trials to community replication. *Prevention Science, 3*, 153–172.

Olivet, J., Grandin, M., & Bassuk, E. (2010). Staffing challenges and strategies for organizations serving individuals who have experienced chronic homelessness. *The Journal of Behavioral Health Services & Research, 37*, 226–238.

Patterson, G. R. (2005). The next generation of PMTO models. *Behavior Therapist, 28*, 25–32.

Prinz, R. J., Sanders, M. R., Shapiro, C. J., Whitaker, D. J., & Lutzker, J. R. (2009). Population-based prevention of child maltreatment: The US Triple P system population trial. *Prevention Science, 10*, 1–12.

Puterbaugh, F. G. (2009). *The impact of the Adolescent Transition Program's parent management curriculum on risk factors for delinquency and perceived parenting efficacy.* Doctoral Dissertation.

Sandler, I. N. (2003). The family bereavement program: Efficacy evaluation of a theory-based prevention program for parentally bereaved children and adolescents. *Journal of Consulting and Clinical Psychology, 71*, 587–593.

Snyder, J., Schrepferman, L., McEachern, A., Barner, S., Johnson, K., & Provines, J. (2008). Peer deviancy training and peer coercion: dual processes associated with early-onset conduct problems. *Child Development, 79*, 252–268. doi:10.1111/j.1467-8624.2007.01124.x.

Thomas, R., & Zimmer-Gembeck, M. J. (2007). Behavioral outcomes of parent–child interaction therapy and triple P—positive parenting program: A review and meta-analysis. *Journal of Abnormal Child Psychology, 35*, 475–495.

Vostanis, P., Grattan, E., & Cumella, S. (1998). Mental health problems of homeless children and families: Longitudinal study. *British Medical Journal, 316*, 899–902.

Webster-Stratton, C., Jamila Reid, M., & Stoolmiller, M. (2008). Preventing conduct problems and improving school readiness: Evaluation of the Incredible Years teacher and child training programs in high-risk schools. *Journal of Child Psychology and Psychiatry, 49*, 471–488.

Zlotnick, C., Kronstadt, D., & Klee, L. (1998). Foster care children and family homelessness. *American Journal of Public Health, 88*, 1368–1370.

Chapter 10
Programs for Homeless Children and Youth: A Critical Review of Evidence

Janette E. Herbers and J.J. Cutuli

Abstract To date, there are few studies that use rigorous research designs to evaluate interventions to address the needs of homeless children. Strengths and noteworthy findings as well as the challenges and limitations of this literature are summarized. The studies reviewed in this chapter represent laudable efforts on the part of researchers, practitioners, and community partners to engage in intervention studies with the challenging and understudied population of children in families experiencing homelessness. However, within the guidelines of the What Works Clearinghouse (WWC) standards for evidence-based practices, none of the interventions represented in these studies have sufficient evidence to be rated as having Positive Effects. Most often, this is due to lack of quality evidence that evaluates the program outcomes. Policymakers, funding agencies, researchers, clinicians, and community practitioners can expand the evidence base for interventions with homeless children through understanding what constitutes quality evaluations and supporting high-quality research. This chapter concludes with recommendations for building a robust and rigorous evidence base of what works to allow stakeholders to improve the well-being of at-risk children, bettering their lives through increasingly effective and efficient programs.

The needs of children experiencing homelessness and recommendations for intervening with these children and families have been well documented (Bassuk, 2010; Hwang, Tolomiczenko, Kouyoumdjian, & Garner, 2005; Rog & Buckner, 2007; Samuels, Shinn, & Buckner, 2010). However, there are surprisingly few studies or reports that document rigorous evaluations of such intervention programs.

J.E. Herbers, Ph.D. (✉)
Department of Psychology, Villanova Univeristy, 800 Lancaster Ave, Villanova, PA 19085, USA
e-mail: janette.herber@villanova.edu

J.J. Cutuli, Ph.D.
Rutgers University, Camden, NJ, USA

M.E. Haskett et al. (eds.), *Supporting Families Experiencing Homelessness:*
Current Practices and Future Directions, DOI 10.1007/978-1-4614-8718-0_10,
© Springer Science+Business Media New York 2014

Among the studies that do exist, there is great variety in the needs targeted by interventions, the services, and methods by which interventions are delivered, the subpopulations of homeless families included, and the methodological and psychometric rigor of the studies. As a result, the research evidence to support intervention effectiveness is difficult to interpret. In this chapter, we review the literature on interventions designed to address the well-being of children experiencing family homelessness, highlighting strengths and weaknesses of the existing evidence for what works. Before reviewing specific studies, we discuss the importance of evidence-based practices in general, noting several standards that exist for establishing well-supported and promising programs and interventions based on evidence. We then use these standards as a context for evaluating the work that has been done, and still needs to be done, to establish a more robust evidence base for various interventions with homeless children.

Children who experience family homelessness have varied needs and experience a number of different risks to healthy development spanning all domains of functioning. See Chaps. 2 (Volk) and 3 (Cowan) for discussions of characteristics of homeless children and youth. Opportunities to intervene are similarly complex and varied. The National Center on Family Homelessness has identified five broad categories of needs that should be addressed in interventions for children from homeless families: housing, maternal well-being, child well-being, family functioning, and family preservation (DeCandia, 2012). These categories emphasize the child's context, acknowledging that as children develop, they are sensitive to their environments at the levels of family, neighborhood, and broader culture and society. Efforts to support the healthy development of children who experience homelessness should attend to the ecology of their experiences and the diverse causes, correlates, and consequences of homelessness (Kilmer, Cook, Crusto, Strater, & Haber, 2012). Because the primary drivers of homelessness are extreme poverty and lack of affordable housing, attending to immediate housing and financial needs would likely prevent children from experiencing additional risks and potentially traumatic events related to living with residential instability (Bassuk, 2010; Burt, Pearson, & Montgomery, 2005; Haber & Toro, 2004). Since most homeless families are headed by young, single mothers who have experienced significant trauma in their own lives, addressing maternal well-being and family functioning can improve child well-being indirectly by fostering more nurturing parent–child relationships and reducing the likelihood of additional trauma within the family (Bassuk, 2010; Kilmer et al., 2012; Paquette & Bassuk, 2009). Finally, child well-being can be addressed directly starting with assessment for early identification of developmental or other health problems, and access to programs or services that can address these needs (DeCandia, 2012).

Evidence-Based Practices

Research evidence is necessary for demonstrating whether different intervention efforts are effective. Across diverse fields including medicine, psychology, education, and public policy, there are increasing demands for prevention and intervention programs that are supported by sound empirical evidence (Levant & Hasan, 2008). The National Institute of Medicine has defined Evidence-Based Practice (EBP) in health care as "the integration of best research evidence with clinical expertise and patient values." Similarly, the American Psychological Association (APA) adopted as policy the definition of Evidence-Based Practices in Psychology (EBPP) as "the integration of the best available research with clinical expertise in the context of patient characteristics, culture, and preferences" (American Psychological Association, 2005). Meanwhile the federal Office of Management and Budget (OMB) has called for expanded capacity and use of rigorous evaluation and evidence in governmental grant-making and other decision-making (Zients, 2012).

Different groups and agencies continue to develop and refine various tiered frameworks to determine the quality of program evaluation studies. For example, at the federal level the Department of Education (Institute of Education Sciences, 2013; What Works Clearinghouse, 2011) and the Substance Abuse and Mental Health Services Administration (SAMHSA) (Substance Abuse and Mental Health Services Administration, 2013) each have explicit review criteria to determine the quality of evidence, while the Top Tier Evidence Initiative of the Coalition for Evidence-Based Policy has established a checklist for reviewing randomized controlled trials (RCT) for social service program evaluation (Coalition for Evidence-Based Policy, 2010) and the APA utilizes a set of criteria to characterize the research support for individual psychological treatments or interventions (American Psychological Association, 2005; Chambless et al., 1998), to name just a few. It is beyond the scope of this chapter to provide a detailed analysis of all such efforts individually. Nevertheless, most frameworks share a number of common elements. Most of these criteria share some recognition that evidence should be considered within the context of the needs and situations of the target populations, and, therefore, should help guide (and not replace) good judgment by clinicians, providers, executive leaders, and other decision-makers. In addition, most emphasize the importance of robust methodology (e.g., by explicitly requiring or favoring certain study designs like RCT), representative samples or population-based approaches with sufficient numbers of participants to detect effects of the expected size, appropriate and rigorous analytical methods, replication (sometimes by independent groups), meaningful effect sizes that are significant with respect to real-world differences (and not just statistically significant), and comprehensive review (e.g., in a peer refereed journal and/or by a specific, independent review process with explicit evaluation criteria).

Applying any of these criteria to the research on prevention and intervention programs for homeless children requires careful consideration of the quality and quantity of existing empirical evidence. For the purposes of this chapter, we use standards from the What Works Clearinghouse (WWC) of the Department of Education's Institute of Educational Sciences (Institute of Education Sciences, 2013; What Works Clearinghouse, 2011). These criteria are sufficiently defined to provide a framework that can be used to evaluate intervention programs across a range of social science disciplines, and they provide guidelines for rating individual studies as well as for rating interventions. According to WWC evidence standards, a study "meets evidence standards" only when it employs an RCT with low attrition rates, the study includes valid and reliable outcomes measures, and measures of effect can be attributed solely to the intervention. A study could "meet evidence standards with reservations" in two different situations; either the study is an RCT with high attrition or a quasi-experimental design (QED), but in either case the groups must be equivalent in relevant characteristics and the study includes valid and reliable outcomes measures with effects attributed solely to the intervention. When any of these criteria are not met, or when a study uses a design other than RCT or QED, the study "does not meet evidence standards" according to the WWC guidelines.

To determine the rating of an intervention, the WWC also provides guidelines for combining findings from multiple studies meeting evidence standards (with or without reservations), which may have conflicting results. The intervention rating scheme is used to categorize interventions as having Positive Effects, Potentially Positive Effects, Mixed Effects, No Discernible Effects, Potentially Negative Effects, or Negative Effects. To be rated as having Positive Effects, an intervention must be supported by two or more studies, one of which must be an RCT, showing statistically significant effects in favor of the intervention and no studies showing statistically significant or substantial negative effects. To be rated as having Potentially Positive Effects, an intervention must be supported by at least one study showing a statistically significant or substantial effect in favor of the intervention, no studies showing significant negative effects, and fewer or the same number of studies showing indeterminate effects as those showing positive effects. An intervention could be rated as having Mixed Effects when either the number of studies with positive and negative effects is equal, or when there are more studies showing indeterminate effects than studies showing significant effects, either positive or negative. An intervention will be rated as having No Discernible Effects when none of the studies show statistically significant positive or negative effects. Finally, an intervention is rated as having Negative Effects or Potentially Negative Effects when a study or studies show statistically significant effects opposed to the intervention, depending upon the strength of evidence.

Like other EBP rating systems for evaluating evidence, the WWC guidelines aim to uphold scientific rigor and reduce potential sources of bias. First and foremost, the WWC standards rely primarily on evidence from RCTs or QEDs. In an RCT, participants (or groups like schools or shelters) are randomly assigned to the intervention condition or one or more alternative conditions. All participants complete the same assessment procedures prior to, during, and following the conditions, and results of the assessments are compared to determine whether the target intervention has effects on relevant outcomes. The alternative conditions can involve assessment with no intervention, a placebo condition, a different intervention, or a wait-list for later participation in the focus intervention. Random assignment dramatically reduces the likelihood that participants in different conditions will differ from each other in ways that could impact the results of the study. For example, if participants are allowed to choose either the target intervention or assessment without intervention, those who choose the intervention might be more open to change and more likely to benefit from any services provided. This characteristic of the participants in the intervention group would then inflate the observed effect of intervention, and the program might be presumed more beneficial than it truly is for the broader population. Alternatively, if participants were placed in different conditions based on their location (e.g., different homeless shelter sites), and there were characteristics of the nonintervention site only that otherwise improved client outcomes, results of the research might underestimate the true impact of a beneficial intervention. In many cases, RCTs are not feasible due to considerations of costs, resources, ethics, or political concerns (Baggerly, 2004; Seibel, Bassuk, & Medeiros, 2012). Costs can prevent the number of participants that can be included, reducing sample sizes and limiting options for comparison groups. More importantly, ethical and political considerations challenge the appropriateness of randomly assigning individuals at risk to conditions of no-treatment, or to conditions which local stakeholders view as suboptimal (whether or not such a view is supported by an evidence base). When randomization is not possible, QEDs can provide valuable evidence under certain conditions. QEDs involve comparison among groups that have not been randomly assigned, such as by participant choice or by shelter site. According to the WWC, QEDs can "meet evidence standards with reservations" when equivalence between groups is established with any necessary statistical adjustments applied (What Works Clearinghouse, 2011), like statistically controlling for established or suspected differences in individual variables or through more complex methodologies like propensity score matching (Heckman, Ichimura, Smith, & Todd, 1998; Heckman, Ichimura, & Todd, 1997; Smith & Todd, 2005).

Clearly WWC standards strongly emphasize RCTs and QEDs to determine whether individual studies meet evidence standards. In addition, the highest rating of "Positive Effects" requires replication of findings. Replication ensures that initial findings are robust and not due to unmeasured factors of a particular sample. Furthermore, when results are replicated by an independent team of researchers, the likelihood that investigator bias impacts the results is reduced (Chambless & Hollon, 1998). Intervention manuals are important not only for enabling replication of intervention research but also for ensuring fidelity in the implementation of interventions that have been supported by research. Practitioners committed to the use of EBPs must have the ability to enact those practices consistent with the specific methods and procedures that the research evidence supports. Finally, inherent in the WWC criteria, the 2005 APA policy statement, and other calls for EBPs described above also are data analysis methodology reflecting best practices for measurement and evaluation (American Psychological Association, 2005; Chambless et al., 1998; Levant & Hasan, 2008; Zients, 2012). These best practices are continually evolving and will vary from field to field as different sorts of data require a host of different considerations. As such, continuing education and ongoing collaborations with experts in data analysis are important in maintaining an up-to-date skill set in this area.

Various organizations including the Department of Education and APA demonstrate a commitment to EBPs by maintaining evolving online lists of EBPs (American Psychological Association, 2005; Coalition for Evidence-Based Policy, 2010; Substance Abuse and Mental Health Services Administration, 2013; What Works Clearinghouse, 2011). While a great deal of evidence exists for a variety of programs that effectively address children's mental health and academic achievement in general (Kazak et al., 2010), very few have been adapted or designed and targeted for use with children experiencing homelessness (Seibel et al., 2012). Next we review the literature on interventions with homeless children in light of the WWC criteria, beginning with the body of descriptive studies then considering studies that use RCTs or QEDs.

Descriptive Projects: Not Meeting Evidence Standards

To date, there are few studies that evaluate interventions for homeless families and even fewer that evaluate child outcomes with rigorous research designs (Bassuk, 2010; Hwang et al., 2005; Samuels et al., 2010). The majority of research on programs is descriptive in nature, without RCTs or QEDs that utilize comparison groups. The interventions represented in the descriptive literature also vary widely in their approaches to improving outcomes for homeless children. Some programs have focused primarily on housing needs of homeless families, while others have targeted maternal well-being, child well-being, family functioning, or a combination of these through case management services or specific therapies and treatments. The existing intervention studies also vary in methods used to assess and describe change that may be associated with their efforts. In this section, we first describe studies on interventions for homeless children without use of RCTs or QEDs. According to the WWC, none of these studies meet evidence standards. We summarize the strengths and noteworthy findings as well as the challenges and limitations of this literature.

Several reports in the literature consider housing programs for families and their effects on residential stability. Interventions specifically designed to address housing needs include subsidized housing, permanent supportive housing, and transitional housing (Samuels et al., 2010). A study in New York City examined differences among 138 families who requested shelter and received housing subsidies compared to 106 who requested shelter and did not receive housing subsidies. Families who requested shelter and received subsidies were over 20 times more likely to achieve stable housing (Shinn et al., 1998) than families who did not receive subsidies. Whether or not families received subsidies was not determined randomly but depended upon the type of shelter, the amount of time the family stayed in shelter, and whether the family circumstances involved domestic violence (Shinn et al., 1998). Because these differences were not accounted for (statistically or otherwise) in the evaluation of housing stability, it is not clear whether stability resulted from the receipt of housing subsidies or because of other factors that distinguish the groups. Another study used administrative data and hazard functions to predict shelter reentry within 2 years among 24,640 families in New York City. Families that left shelter to enter subsidized housing were much less likely to return to shelter (Wong, Culhane, & Kuhn, 1997). Similarly, families were not assigned to different housing conditions, and there were differences among groups in important characteristics that were not accounted for in the models.

While affordable, stable housing is clearly important, families might to benefit more when they are able to connect with additional services (Samuels et al., 2010). In the Homeless Families Program, 1,298 families across nine sites received Section 8 vouchers, some level of case management, and access to services (Rog, McCombs-Thornton, Gilbert-Mongelli, Brito, & Holupka, 1995). Analyses of housing stability at follow-up revealed that families who received more intensive service packages in addition to Section 8 subsidized housing certificates fared better in terms of housing stability than families who received fewer services. However, the families included in the study were not representative of homeless families in general, and there were considerable differences in recruitment strategies, selection criteria, and referral sources across the nine sites such that groups being compared were not equivalent and results cannot be attributed to differences in services (Rog et al., 1995). The Sound Families Project involved funding housing units with services available in three counties in Washington State, with intensive case management including referrals for substance use problems, mental health issues, and education or job training for homeless mothers (Bodonyi, 2008). Data from ten case study sites suggested that most families moved to permanent housing within about a year, that many parents increased their employment and incomes, and that children improved their school attendance and stability (Bodonyi, 2008).

Several other studies have documented intervention efforts towards improvements in housing stability and other outcomes in contexts of supportive or transitional housing programs, with intensive case management and a range of services and opportunities available (Fischer, 2000; Medeiros & Vaulton, 2010; Murrell et al., 2000; Swann-Jackson, Tapper, & Fields, 2010). For example, Keeping Families Together (KFT) was a pilot program that provided permanent supportive housing with intensive services to 29 families in New York City that had been homeless for at least 1 year and had at least one case of child abuse or neglect open with the city's Administration for Children's Services (Swann-Jackson et al., 2010). In addition to supportive housing, families received flexible spending grants for one-time expenses to promote positive family functioning and individual case management services from on-site social workers, including referrals and access to additional services both on-site and through community providers. Twelve adults in the program participated in substance abuse treatment programs and seven received psychiatric treatment for mental illness. Results of the program were evaluated using data on housing stability, welfare involvement, and children's school attendance and academic achievement. Compared to 15 families who were eligible for the program but chose not to participate, the KFT families maintained superior housing stability. Over the course of the 3-year program, over half of the open child welfare cases were closed for the KFT families, and all children who were in foster care with the goal of reunification were reunified with their families. Children involved in KFT significantly improved their school attendance. Parents in KFT also reported that the program helped them to rebuild social supports and enhanced their desire to become better parents (Swann-Jackson et al., 2010).

Other intervention efforts involve more targeted programs to improve maternal well-being. The AfterCare project was designed to provide support, education, and connections to health-care services for mothers currently homeless or at risk based on previous homelessness (Murrell et al., 2000). The 79 mothers who participated were either pregnant or had an infant 6 months or younger. They received case management services and home visits from nurses, and they participated in a women's support group. Survey data indicated high rates of prenatal care and successful births among the mothers (Murrell et al., 2000), but effects were not compared to any comparison group. Another program targeted young, unmarried first-time mothers of infants to provide transitional housing with available day care, transportation, counseling, parent training, educational opportunities, and job-related skills (Fischer, 2000). Qualitative evaluations indicated some improvements in housing, employment, and self-sufficiency, though most of the mothers were still dependent on welfare following participation in the program (Fischer, 2000). Without a comparison group or any rigorous analysis, it is unclear what impact this program may have had.

Efforts to improve maternal well-being, family functioning, and child behavior also take the form of interventions targeting parenting skills. Because parenting interventions are discussed in detail in Chap. 9 of this volume (Gewirtz et al.), we review them here only briefly. Many of these programs are evaluated using a pre–post design that tests for within-individual change before and after the intervention. While pre–post designs provide meaningful evidence, they fall short of the level of rigor that comes with random assignment or QED approaches. One study evaluated the Adolescent Transition and Parent Management Curriculum for mothers of adolescents at risk for behavior problems living in long-term shelter (Puterbaugh, 2009). Results indicated changes from pretest to posttest on two parent-report measures of child behavior (Puterbaugh, 2009). Another study described the implementation of the evidence-based intervention, Parenting Through Change, for ten mothers living with their children in domestic violence shelters, with initial findings indicating good attendance at sessions and mothers reporting that they enjoyed sessions and felt that their parenting skills were improving (Gewirtz & Taylor, 2009). Kelly, Buehlman, and Caldwell (2000) trained parent–child advocates to deliver early intervention services to homeless mothers, with the goal of improving parent–child interactions. Observational ratings of parent–child interactions indicated that parent teaching behaviors increased significantly following intervention. Another study (Davey, 2004) involved the use of a retreat to target role clarification and communication among family members, with results of a brief survey suggesting that families enjoyed the retreat and parents felt it helped families feel more positive about themselves and deal with stress. Using a therapeutic nursery program with services for parents in shelter, Norris-Shortle and colleagues implemented an intervention called Wee Cuddle and Grow, which utilizes video-taped interactions to provide feedback to caregivers (Melley et al., 2010; Norris-Shortle et al., 2006). The program involved individual parent–child therapy, structured activities, and parent support groups in which parents were coached to respond to their children's cues, teach skills, develop family routines, and engage in child-centered play. Results of pre–post analyses suggested that children improved in all domains assessed by the Nursing Child Assessment Satellite Training tool, and amount of participation in interventions was related to improvements (Melley et al., 2010; Norris-Shortle et al., 2006). The project had a large sample of 99 mothers but no comparison group. Finally, a program targeting homeless fathers with children under the age of 5 required fathers to participate in the evidence-based program Parents as Teachers in order to obtain supporting housing (Ferguson & Morley, 2011). Fathers participated in a curriculum about early childhood development and weekly individual sessions and support groups. Unfortunately, evaluation of this program consisted only of qualitative reports from a focus group of four fathers, and there was no information regarding fidelity of implementing the Parents as Teachers program.

Programs also have been designed to target child behavior and well-being directly. An early study described providing day care for 87 preschool children who were staying with their mothers at a "welfare hotel" (Grant, 1991). Based on observations by the childcare providers, it was reported that most children in the intervention were functioning at age level by the end (Grant, 1991). However, it is unclear whether outcomes were based on any sort of psychometrically supported assessment. A more recent intervention engaged children ages 5–11 in child-centered group play therapy with the goal of improving self-esteem and symptoms of anxiety and depression (Baggerly, 2004). Pre–post design results from the 25 children who completed therapy and standardized assessments indicated some improvement in self-concept but mixed results for anxiety and depression (Baggerly, 2004).

Finally, several intervention programs have targeted parent well-being, child well-being, and family functioning with separate components delivered simultaneously. A camp-based program involved 42 mothers and their children in outdoor activities for families. In addition, caregivers participated in discussion groups related to parenting while children engaged in groups for behavior management. Qualitative interviews indicated that parents enjoyed some aspects of the programming, but no psychometrically established assessment was reported (Kissman, 1999). In a different school-based summer program, 20 homeless children and 33 low-income children participated in mental health services and parents received training in behavior management (Nabors et al., 2004; Nabors, Proescher, & DeSilva, 2001). Parents in both homeless and non-homeless, low-income groups reported decreases in total behavior problems, with larger changes among the homeless group. Teacher reports indicated improvement in social skills for both groups as well (Nabors et al., 2001, 2004). In a large, 5-year study called Strengthening At Risk and Homeless Youth, Mothers, and Children, a range of services were provided to mothers aged 18–25 and their children in four different sites across the country to address homelessness, residential instability, and developmental issues of the children (Medeiros & Vaulton, 2010). While some services differed by site, all programs included intensive case management, housing assistance and supports, counseling for parents and children as well as therapy to improve the parent–child relationship, and regular developmental screenings. Overall, results from the four sites indicated that with housing assistance, about 80 % of the mothers were stably housed in their communities, and that the cost of the intervention was less than the cost of emergency housing for the same number of families in the those communities (Medeiros & Vaulton, 2010).

In the process of conducting each of these descriptive studies, the researchers and practitioners gained insight into the challenges associated with intervening with children and families experiencing homelessness. Several reports noted the impact of high attrition rates and time limitations associated with highly mobile families staying in emergency shelter for short periods of time (Davey, 2004; Fischer, 2000). Others noted cost concerns arising from training of staff and best use of resources in a context of high need (Baggerly, 2004; Gewirtz & Taylor, 2009). Emphasis was placed on the importance of collaborations among researchers, practitioners, schools, and community providers in the development and implementation of intervention programs (Gewirtz & Taylor, 2009; Nabors et al., 2004; Swann-Jackson et al., 2010). Several reports also noted that children and families were generally receptive to intervention programs and reported enjoying a variety of intervention activities (Davey, 2004; Fischer, 2000; Gewirtz & Taylor, 2009; Kissman, 1999), which speaks to feasibility of implementation. Several studies made use of measures with good psychometric properties (Baggerly, 2004; Medeiros & Vaulton, 2010; Nabors et al., 2004; Swann-Jackson et al., 2010), and some included manuals or based their interventions on existing EBPs (Ferguson & Morley, 2011; Gewirtz & Taylor, 2009; Nabors et al., 2004). Most of the studies were embedded and delivered in the contexts of the children's daily lives, such as shelters and schools.

While each of the studies described above provides useful information about the feasibility of interventions with homeless families, none have sufficiently rigorous designs to test efficacy or effectiveness. Few of the studies evaluated their programs using psychometrically established, quantitative assessments. Even among the studies that measure outcomes and report positive pre-intervention to post-intervention changes, the effect of these services is unclear because studies did not include comparison groups assigned to different programs. With the exception of the housing outcomes in the KFT intervention, there were no comparison groups that did not receive the intervention being evaluated. Single-group designs that consider only individuals receiving an intervention can provide preliminary insight into the feasibility and likely value of further pursuing the more rigorous evidence that comes with an RCT or QED approach for any particular program, recognizing that these comparison-group designs often carry additional logistic, cost, ethical and political investment and challenges. Nevertheless, rigorous evidence requires RCT or QED methodologies to adequately control for various forms of bias that usually cannot be detected nor accounted for in single-group designs.

RCTs and QEDs: Potentially Meeting Evidence Standards

RCTs or QEDs more rigorously evaluate the potential benefits of their programs. Based on WWC guidelines, these studies have the potential to meet evidence standards with or without reservations depending upon other aspects of the methods and findings. As with the variety of approaches represented in the descriptive studies, the following intervention studies range from specifically targeted to broad-based and address different categories of needs. We review each study in detail, discuss strengths and weaknesses, then summarize the findings overall with respect to WWC guidelines.

Tischler, Vostanis, Bellerby, and Cumella (2002) evaluated an intervention with UK families residing in emergency hostels providing mental health outreach services to families with children ages 3–16 with an identified need. Services included counseling for children and support provided to parents to engage other agencies, such as finding child care and participating in child protection conferences. The intervention group involved 23 families with 27 children who were compared to a group of 31 families with 49 children staying at other hostels that did not provide mental health outreach services. Parents in the intervention group reported a greater reduction in children's symptoms from baseline to a 6-month follow-up on the Strengths and Difficulties Questionnaire for the intervention group, with no significant differences in parents' self-reported symptoms on the General Health Questionnaire (Tischler et al., 2002). However, the authors noted that there was higher attrition and lack of follow-up in the control group than the intervention group. Strengths of the study include a QED with use of sound quantitative measures. Based on recruitment of the experimental and control groups, however, it seems likely that site differences could influence the results. It is also not clear how intervention participants were initially screened, as authors indicate that about 29 % of otherwise eligible families were not recruited because they did not need a mental health intervention (Tischler et al., 2002). Furthermore, the services provided had no manual, and the level of services families received varied considerably in the intervention group, ranging from 1 to 24 appointments with an average of six sessions. While the results of the study suggest that mental health outreach services could provide benefit, methodology issues limit the strength of the findings and the study would be difficult to replicate. As such, the study would be considered not meeting evidence standards by WWC.

Beharie and colleagues (2011) conducted a family-focused intervention with homeless youth and their parents to prevent HIV/AIDS and substance abuse, to strengthen family communication, and to improve mental health. The HOPE Family Project involved an eight session curriculum that was based on material from three different EBPs: the Strengthening Families Program, which involves parent skills, child skills, and family life skills; the SISTA Project, a prevention program developed by the CDC to increase safe sex behaviors; and the CHAMP Program, an HIV prevention program for youths and families. With close community partnerships, the intervention was delivered to 102 caregivers and 122 youth ages 11–14 in six urban shelters. For comparison, a group of families participated in a three-session group discussion of HIV and drug use, with caregivers and youth in separate groups with no combined activities. Assessments occurred at pretest, posttest, 6-month follow-up, and 12-month follow-up, and included a number of psychometrically established measures (the Parenting Skills Questionnaire for parental monitoring and supervision, the Children's Depression Inventory for youth mental health, the Brief Symptom Inventory for parent mental health) as well as questions designed to assess family support, parent–child communication, youth substance use, and youth sexual behavior. Results indicated increased knowledge of HIV at posttest and 6 and 12 months follow-up for both the intervention and comparison group. Also, there were statistically significant increases in parent–child communication for the HOPE Family group compared to the HOPE Health group at posttest, 6-month, and 12-month follow-up, and there were significant decreases in suicidal ideation for teens in the HOPE Family group (Beharie et al., 2011). Unfortunately, no information was provided regarding the number of families who participated in the comparison condition, how families were placed in groups, or whether there were differences between the intervention and comparison groups at baseline. Thus, despite some apparent strengths in methodology (e.g., use of psychometrically strong measures and use of a comparison group) the information provided is not sufficient for determining whether this study meets evidence standards.

Another program focused on teaching parents to emphasize preschool child language development (O'Neil-Pirozzi, 2009). Sixteen single parents residing with their children in Boston family homeless shelters were randomly assigned to either the intervention group (12 parents) or the control group (4 parents). These families represented 84 % of eligible families in shelter at the time. Parents in the intervention group attended four weekly, 90-min small-group program sessions focused on understanding, discussing, and learning about language development in preschool children and methods for encouraging it. They also were given two children's books to read with their children between sessions. The control group parents participated in a social group and also received books for their children. Both groups were asked to keep track of reading activities with their children. Measures included parent receptive vocabulary skills with the Peabody Picture Vocabulary Test, attendance, parent-recorded reading practices, and observations of how parents facilitated their children's use of language during shared book reading both before and after intervention participation. Parents in the intervention group facilitated child language use more at posttest than parents in the control group (O'Neil-Pirozzi, 2009), although these differences were not statistically significant. Strengths of this study include its RCT design and measurement of relevant outcomes. By comparing the intervention group to a group who participated in assessments and received books but did not receive the instruction sessions, the researchers could be more confident that observed differences were due to the intervention itself. This intervention also was designed specifically to improve parent facilitation of preschool children's language development, and the study design and measures matched this specificity. However, the study was limited by a small sample size, particularly with regard to the control group of only four parents. It is possible that with a larger sample size, the differences would emerge as statistically significant. Only short-term outcomes were examined, and there were no measures of child outcomes to verify that enhancing parents' skills in facilitative language would benefit child language development. Also, it was not clear whether a manual was developed to enable replication or dissemination of the program. Based on all these considerations, this study likely would not meet evidence standards despite the strengths of its RCT design.

Project Support is a program designed specifically for mothers and their children ages 4–9 in domestic violence shelters who had experienced violence by male partners during the previous 12 months. It was evaluated as an RCT. This program focused on mothers, but with an emphasis on behavior management skills for reducing child conduct problems as well as instrumental and emotional support during transition out of shelter (Jouriles et al., 2009). In order to be eligible to participate, mothers had to have at least one child meeting criteria for oppositional defiant disorder (ODD) or conduct disorder (CD), could not be receiving other services for child behavior problems, and could not have significant mental health issues or substance use problems. The manual for Project Support was based on research and treatment studies showing that reducing inconsistent and harsh parenting can reduce child conduct problems and that targeting parent adjustment and psychiatric symptoms can improve treatment impacts, particularly with mothers who have experienced interpersonal violence. The child management portion of the intervention was modeled after other behavioral training programs (Jouriles et al., 2009). Following an initial, promising randomized clinical trial with a small sample of 36 families (Jouriles et al., 2001; McDonald, Jouriles, & Skopp, 2006), researchers conducted a second randomized clinical trial with 66 families. Families were screened first in shelter then again after leaving shelter before being randomly assigned to program ($N = 32$ families) and comparison ($N = 34$) conditions. Trained therapists worked with mothers in the intervention condition, and mothers in the comparison condition received only instrumental and emotional support by phone. Mothers in the comparison condition were encouraged to seek other community resources if needed. Baseline and outcome assessments involved psychometrically established measures, including the Child Behavior Checklist (CBCL) and the Eyberg Child Behavior Inventory (ECBI) for child conduct problems, the Parenting Dimensions Inventory (PDI) and the Revised Conflict Tactics Scale-Parent–child as measures of their inconsistency and acts of aggression, and the SCL-90-R as a measure of psychiatric symptoms. Finally, mothers' negative affect and harsh parenting behavior were observed and coded by trained raters with good reliability. Results indicated significant reductions in conduct problems on the CBCL and ECBI and in inconsistent and harsh parenting, with greater effects in the Project Support group than the comparison group.

Overall, the Project Support study design was methodologically strong with random assignment to groups, measures with sound psychometric properties and multiple methods, and long-term follow-up in addition to immediate posttreatment assessment. The researchers considered both statistical and clinical significance of findings. Furthermore, the detailed treatment manual enables attempts at replication and dissemination of the intervention. Limitations of the study and its findings include a reliance on mother's report for most outcomes, particularly child externalizing behavior. Because the intervention targeted mother behavior and symptoms, it is possible that participation in the Project Support intervention would impact how mothers reported on their parenting and their children's behavior without altering these behaviors in actuality, introducing bias. The findings would be strengthened if intervention impacts were apparent in reports of child behavior from other sources, such as teachers or other caregivers. Similarly, differences in mother-reported parenting behaviors were significant, whereas differences in observed parenting behavior were not. Finally, the inclusion criteria for the study based on level of child behavior problems and lack of mother's mental health or substance use problems were quite strict such that less than half of families screened for the intervention were eligible, and an even smaller percentage were followed out of shelter, producing high attrition rates. This suggests that the families in the study are not representative of the general population of families staying in domestic violence shelters and limits the extent to which the findings can be generalized more broadly. Thus, the study could meet standard with reservations, based on an RCT with high attrition but equivalence, allowing the intervention to be considered to have Potentially Positive Effects.

In contrast, another program focused on mothers with substance abuse issues who were either homeless or at-risk for homelessness. Using a QED, Sacks and colleagues (2004) examined the impact of a residential therapeutic community (TC) with additional components designed for needs of homeless mothers. A therapeutic community refers to a comprehensive psychosocial intervention with documented effectiveness for treating substance abuse problems and improving both psychological functioning and social behavior (De Leon, 2000; Sacks et al., 2004). In addition, the homeless parents' therapeutic community intervention (HP-TC) emphasized parenting, world of work, housing stabilization, and building a supportive community. Parenting aspects included a parents' group and family counseling, as well as child-focused activities such as daily child care, assessment with referral for early intervention, a children's group for age-appropriate substance abuse prevention activities, and prevention activities for visiting children not currently residing with the family in the therapeutic community. Work intervention activities included education preparation, work readiness seminars, assistance with job searches, and goal-setting and self-monitoring. Housing stabilization efforts involved case assistance and groups focused on applications, leases, and reentry into the community. Families were recruited for participation at two HP-TC sites (intervention group, 77 families) and two traditional TC sites (comparison group, 71 families). Because intervention participation was not random but was based on geographical location, researchers used propensity scores and statistical control techniques to account for preexisting differences between groups. Outcomes were measured primarily by parent-report across domains of parenting (including the Parenting Stress Index), housing stabilization, substance use/abuse, criminality, HIV risk behavior, employment, trauma, psychological distress (including the Beck Depression Inventory-II and the Symptom Check List 90-Revised), community, and health/treatment. Results indicated significant improvements in psychological distress and health for the HP-TC intervention group relative to the TC comparison group. There were no significant differences in other domains including parenting, substance use, and housing stabilization.

When an RCT is not possible, the sort of QED used in the TC study provides the next best evidence for evaluating an intervention's effectiveness, provided that sources of bias are controlled and groups can be considered equivalent on relevant domains. Another strength of the HP-TC study is that the novel intervention was compared to an established intervention, the traditional TC. The lack of difference between the intervention and comparison groups on mothers' substance use outcomes may indicate that both the HP-TC and traditional TC interventions were equally effective in improving substance use issues. It is noteworthy, however, that parenting and housing stability were not better among mothers who received the HP-TC intervention, despite being outcomes specifically targeted by the HP-TC protocol. Without a no-intervention comparison group, it is not clear whether both intervention conditions improved these outcomes or whether these outcomes were unaffected. The HP-TC study also relied on parent report for most outcomes. The HP-TC study failed to measure child outcomes, so there is no evidence for impacts of the program on child behavior, mental health, or general well-being. With regards to child outcomes, the study does not meet evidence standards. For parent outcomes of health and psychological distress, the study may meet evidence standards with potentially positive effects. In contrast to targeted interventions, the HP-TC intervention involved multiple components to address a range of goals, with case management, parent-directed programming, and child-directed programming. When several components are tested simultaneously in the same individuals, it is not clear whether all components are necessary, or if certain components are responsible for the effects. The two RCTs described next were similarly broad in their approaches.

Buckner and colleagues conducted a large, eight-site study to examine the effectiveness of a mother-focused intervention for improving behavior of children experiencing homelessness (Buckner, Weinreb, Rog, Holupka, & Samuels; Rog & Buckner, 2007). The intervention, the CMHS/CSAT Homeless Families Program, introduced an array of services to mothers such as mental health and substance abuse treatment, trauma recovery services, assistance in securing housing, and parent training. The study design was based on the assumption that improvements in maternal functioning would indirectly benefit children, improving their behavior and well-being. Furthermore, the study was designed for longitudinal follow-up to examine long-term impacts of intervention and changes in behavior problems over time. Over 1,500 families were involved in the study, and 1,103 children ranging in age from 2 to 16 years had assessment data for behavior problems, with initial assessments and three follow-up assessments at 3, 9, and 15 months. At each site in the intervention study, about half of the families were assigned to the target intervention group or comparison group with either randomized or QEDs. The comparison group received services within the shelters and community that were considered "services-as-usual" rather than the specialized package of services designed as the target intervention at each site. Because sites differed somewhat in the services that were included and emphasized in their target intervention packages, treatment status and programmatic emphases were both considered in analyses. Results across sites indicated that although behavior problems improved for children over time, there were no significant differences based on intervention status or programmatic emphases (Rog & Buckner, 2007).

The Family Critical Time Intervention (FCTI) was implemented in Westchester County, New York to target the well-being of homeless mothers with mental illness or substance abuse problems for rapid rehousing and intensive case management services (Samuels et al., 2010; Samuels, Shinn, & Fischer, 2006). The intervention was based on the Critical Time Intervention, a distinct evidence-based and manualized treatment that originated with single homeless men in New York City (Herman et al., 2000). For FCTI, families were stratified by size then randomized into an intervention group (97 families receiving FCTI) and a comparison group (113 families) who received services-as-usual. Families in the intervention group received intensive case management to connect the mother with appropriate services in the community and then encourage increasing independence within a network of community supports (Samuels et al., 2010, 2006). Child outcomes were measured at baseline and at 3, 9, 15, and 24 months in three broad domains of mental health, school functioning, and stressful life events. For mental health outcomes, parents completed the Child Behavior Checklist (CBCL), youth ages 11–16 completed the Youth Self-Report (YSR), and youth ages 6–16 completed the Children's Depression Inventory (CDI). School outcomes were measured based on parent and child report of attendance and parent report of the child's attitude towards school or childcare, experience of school or childcare, and troubles with school or childcare. Children also reported on their troubles with school and their level of effort in school. Finally, youth completed a measure to report whether they had experienced items from a list of 24 negative life events. Results of the study indicated that children in the FCTI intervention group had "modestly" better scores on mental health and school outcomes, but that these improvements were less stable than the general improvement observed in both groups over time, as families stabilized (Samuels et al., 2010, 2006).

Both the CMHS/CSAT Homeless Families Program overall and the Family Critical Time Intervention study included strong research designs with large samples across different geographical sites or shelters, well-validated measures assessing child behavior problems, and longitudinal follow-up to assess possible impacts over time. The intervention groups were compared to families receiving a different set of services rather than a no-treatment control. This created a stringent test of intervention effects above possible benefits afforded by receiving any services. Interestingly, both studies found no significant effects of the interventions on child outcomes. Because both groups were receiving services, it is possible that both packages of services, the intervention and "services-as-usual," provided benefit to families and that the intervention had no added effect beyond services-as-usual. This could only be explored with the use of an assessment-only comparison group, which is impossible for both ethical and practical reasons (Seibel et al., 2012). However, if both sets of services are producing equal benefit, other considerations such as the resources needed and costs of both programs could be considered to determine which condition provides benefit most efficiently. Overall, the studies of the CMHS/CSAT Homeless Families Program and the Family Critical Time Intervention meet evidence standards based on RCT or QED design; however the interventions themselves would be considered to have No Discernible Effects at this time, based on the lack of findings in either a positive or negative direction. In other words, these studies have produced quality evidence that the interventions produced no meaningful effects on the considered outcomes. Furthermore, additional studies could consider individual components of the programs in isolation to determine whether and which services within the broad packages account for positive change.

Summary and Conclusion

The studies reviewed in this chapter represent laudable efforts on the part of researchers, practitioners, and community partners to engage in intervention studies with the challenging and understudied population of children in families experiencing homelessness. Challenges associated with intervening with this population are well documented in these studies, including issues of great heterogeneity in the needs and characteristics of families experiencing homelessness, cultural sensitivity, trauma-informed care, high mobility, and ongoing stressors in the lives of these families (see Chap. 9 of this volume for a discussion of similar issues in relation to programs designed to promote positive parenting). In response to the varied challenges, these studies also have provided insight about what works to engage stakeholders, communities, practitioners, and families. Wisdom and experience acquired through these initial efforts is valuable as it provides clinical expertise in the context of client characteristics, values, and preferences. According to the Institute of Medicine and APA, such expertise in context is essential for developing EBPs. Also essential, however, is the integration of best available research evidence (American Psychological Association, 2005; Kazak et al., 2010; Seibel et al., 2012). Based on our review of existing studies within the guidelines of the What Works Clearinghouse (WWC) standards for EBPs (What Works Clearinghouse, 2011), none of the interventions represented in these studies have sufficient evidence to be rated as having Positive Effects. In most cases, this is because quality evidence that supports the program effects does not exist.

First and foremost, more studies with rigorous methodology including RCTs or QEDs are critical for advancing the evidence base for interventions with homeless children. Studies that do not include equivalent comparison groups simply cannot demonstrate that positive changes result from the intervention itself rather than other factors. In particular, families who experience homelessness tend to improve in functioning over time (Samuels et al., 2010), making it particularly important to demonstrate that intervention efforts produce benefits beyond those experienced by families receiving no intervention or care as usual. Descriptive studies alone are not sufficient for providing this information. In the context of well-designed RCTs and QEDs, it also is essential that studies include valid and reliable outcome measures, low attrition rates or equivalent groups despite attrition, statistical adjustments for pre-intervention differences in a QED, and specificity such that interventions are not combined and tested simultaneously (What Works Clearinghouse, 2011). To build an evidence base such that an intervention can be considered to have Positive Effects, results in favor of the intervention must be replicated in multiple studies and conducted with fidelity to the intervention, which requires that interventions have manuals (Chambless & Hollon, 1998; What Works Clearinghouse, 2011).

Next steps in developing evidence-based interventions with homeless families must combine the wisdom and expertise gained by efforts represented in this review with empirical studies that meet evidence standards. Interventions that are represented in descriptive studies but have not been tested with RCTs or QEDs may indeed produce positive effects, and thus the intervention developers are encouraged to rigorously evaluate their programs with strong designs and valid, reliable assessments. Other efforts may involve adapting existing EBPs for use with children experiencing homelessness (Bassuk, 2010; Gewirtz & Taylor, 2009; Samuels et al., 2010). Examples of such efforts currently underway include using Trauma-Focused Cognitive Behavioral Therapy (Cohen, Mannarino, Berliner, & Deblinger, 2000), Parenting Through Change (Forgatch & DeGarmo, 1999; Gewirtz, Forgatch, & Wieling, 2008), Early Risers (August, Realmuto, Hektner, & Bloomquist, 2001) through the Healthy Families Network (Gewirtz, 2007), and the Building on Strengths and Advocating for Family Empowerment (BSAFE), an adaptation of the Critical Time Intervention developed by the National Center on Family Homelessness (Bassuk, 2010). Of course, adaptations of EBPs or even EBPs implemented without adaptation should be rigorously evaluated for homeless families, as contextual differences may impact the effectiveness of any intervention. Finally, attention should be paid to the specificity of interventions. Given the heterogeneity among families experiencing homelessness and the diverse needs of this extremely high-risk population, programs combining multiple interventions or components may be most likely to be effective. However, such programs also are likely to be more expensive. Individual components must be tested separately and even compared to determine which produce positive effects most efficiently. Such efforts would be best served by programs of research and multiple studies that could examine intervention components individually and in combination.

Conducting empirical investigations that meet evidence standards may be costly in terms of training, resources, and time. States and municipalities have begun developing and investing in ways to routinely evaluate their programs and services in rigorous-but-cost-effective ways, such as through integrated administrative data systems (Culhane, Fantuzzo, Rouse, Tam, & Lukens, 2010). Without an investment in quality evidence, however, little can be learned beyond what we already know regarding the best practices for intervening with children experiencing homelessness, and what we already know is largely not based on rigorous evidence. Policymakers, funding agencies, researchers, clinicians, and community practitioners can expand the evidence base for interventions with homeless children through understanding what constitutes quality evaluations and supporting these efforts. Building a robust and rigorous evidence base of what works will allow stakeholders to improve the well-being of at-risk children, bettering their lives through increasingly effective and increasingly efficient programs.

References

American Psychological Association. (2005). *Policy statement on evidence-based practice in psychology.* http://www.apa.org/practice/ebpreport.pdf
August, G. J., Realmuto, G. M., Hektner, J. M., & Bloomquist, M. L. (2001). An integrated components preventive intervention for aggressive elementary school children: The early risers program. *Journal of Consulting and Clinical Psychology, 69,* 614–626.

Baggerly, J. (2004). The effects of child-centered group play therapy on self-concept, depression, and anxiety of children who are homeless. *International Journal of Play Therapy, 13*(2), 31–51.

Bassuk, E. L. (2010). Ending child homelessness in America. *American Journal of Orthopsychiatry, 80*, 496–504. doi:10.1111/j.1939-0025.2010.01052.x.

Beharie, N., Kalogerogiannis, K., McKay, M. M., Paulino, A., Miranda, A., Rivera-Rodriguez, A., et al. (2011). The HOPE Family Project: A family-based group intervention to reduce the impact of homelessness on HIV/STI and drug risk behaviors. *Social Work with Groups, 34*, 61–78. doi:10.1080/01609513.2010.510091.

Bodonyi, J. (2008). Evaluation of the sound families initiative: Final findings report: A comprehensive evaluation of the sound families initiative. Retrieved from http://www.buildingchanges. org/images/documents/library/2008%20Sound%20Families%20Final%20Findings%20 Report.pdf

Buckner, J. C., Weinreb, L. F., Rog, D. J., Holupka, C. S., & Samuels, J. *Predictors of homeless children's problem behaviors over time: Findings from the CMHS/CSAT homeless families program.* Unpublished manuscript.

Burt, M. R., Pearson, C., & Montgomery, A. (2005). *Strategies for preventing homelessness.* Washington, DC: Department of Housing and Urban Development.

Chambless, D. L., Baker, M. J., Baucom, D. H., Beutler, L. E., Calhoun, K. S., Crits-Christoph, P., et al. (1998). Update on empirically validated therapies, II. *Clinical Psychologist, 51*(1), 3–16.

Chambless, D. L., & Hollon, S. D. (1998). Defining empirically supported therapies. *Journal of Consulting and Clinical Psychology, 66*(1), 7–18.

Coalition for Evidence-Based Policy. (2010). Checklist for reviewing a randomized controlled trial of a social program of project, to assess whether it produced valid evidence. Retrieved December 12, 2012, from http://toptierevidence.org/wp-content/uploads/2010/02/Top-Tier-Checklist-for-Reviewing-RCTs-Updated-Jan10.pdf

Cohen, J. A., Mannarino, A. P., Berliner, L., & Deblinger, E. (2000). Trauma-focused cognitive behavioral therapy for children and adolescents an empirical update. *Journal of Interpersonal Violence, 15*(11), 1202–1223.

Culhane, D. P., Fantuzzo, J., Rouse, H. L., Tam, V., & Lukens, J. (2010). Connecting the dots: The promise of integrated data systems for policy analysis and systems reform. *Intelligence for Social Policy, 1*(3), 1–22.

Davey, T. L. (2004). A multiple-family group intervention for homeless families: The weekend retreat. *Health & Social Work, 29*(4), 326–329.

De Leon, G. (2000). *The therapeutic community: Theory, model, and method.* New York, NY: Springer Publishing Company.

DeCandia, C. J. (2012). Designing developmentally-based services for young homeless families. *Strengthening at risk and homeless young mothers and children.* Retrieved January 13, 2012, from www.familyhomelessness.org/media/313.pdf

Ferguson, S., & Morley, P. (2011). Improving engagement in the role of father for homeless, non-custodial fathers: A program evaluation. *Journal of Poverty, 15*(2), 206–225.

Fischer, R. L. (2000). Toward self-sufficiency: Evaluating a transitional housing program for homeless families. *Policy Studies Journal, 28*(2), 402–420. doi:10.1111/j.1541-0072.2000. tb02038.x.

Forgatch, M. S., & DeGarmo, D. S. (1999). Parenting through change: An effective prevention program for single mothers. *Journal of Consulting and Clinical Psychology, 67*(5), 711–724.

Gewirtz, A. (2007). Promoting children's mental health in family supportive housing: A community-university partnership for formerly homeless children and families. *Journal of Primary Prevention, 28*, 359–374. doi:10.1007/s10935-007-0102-z.

Gewirtz, A., Forgatch, M., & Wieling, E. (2008). Parenting practices as potential mechanisms for child adjustment following mass trauma. *Journal of Marital and Family Therapy, 34*(2), 177–192. doi:10.1111/j.1752-0606.2008.00063.x.

Gewirtz, A., & Taylor, T. (2009). Participation of homeless and abused women in a parent training program: Science and practice converge in a battered women's shelter. In M. F. Hindsworth & T. B. Lang (Eds.), *Community participation and empowerment* (pp. 97–114). Hauppage, NY: Nova.

Grant, R. (1991). The special needs of homeless children: Early intervention at a welfare hotel. *Topics in Early Childhood Special Education, 10*(4), 76–91.

Haber, M. G., & Toro, P. A. (2004). Homelessness among families, children, and adolescents: An ecological-developmental perspective. *Clinical Child and Family Psychology Review, 7*(3), 123–164. doi:10.1023/B:CCFP.0000045124.09503.f1.

Heckman, J. J., Ichimura, H., Smith, J., & Todd, P. (1998). Characterizing selection bias using experimental data. *Econometrica, 66*(5), 1017–1098.

Heckman, J. J., Ichimura, H., & Todd, P. E. (1997). Matching as an econometric evaluation estimator: Evidence from evaluating a job training programme. *The Review of Economic Studies, 64*(4), 605–654.

Herman, D., Opler, L., Felix, A., Valencia, E., Wyatt, R. J., & Susser, E. (2000). A critical time intervention with mentally ill homeless men: Impact on psychiatric symptoms. *The Journal of Nervous and Mental Disease, 188*(3), 135–140.

Hwang, S. W., Tolomiczenko, G., Kouyoumdjian, F. G., & Garner, R. E. (2005). Interventions to improve the health of the homeless. *American Journal of Preventive Medicine, 29*(4), 311–319.

Institute of Education Sciences. (2013). *What works clearinghouse.* Retrieved December 12, 2012, from http://ies.ed.gov/ncee/wwc/default.aspx

Jouriles, E. N., McDonald, R., Rosenfield, D., Stephens, N., Corbitt-Shindler, D., & Miller, P. C. (2009). Reducing conduct problems among children exposed to intimate partner violence: A randomized clinical trial examining effects of project support. *Journal of Consulting and Clinical Psychology, 77*(4), 705–717.

Jouriles, E. N., McDonald, R., Spiller, L., Norwood, W. D., Swank, P. R., Stephens, N., et al. (2001). Reducing conduct problems among children of battered women. *Journal of Consulting and Clinical Psychology, 69*(5), 774–785. doi:10.1037/0022-006X.69.5.774.

Kazak, A. E., Hoagwood, K., Weisz, J. R., Hood, K., Kratochwill, T. R., Vargas, L. A., et al. (2010). A meta-systems approach to evidence-based practice for children and adolescents. *American Psychologist, 65*(2), 85–97.

Kelly, J. F., Buehlman, K., & Caldwell, K. (2000) Training personnel to promote quality parent-child interaction in families who are homeless. *Topics in Early Childhood Special Education, 20*(3), 174–185.

Kilmer, R. P., Cook, J. R., Crusto, C., Strater, K. P., & Haber, M. G. (2012). Understanding the ecology and development of children and families experiencing homelessness: Implications for practice, supportive services, and policy. *American Journal of Orthopsychiatry, 82*(3), 389–401.

Kissman, K. (1999). Time out from stress: Camp program and parenting groups for homeless mothers. *Contemporary Family Therapy, 21*(3), 373–384. doi:10.1023/A:1021964416412.

Levant, R. F., & Hasan, N. T. (2008). Evidence-based practice in psychology. *Professional Psychology: Research and Practice, 39*(6), 658–662.

McDonald, R., Jouriles, E. N., & Skopp, N. A. (2006). Reducing conduct problems among children brought to women's shelters: Intervention effects 24 months following termination of services. *Journal of Family Psychology, 20*(1), 127–136.

Medeiros, D., & Vaulton, W. (2010). Strengthening at-risk and homeless young mothers and children. *Zero to Three, 30*(3), 27–33.

Melley, A. H., Cosgrove, K., Norris-Shortle, C., Kiser, L. J., Levey, E. B., Coble, C. A., et al. (2010). Supporting positive parenting for young children experiencing homelessness: The PACT therapeutic nursery. *Zero to Three, 30*(3), 39–45.

Murrell, N. L., Scherzer, T., Ryan, M., Frappier, N., Abrams, A., & Roberts, C. (2000). The AfterCare project: An intervention for homeless childbearing families. *Family & Community Health, 23*(3), 17–27.

Nabors, L. A., Proescher, E., & DeSilva, M. (2001). School-based mental health prevention activities for homeless and at-risk youth. *Child and Youth Care Forum, 30*(1), 3–18.

Nabors, L. A., Weist, M. D., Shugarman, R., Woeste, M. J., Mullet, E., & Rosner, L. (2004). Assessment, prevention, and intervention activities in a school-based program for children experiencing homelessness. *Behavior Modification, 28*(4), 565–578. doi:10.1177/0145445503259517.

Norris-Shortle, C., Melley, A. H., Kiser, L. J., Levey, E., Cosgrove, K., & Leviton, A. (2006). Targeted interventions for homeless children at a therapeutic nursery. *Zero to Three, 26*(4), 49–55.

O'Neil-Pirozzi, T. M. (2009). Feasibility and benefit of parent participation in a program emphasizing preschool child language development while homeless. *American Journal of Speech-Language Pathology, 18*(3), 252–263.

Paquette, K., & Bassuk, E. L. (2009). Parenting and homelessness: Overview and introduction to the special section. *American Journal of Orthopsychiatry, 79*(3), 292–298.

Puterbaugh, F. G. (2009). *The impact of the adolescent transition program's parent management curriculum on risk factors for delinquency and perceived parenting efficacy.* Doctoral Dissertation, Alliant International University, Fresno, CA.

Rog, D. J., & Buckner, J. C. (2007). Homeless families and children. In D. Dennis, G. Locke, & J. Khadduri (Eds.), *Toward understanding homelessness: The 2007 national symposium on homelessness research.* U.S. Department of Housing and Urban Development: Washington, DC.

Rog, D. J., McCombs-Thornton, K. L., Gilbert-Mongelli, A. M., Brito, M. C., & Holupka, C. S. (1995). Implementation of the homeless families program: 2. Characteristics, strengths, and needs of participant families. *American Journal of Orthopsychiatry, 65*(4), 514–528.

Sacks, S., Sacks, J. A. Y., McKendrick, K., Pearson, F. S., Banks, S., & Harle, M. (2004). Outcomes from a therapeutic community for homeless addicted mothers and their children. *Administration and Policy in Mental Health and Mental Health Services Research, 31*(4), 313–338.

Samuels, J., Shinn, M., & Buckner, J. C. (2010). *Homeless children: Update on research, policy, programs, and opportunities: Prepared for the Office of the Assistant Secretary for Planning and Evaluation. U. S. Department of Health and Human Services.* Delmar, NY: Policy Research Associates, Inc.

Samuels, J., Shinn, M., & Fischer, S. (2006). *The impact of the Family Critical Time Intervention on homeless children.* Final report to the National Institute of Mental Health

Seibel, N. L., Bassuk, E., & Medeiros, D. (2012). Using evidence-based programs to support children and families experiencing homelessness. *Zero to Three, 32*(4), 30–35.

Shinn, M., Weitzman, B. C., Stojanovic, D., Knickman, J. R., Jimenez, L., Duchon, L., et al. (1998). Predictors of homelessness among families in New York city: From shelter request to housing stability. *American Journal of Public Health, 88*(11), 1651–1657.

Smith, J., & Todd, P. (2005). Does matching overcome LaLonde's critique of nonexperimental estimators? *Journal of Econometrics, 125*(1), 305–353.

Substance Abuse and Mental Health Services Administration. (2013). Prevention training and technical assistance. From http://captus.samhsa.gov/prevention-practice/defining-evidence-based/samhsa-criteria

Swann-Jackson, R., Tapper, D., & Fields, A. (2010). *Keeping families together: Program evaluation overview.* New York, NY: Corporation for Supportive Housing.

Tischler, V., Vostanis, P., Bellerby, T., & Cumella, S. (2002). Evaluation of a mental health outreach service for homeless families. *Archives of Disease in Childhood, 86*(3), 158–163.

What Works Clearinghouse (2011). *What works clearinghouse procedures and standards handbook* (Version 2.1). Retrieved January 9, 2013, from http://ies.ed.gov/ncee/wwc/pdf/reference_resources/wwc_procedures_v2_1_standards_handbook.pdf

Wong, Y. L. I., Culhane, D. P., & Kuhn, R. (1997). Predictors of exit and reentry among family shelter users in New York city. *The Social Service Review, 71*, 441–462.

Zients, J. D. (2012). *Memorandum to the heads of executive departments and agencies: Use of evidence and evaluation in the 2014 budget.* Retrieved from http://www.whitehouse.gov/sites/default/files/omb/memoranda/2012/m-12-14.pdf.

Chapter 11
Primary Stakeholders' Perspectives on Services for Families Without Homes

Ralph da Costa Nunez and Matthew Adams

Abstract This chapter presents the perspectives of 12 stakeholders on the current state of family homelessness. To prepare the chapter, the authors conducted interviews with two policymakers, three advocates, three researchers, three shelter providers, and one formerly homeless parent. This qualitative method was selected in order to collect in-depth information from a wide range of people who have first-hand knowledge regarding family homelessness. The first half of this chapter relates the effects of homelessness that inhibit parents' ability to provide adequate care for their children. The second half of the chapter focuses on the federal policies that positively and negatively impact homeless parents and their children.

This chapter presents the perspectives of 12 stakeholders—two policymakers, three advocates, three researchers, three shelter providers, and one formerly homeless parent—on the current state of family homelessness. In-depth, key informant interviews were individually conducted to understand the effects of homelessness on parents and their children. Interviewees also were asked to discuss federal policies and programs that have positive impacts on families experiencing homelessness as well as those that hinder their success. What follows in this chapter is a structured presentation of discussions with these key stakeholders.

The first half of this chapter relates the effects of homelessness that inhibit parents' ability to provide adequate care for their children. Families experience these negative impacts outside of shelters and within homelessness shelters, with serious implications for children. To avoid shelter, parents often exhaust their network of family and friends for places to stay. These "doubled-up" situations are characterized by frequent moves, conflicts with leaseholders, and fear that arrangements may end abruptly and unpredictably. Moreover, parents may have insufficient access to basic necessities and supportive services to place them on a path to stable housing.

R. da Costa Nunez, Ph.D. • M. Adams (✉)
Institute for Children, Poverty, and Homelessness, New York, NY, USA
e-mail: madams@icphusa.org

M.E. Haskett et al. (eds.), *Supporting Families Experiencing Homelessness:*
Current Practices and Future Directions, DOI 10.1007/978-1-4614-8718-0_11,
© Springer Science+Business Media New York 2014

In the worst cases, homeless mothers in particular can endure relationship violence or participate in illegal schemes to maintain these tenuous living conditions.

Once a family enters shelter, a homeless parent's experience is significantly shaped by two factors: the building's physical structure and the provider's philosophy toward service provision. Congregate facilities, where many families sleep together in large rooms, create more stress and offer little privacy compared with shelters that have individual rooms. Similarly, the organizational attitude toward administering services varies; some staffs foster nurturing and encouraging environments, while others generate atmospheres of fear. Staff, for example, can create tension by undermining parents' authority or indiscriminately threatening them with child protective service involvement. Additional negative effects of living in shelter can include disruptions of essential family routines and rituals, intensified stress due to parents' inability to provide for their own children, and anxiety from constantly being watched and monitored by staff and other parents.

Children ultimately suffer from the cumulative negative effects of homelessness on their parents. Shelters direct attention to resolving parents' barriers to self-sufficiency but, in doing so, often neglect children's experiences of trauma and their unique service needs. Homeless children can experience depression, low self-esteem, developmental delays, behavioral issues, difficulties in school, and low executive functioning, which can affect them for the rest of their lives. For a detailed discussion of characteristics of youth who experience homelessness, see Chaps. 2 and 3 of this volume.

The second half of this chapter focuses on the federal policies that positively and negatively impact homeless parents and their children. Stakeholders' opinions on policies detrimental to homeless families followed three primary themes. First, four interviewees cited the interrelated and long-standing set of policies that have resulted in a lack of affordable housing and an increasing number of families with extremely low incomes. Simply put, families cannot prevent or end their homelessness if homes that they could afford do not exist. Second, seven stakeholders noted that the federal government has focused political capital and fiscal resources on the needs of chronically homeless single individuals and veterans; families have not been afforded the same degree of attention or support. As a by-product, emphasis has been placed on rapidly moving homeless individuals and families alike into permanent housing. If, however, families are not offered appropriate preparation and supports, the stakeholders expressed fear that families will return to shelter and perpetuate a cycle of housing instability. Key informants discussed some bureaucratic impediments to serving families, including conflicting federal definitions of homelessness, which hinder providers' ability to serve families in need of assistance. While three stakeholders were unable to identify positive policies, other key informants were able to agree upon one key federal program that benefits homeless families: the comprehensive services provided to homeless students through the US Department of Education's Education for Homeless Children and Youth program. As mandated by the McKinney–Vento Homeless Assistance Act, there is a liaison in every school district nationwide to alleviate obstacles that threaten homeless students' equal access to education.

Methodology and Selection of Key Informants

Key informant interviews were conducted to ascertain the current state of family homelessness and directions for future research, policy, and practice. This qualitative method was selected in order to collect in-depth information from a wide range of people who have firsthand knowledge regarding family homelessness. The key informants, or principal stakeholders, interviewed are divided into five groups, although it is acknowledged that their experiences and work may span across several categories: policymakers, advocates, researchers, family service providers, and homeless families. In the selection of key informants, consideration was given to multiple domains, including level of authority, area of expertise, and geographic representation, to ensure that a wide range of views would be represented. There are very few policymakers, advocates, and researchers focused on the issue of family homelessness; therefore, selection was straightforward. On the other hand, the number of service providers and families experiencing homelessness is substantial. The authors used their knowledge and experience in the field to carefully select providers. Lastly, one formerly homeless parent was identified who the authors felt could offer a holistic perspective given the nature of the research; the parent experienced homelessness approximately a decade ago and is presently involved in the delivery of family homelessness services.

Semi-structured, 30-min phone interviews were conducted with the 12 key informants between November 27th and December 20th of 2012. Stakeholders were asked a set of five broad questions developed to guide each conversation. The authors sometimes asked follow-up questions to obtain more detail or provide clarity. All interviews were digitally recorded. Transcripts were produced from the audio recordings, then iteratively combined, and thematically organized.

Twelve interviews were sufficient to reach saturation, or the point at which additional data did not appear to yield new insights, and identify primary themes. The following analysis synthesizes and presents the stakeholders' informed opinions. The names and affiliations of the key informants, along with the categories assigned to each, are listed below. Names have been disclosed here to lend a level of authority and context to this analysis. Subsequently, names are withheld in order to provide some degree of anonymity when relating responses, but stakeholder categories are provided for context. The authors thank the interviewees for their participation in this study.

Policymakers

- Jennifer Ho is the Deputy Director of the US Interagency Council on Homelessness and is the point person on issues related to family homelessness. The council is an independent agency within the federal executive branch, consisting of 19 federal Cabinet secretaries and agency heads who coordinate the federal response to homelessness.

- Ellen Howard-Cooper is the Deputy Commissioner of Prevention, Policy, and Planning for the New York City Department of Homeless Services (DHS). The largest provider of family shelter nationwide, DHS serves over 30,000 parents and their children daily.

Advocates

- Barbara Duffield is the Policy Director of the National Association for the Education of Homeless Children and Youth (EHCY), a national grassroots membership association that connects educators, parents, advocates, researchers, and service providers to support the academic success of children and youth experiencing homelessness.
- Diane Nilan is the Founder and President of HEAR US, a national advocacy project that produces films and books to give a voice to and raise awareness of children and youth experiencing homelessness.
- Joe Willard is the Vice President of Policy at the People's Emergency Center, an organization focused on sheltering homeless families and strengthening neighborhoods in Philadelphia.

Researchers

- Doug Rice is a Senior Policy Analyst at the Center on Budget and Policy Priorities, a national policy organization working on federal- and state-level fiscal policy and public programs that affect low- and moderate-income families and individuals. His work focuses on the impact of federal housing policy on low-income families.
- Jeremy Rosen is the Policy Director at the National Law Center on Homelessness and Poverty, an organization that serves as the legal arm of the nationwide movement to end homelessness through impact litigation, policy advocacy, and public education.
- Beth Shinn is a Professor and the Chair of the Department of Human and Organizational Development at Vanderbilt University's Peabody College. Her research focuses on persons who face social exclusion due to poverty, homelessness, and/or mental illness; how social settings influence individual well-being; and how settings can be modified to foster individual welfare.

Family Service Providers

- Mattie Lord is the Chief Program Officer for UMOM New Day Centers in Phoenix, the largest provider of shelter for homeless families in Arizona.

- Kelly Wierzbinski is the Director of Children, Youth, and Family Services for the Family Connection Program at Rainbow Days. The program provides support groups; supportive, drug-free alternative activities; and life-enrichment services for homeless children and families in Dallas.
- Aurora Zepeda is the Executive Vice President for Homes for the Homeless (HFH), a nonprofit organization that shelters over 500 families each day in New York City. In the interest of full disclosure, HFH is a sister organization of the Institute for Children, Poverty, and Homelessness, with which the authors are affiliated.

Formerly Homeless Parent

- A parent, whose name and further identifying details have been omitted to protect her privacy, spent 9 months in a New York City shelter more than 10 years ago as a young single mother with her 10-year-old boy. As part of her Master of Social Work program, she is currently interning at the same shelter.

Part I: Effects of Homelessness on Parents and Their Children

Individual Challenges to Parenting Prior to Shelter

Homeless parents often arrive at shelter with multiple personal obstacles preventing them from parenting effectively. See Chap. 4, this volume, for a review of research on parenting in the face of homelessness and Chap. 9 for a review of research on programs to support homeless parents. While nearly all interviewees named these barriers simply as prior "trauma" and the negative consequences of "poverty" and "mobility," conversations with two providers and two advocates provided a clearer picture. Negative childhood experiences lay the foundation for future challenges. These issues are exacerbated by individuals becoming single parents at young ages, when they lack the education and skills necessary for self-sufficiency. Additional stress induced by unstable and sometimes violent living situations ultimately leaves homeless parents without basic parenting skills. "The odds are really stacked against any parent who in the best of all worlds really feels like she—and it's usually single mothers—wants to do well by her kids," explained one of the providers.

The individual challenges that homeless parents face often stem from negative experiences in their own childhoods. Homeless parents often lacked positive role models to demonstrate how to properly care for their own children. One provider observed,

> Many of them did not have an experience of being parented very completely themselves. Many of them had out-of-home experiences, meaning not living with their parents. They were living with, at best, relatives. [Less optimally,] they were living with extended family or friends. A lot of them had interruptions in their own childhoods by either being homeless or being uprooted suddenly. So there's not a lot of modeling in terms of what good parenting

might have been. They're subject to whatever happened to their own parents, but sometimes there were truly crises that happened that ripped the families apart. These parents didn't have good role models of what good parenting was and what good childhood experiences were.

An advocate added, "Young parents have never had a stable life; we cannot assume that as adults they should act like [adults]."

At the young ages at which homeless parents have children, their own development is often incomplete and they are not yet self-sufficient. As a provider explained,

They jump out of the gate with a lot of struggles. They didn't have a full kind of youth, going out and doing all the things that young kids do—going to high school and to games and proms and dating and socializing—they didn't do that. They jumped into parenthood very early. A lot of them have children before the age of 21, 22. So they're trying to have this youthful life and then suddenly they have this kid. [...]. They don't have, a lot of them, complete education or any work experience. They immediately are smacked with all the economic struggles that young parents face. Kids are expensive and they have to make tough choices about where they spend their limited resources.

As families lose their own housing, they frequently live doubled-up with family or friends before resorting to shelter, bringing more stress to already vulnerable young parents. According to an advocate, at the time they entered shelter,

...almost 100 % of the families were living doubled-up and have been bouncing around for three to five months at a time. It has to be a tremendous burden on being a good parent when you are moving your child that many times from place to place. The stress on the mom and on the dad for those instances, to feel that they are being a good parent and providing the children everything that they need.

As the advocate related, most homeless families are headed by single mothers, which adds yet another layer of complexity to already tenuous doubled-up living environments: domestic violence. "Often mom goes from abusive relationship to abusive relationship in doubled-up situations just because she doesn't want to come in to shelter," one provider explained. Another provider observed that "women will put up with everything that they have to put up with to keep their kids [relatively safe] or with a roof over their heads." As a result, "a lot of domestic violence and relationship violence is tolerated, with the fear that they'll get thrown out."

Due to unstable childhoods, lack of parenting role models, and the trauma of temporary and violent living arrangements, parents often enter shelter without basic parenting skills. In one advocate's view, homeless parents require "life skills training, such as how to cook when you have a toddler who is needy and demanding, how to cook quality food that is nutritious, how to remain on a budget and the importance of having a set pattern throughout the day."

Furthermore, as a policymaker summarized, "For any family to become homeless and need to seek shelter, that family is under an extraordinary amount of stress already walking into that situation, which is going to be incredibly variable based on what the short- and medium-term prospects are [for exiting homelessness]."

Additional Stress of Shelter Life Negatively Affects Parenting

Key informants, with the exception of two who lacked direct experience in family shelter settings, unanimously agreed that shelters are rarely conducive to positive parenting and family well-being.

Separation

During the intake process, some parents must choose between splitting up their families or not entering shelter due to shelter rules and regulations. A researcher explained that a lot of families are separated by shelter rules, "either because of rules prohibiting all men or because of rules about married men." The researcher also indicated that many shelters prohibit teenage boys and adult children from remaining with their families, a necessary rule when many families live in the same space: "One of the things that we can do to try to support families is to not tear them apart. It's an inherent problem when you put disparate people with different needs in a tight space. It's not that shelters are out to get families and to rip them apart. It's that [each mother is] worried about the safety of [her own daughter]; 'my husband or father is your strange man in the next bed.'"

Uncertainty

As soon as parents arrive in shelter, uncertainty over the length of time they can stay and where their children will go to school causes anxiety. A researcher noted,

> I think you have challenges just because the situation is not permanent. Parents know this; kids know this. There's going to be a great sense of uncertainty, and for children that usually results in high stress levels,[which makes them] more difficult to deal with [for parents]. The school situation is potentially uncertain. Are they going to go to a new school by the shelter? Are they going to go back to their old school? If they decide to go back to the old school because they really like that setting, are there going to be significant transportation challenges that prevent that from happening?

According to an advocate, the initial stress over time limits "looms" over families throughout their stay, particularly in cases where parents must exit within as little as 30–60 days.

Varieties in Shelter Space and Service Style

Once families locate shelter programs for which they are eligible, potentially make difficult choices to separate their families, and determine school arrangements and length of stay, their future parenting success largely depends upon two factors: the physical structure and the management of the shelter. Four stakeholders, three advocates, and a researcher noted that the term "shelter" refers to many different physical settings, which have progressively negative consequences to family and child well-being. Ideally, each family has its own private room. A less desirable scenario is one in which two to three families share a living space. At worst, all families live together in a large, congregate, barracks-style setting.

Congregate shelters present the most difficulty for parents to care for their children. They create tension with shelter staff and other residents due to "the close quarters, the noise level, and the influence of others," as summarized by a provider. One advocate illustrated the inherent difficulties of parenting within a congregate shelter:

> So a parent of a young child would complain that the little kids aren't allowed to run around and make noise the way little kids ordinarily do. And the parent of a teenage child would say, 'My kid can't get her homework done when there are all these little kids running around and making noise.' So it's very difficult in the congregate situation to support all the families' routines and to create environments where parents can do what they think works for their kids.

Another advocate described this environment as a "cesspool of human behavior" that includes "family rivalries, territories, and bullying." The advocate went on to explain that "fear is a major issue"; this includes the "fear of being kicked out for children's behavior" and of health and hygiene issues such as head lice or influenza.

In less positive shelter environments, staff can create "highly anxiety-provoking and unhelpful" fear among parents. According to a researcher:

> There were some places where multiple families told us that staff routinely threatened parents with child protective service involvement and those same parents didn't have those experiences in other places. So I don't think it's all about the parents. I recognize that there are some times when these services should be invoked. But because it seemed to be associated more with the places than with the parents, it seemed that some places were using that as a way to try to get parents' attention, to get them to take seriously the perspective of the providers.

In describing tension felt by these parents, an advocate stressed the need for "respect and open communication." A researcher offered more clarity on how to better prepare families for independent living while they are in shelter: "So the kinds of things that work ... [are] clear expectations and rules, programs that try to work with families to maintain family routines and rituals, programs that think about families as families and not just as parents and as children, but to try to help families be the families that they were."

Loss of Authority and Privacy

Even in ideal shelter environments, parents may lose some of their authority due to their inability to effectively provide for their children. According to an advocate, "When parents are in a shelter they're not really the parent anymore. I think that is a tremendous challenge to have lost whatever authority or legitimacy as a caregiver for your child when you can no longer provide even a roof over their head and to have their very role be in question and by having to follow somebody else's rules."

Staffs in less positive shelter environments further undermine parents' authority as caregivers. As one researcher related,

> There is a tendency in at least some programs to try to influence parents' parenting right at the time they were doing it in front of their kids. So a staff member would correct the parent, confusing the kid—'Who's in charge and what's right here?'—humiliating the parent and setting up an opposition between the parent and the provider. Whereas had that same inter-action taken place privately later, the parent would've been much more likely to hear what the provider had to say.

This scenario exemplifies the close relationship between parents' loss of control and the uncomfortable reality of being constantly watched and evaluated. One advo-cate explained,

> There's a whole public aspect of whatever parenting they are doing, which they had done in the privacy of their home, is now done in a very public setting. I know there are a variety of shelters, some of which are more heavy-handed and force parents to take parenting skills as if the reason they're homeless is because they weren't good parents, to those that are more encouraging.

The formerly homeless mother also described the loss of privacy in shelter: "All the time, anything that you do. Once you come out of your room, someone's always watching you. If it's not the staff or the security guards, it's other residents. You're always being monitored by someone."

Conflicts Between Shelter Schedules and Family Routines

Operating shelters requires establishing set times for meals and supportive services, which can conflict with the type of structure parents would like to provide for their children. The formerly homeless mother offered an example: "If [your kids] were hungry in the middle of the night, you can't get up and just make them a meal. It was different for me because my son was older, so you eat when I eat and then we did snacks in-between. But I do know a lot of people who had babies, toddlers, and that was the hardest thing, not being able to just grab something quick." A researcher further explained, "It is very hard for parents to maintain these family routines and rituals. They have schedules to keep, they have mandated services that they have to go to, and they have to demonstrate to program staff that they are making efforts to improve their situation in various ways."

Difficulties coordinating family and shelter schedules were described by one pro-vider using the example of a single mother with a preschool and school-aged child:

> Families are very fluid, and a shelter system doesn't really allow for that. Kids have the best situation if they can go to child care on-site. But if they have to go to off-site, that requires sometimes parents getting up really early in the morning—4:30, 5, 5:30—to get their kid to child care so they can get to a job. The problem is then they have to leave the facility without having breakfast because there's only a certain window for mealtime. So often mom has to go get her preschool-aged child to day care, drags the school-aged child with her, and then goes off to do as she needs to do. Same thing's true for an afterschool program. Ideally we have afterschool programs in our facilities but then mom's up against difficult choices.

> Does she have her child go to the afterschool in school and then coordinate the logistics of picking up any other children? Or bring them back to the shelter? Again, mealtime is at the shelter, do you separate the child from their friends at school? There's a lot of pressures on that family, and it creates and adds layers of tension.

Children's development is best fostered with routine and set schedules, which shelter rules and programming can interrupt.

Although shelters are not ideal environments, some aspects of families' shelter stays are positive. According to the formerly homeless mother, the experience of hardship brought her and her son closer together. She also noted that she and her child each made two lifelong friends while in shelter. A formerly homeless child known by an advocate also forged friendships and actually achieved an important sense of stability while in shelter. According to the advocate, this child "didn't spend an entire year in school until she got into a shelter. That was the greatest stability she'd ever had in her life, was when she went into a shelter. Before that, it was moving, moving, moving. The first friend she ever had was when she went into a shelter." For some homeless families, shelters can be stabilizing environments, filling gaps and fulfilling needs that were unmet in their previous living situations and routines.

Parents Need Knowledge and Support to Advocate for Their Families

Despite the myriad challenges that homeless families face, parents have some opportunities to advocate for themselves, according to three providers, two advocates, two researchers, a policymaker, and the formerly homeless mother. Staff in an empowering shelter can arm parents with the knowledge necessary for them to flourish; however, case managers are often overworked and are therefore sometimes insensitive to the needs of their traumatized clients. Families must do their part in this relationship as well by demonstrating their efforts toward reaching self-sufficiency. Creating open and honest communication between parents and shelter staff, allowing parents to participate in setting their own goals and service plans, and establishing processes for parents to voice grievances are all necessary to best position families to attain housing stability.

If parents are unaware of their legal rights as homeless parents or afraid to exercise them, they are less likely to be able to advocate for improved conditions for themselves and their children, as a provider, an advocate, and a researcher all emphasized. As the advocate explained,

> So much of the ability to advocate for yourself depends on how you're made to feel and the access to information that you have. Particularly if there's that fear of 'If I break a rule, we're out again, and where will I go?' Shelters have to create an environment where parents are not dehumanized, where their role as parent is respected, and they are given information that will help them better advocate for themselves.

Shelter providers must not only make pertinent information readily accessible to parents but must also ensure that the shelter's policies do not infringe upon parents' rights. One example the advocate offered was a potential conflict in a child's right to participate in afterschool activities outside the shelter, despite shelter rules that may require all residents to attend mealtimes.

Mutual respect and open dialogue between parents and case managers are essential for parents to effectively advocate for themselves and their families. Challenges arise, however, from both sides. Parents, often traumatized and guarded around shelter staff, can be difficult to work with, and case managers are overworked. According to a researcher, "Most shelter staff are dealing with a lot of clients, they're doing triage rather than having the luxury of being able to spend huge amounts of time with every person, every family." This point was supported by a provider as well, who, along with an advocate and the formerly homeless parent, also related the difficulties of working with families who are already in crisis. The provider explained:

> A lot of times caseworkers forget that. They get upset because it feels like they have to say things over and over again, but [families are] in trauma and they're in emergency situations, so caseworkers need to know that they need to be told over and over again what to do and provide stability for their parents, saying to them 'you know I know you've got a lot of stress, but you need to spend some time with your kids, some quality time.'

The advocate added, "When so many systems have failed these parents for so long, how do you build trust?" and suggested that, as a consequence, parents often resort to "belligerent" behavior to have their needs met.

Ultimately, both sides must assume responsibility, explained a researcher:

> To the extent that parents show service providers that they're trying to work towards self-sufficiency and trying to be good parents and trying to cooperate, things tend to go better for them. But it is a two-way street and the service providers have a lot of the power, so to the extent that the service providers can also show the parents that they're ready to collaborate, both sides [are helped].

Two providers noted that parents are best equipped to advocate for their families when they play active roles in goal-setting and developing their own case plans. Motivational interviewing, which places the onus on the parent rather than the case manager to identify solutions, can be used to build trust with and engage homeless parents. One provider discussed how this technique empowers homeless families in practice:

> The first thing we talk to them about is 'Welcome. What are your short- and long-term goals for yourself and how can we help you get there? You can't live here, where is it you want to live and how can we help you to achieve that?' They're then forever advocating for what's best for them because they're setting the goals, they're driving their own case plan.

Holding structured group family meetings and establishing formal complaint systems can help give parents their own voice. A provider and an advocate emphasized the benefits of organizing group meetings for parents to discover and discuss their shared challenges. Another provider and a policymaker indicated that when parents and case managers cannot otherwise mediate conflict, having a formal grievance process—even one as simple as a "complaint box"—can strengthen parents' sense of self-sufficiency and help them in achieving their goals.

Doubled-Up

Thus far, this chapter has limited the definition of homelessness to families living in shelter. Some federal agencies, however, consider families living doubled-up with family or friends to also be homeless. While these regulatory discrepancies will be explored in greater detail later in this chapter, stakeholders emphasized that the various stresses of living doubled-up extend beyond the negative effects of short stays, multiple moves, and relationship violence.

All three providers and advocates as well as two researchers perceived doubled-up situations as far worse for family well-being. One provider described these conditions as "chaotic." An advocate explained that families living doubled-up feel like they cannot relax and are "walking on egg shells."

While families may face anxiety in shelter over the amount of time they may stay, three stakeholders noted that this fear is exacerbated in a doubled-up arrangement. According to a researcher,

> A shelter may be known as not being permanent, but if you go to a shelter you will have a certain amount of time. I think one of the biggest challenges of doubled-up situations is the most simple one—uncertainty and the reality that the situation could literally end at any time. Things could be going great and suddenly one day an incident occurs and the people you're staying with just inform you that you need to leave on a moment's notice.

Families living doubled-up may also be less likely to have access to basic necessities or supportive services. Describing doubled-up households, a provider observed, "It's like a lower level of a shelter where they're just not getting their needs met: food, school, clothes, all those needs." For example, an advocate posited that families may have a "fear of eating because you don't want to use up the resources that are being extended to you" and then be asked to leave. Another provider expressed concern that these families "don't know how to access the services without having a direct link to a case manager, someone who's inside the system and knows how to navigate proper channels to get the resources. They're outside the system, and therefore they're limited in the resources they can access to end their homelessness."

Parents may also face tensions with primary leaseholders, similar to those witnessed in shelters with staff, which inhibit their ability to parent effectively. "Often the leaseholder might conflict with the parent" over "disciplinary requirements or plans or processes," according to a researcher. An example provided was that the leaseholder may give the children dessert when the parent had already taken it away as a disciplinary measure. As the researcher stated, "Everybody criticizes everybody else's parenting," making doubled-up living environments particularly challenging.

In addition to undermining doubled-up parents' authority, leaseholders may require parents to provide services in exchange for a place to stay. For example, a parent may be "expected to take care of not only her kids, but also the kids of the person that she was living with," according to a researcher. Sometimes, a provider noted, more extreme cases occur: "We hear everything. Everything from prostitution rings to number-running to card dealing to all kinds of frauds, scams, stuff like that. Sometimes that's why people allow other people to come into their home—because it becomes extra labor."

Stress associated with unstable and uncomfortable living arrangements, lack of access to basic requirements and needed services, and limitations on parents' ability to independently care for their children all negatively impact child development, a point all stakeholders stressed. A provider explained, "There's just not a sense of stability … There's just that inconsistency of structure that children need so much. They seem to struggle a lot more … to be very tired, confused, and just out of sorts." Another provider stated, "I worry about the kids who are in those circumstances because the kids that are [in shelter] have 24/7 staff who are keeping eyes on them and making sure they're healthy and safe and fed and cared for, and the kids in doubled-up situations don't have that. A lot of the doubled-up children are even more vulnerable than those that we have in shelter."

Children Suffer

This analysis has primarily focused on the effects of homelessness on parents, their ability to care for their children, and barriers to resolving their housing instability. An important and significant by-product, however, is the negative impact on children, as emphasized by all three providers and advocates as well as a researcher and the formerly homeless parent. Shelters rightly focus their attention on resolving parents' barriers to self-sufficiency, but this sometimes results in the neglect of the children's needs that arise due to their homelessness.

The detrimental effects of shelter on children's well-being are centered around this lack of consideration of their needs, a view strongly held by two providers, two advocates, and a researcher. One advocate explained, "Children are not seen as clients in too many shelter settings. Because the parent is the reason that the family is homeless, it's almost like the kids are suitcases or appendages, something that come with the parent and are not seen as little human beings with their own set of needs and conditions." Shelters often lack a holistic approach to care that incorporates the needs of the entire family unit, which leaves children "invisible" and "the real victims of all of the funding issues, barrier issues, and lack-of-awareness issues, as they're the least able to advocate for themselves."

Children often do not have access to basic resources, such as places to play, explained an advocate and a researcher. The researcher elaborated,

> Shelters are not necessarily in the type of area that's right down the street from a great big beautiful park or other types of facilities where kids can go out and play. So in many shelter situations you're simply stuck keeping your kids in whatever room you have, you can't really let them go outside or do anything outside of the facilities. Keeping kids cooped up is a major challenge.

A provider and an advocate stressed the importance of increased access to high-quality early childhood development programs for younger children and afterschool programs for students that extend beyond educational enrichment to include cultural and recreational activities. School-aged children, as the provider related, require "more after school enrichment, and that doesn't just mean homework help; it means truly taking advantage of the educational and cultural experiences, as well as recreation and sports. Kids don't get a chance to be kids! And they need to."

Parents also often fail to adequately address their children's needs due to their own traumatic experiences of homelessness. One provider, for example, expressed frustration over parents' inability to utilize existing transportation arrangements for their children to regularly attend school:

> That's really frustrating for us […]. [We work so hard with the homeless liaisons to make sure that they have transportation,] but then that parent doesn't get them out of bed to go to the bus right in front of the shelter. We do track that and follow up, but we can't make them do it; they're adults in their own right. The kids suffer from the parents' inability to function.

Another provider was similarly concerned about children's poor school attendance rates, having frequently witnessed children in shelters during the school day.

The lack of attention to and resources for children who experience homelessness can contribute to adverse developmental outcomes. As one advocate explained, children "suffer" and become "feral" in these "unnatural environments," "just focused on the need to survive." The formerly homeless mother, who continues to provide services within a shelter, sees "depression" and "low self-esteem" among the children in shelter. A provider noted, "We have quite a few significant delays. We have behavioral issues. Their executive functioning is very low. They struggle in school. For the families that we're most worried about, we see recurrent patterns between the parents and the kids with delays, behavior, and mistrust of other people." These negative short-term consequences, as a provider and an advocate explained, can have detrimental long-term effects as well; these experiences can lead to intergenerational homelessness once homeless children reach adulthood.

Interrelated Challenges to Maintaining Stable Housing

Parents experiencing homelessness not only face personal barriers to meeting their families' needs but also encounter institutional and structural challenges. Some of these challenges are discussed in Chap. 1 of this volume. Independent, stable housing is the most essential ingredient to promote families' well-being, maintain healthy parenting practices, and foster positive child development. As one policymaker explained, "Housing stability is critical to school stability, is critical to family stability, is critical to a parent being able to get education and training and go back to work. We can't pretend that we can accomplish the other outcomes in these other systems if families don't have homes." Interviewees were asked to identify the other primary unmet needs of homeless parents and the barriers to meeting those needs. Three additional needs critical to homeless parents' self-sufficiency were named: child care, employment, and education. Eight key informants, covering all five groups of stakeholders, discussed the complex and interrelated challenges to gaining and maintaining access to these basic necessities, which are explored in turn below. In doing so, they stressed the importance of simultaneously balancing and preserving all three, as failing to secure or losing access to one can threaten access to the others.

Unemployed or underemployed homeless single parents cannot search for work and attend job interviews without others to care for their children. If they find employment, the low-wage jobs that these parents typically qualify for often have inflexible and unpredictable work schedules, causing a mismatch between set child care hours and employer expectations. Gaining access to employment that pays a living wage and offers more accommodating hours requires higher educational attainment than most homeless parents have. Parents cannot improve their employability and further their careers without access to child care and either stable low-wage jobs or income supports. Implicit in maintaining the delicate balance among child care, employment, and education lies yet another basic requirement: transportation. Without transportation, parents cannot get to and from work, skills-training sites, child care facilities, and their homes, whether in a shelter or an independent housing. This complex interplay was well summarized by one researcher:

> There's often a 'Catch-22' where you can't get child care until you have a job, but you can't very well get a job if you have your kids in tow when you go to the interview. And you need the job to decide where to live because you don't have a car and you're going to have to get there by public transportation. But until you have a job then you're not eligible for rental assistance because you have to establish an income... it goes on and on and on.

In many ways, access to child care is the first and most important need for families aside from their own housing. "Homelessness is highest among people who are less than 1 year of age, remains high through the preschool years, but not as high, and goes down a lot by the time the kids are ready for elementary school," explained a researcher. Gaining access to child care, according to the same researcher, a provider, and a policymaker, is essential for parents of young children to search for, secure, and maintain employment. The availability of child care, however, is often limited by capacity or funding constraints. For example, Head Start and Early Head Start, which offer high-quality early childhood development programming for low-income children and their families, are oversubscribed or under-resourced according to one provider and an advocate. Further complicating access are barriers inherent to their homelessness; the advocate said, "If you're homeless and you're mobile, you often can't meet the requirements or you go to the bottom of the waiting list."

Even when child care is available, homeless parents struggle to find employment. Four interviewees viewed homeless parents' low levels of educational attainment, a decrease in the availability of low-wage jobs, and high unemployment as factors that inhibit their success.

The majority of homeless parents arrive at shelter without a high school diploma or equivalent. "A lot of people come with 5th grade reading level," said one advocate. "Our high school system is just deplorable, like 40 % of kids don't graduate on time. That's the pool of kids that we get, that become homeless in a couple of years when they show up on our front door." The advocate attributed deficiencies in the public school system to a lack of accountability in spending for low-income students, insufficient tutoring and other supports, and high truancy.

The same advocate and a researcher also see a decline in the number of low-wage jobs available. This increases competition and places homeless parents at a disadvantage compared with their housed peers. "The unemployment rate is high and even when it's not, unemployment among minority groups is higher than among whites, among people who have not such a great education is higher than among college graduates, so the folks who become homeless are in a demographic group where unemployment is high," said the researcher.

If some families can secure child care and low-wage employment, homeless parents with young children often encounter difficulty maintaining both due to inflexible schedules. As a researcher expressed, homeless parents are

> getting the kinds of jobs that if you miss because your kid is sick and you have to take care of your sick child, you're likely to get fired. You don't get vacation and sick days. You may have shifts that change without being predictable. And so you have to stay late and then your child care provider quits on you because your job has made you late to pick up your kid and then you lose your job because then you have to take care of your kid. So that the nexus of low-wage work and child care is a huge problem.

These challenges cited by the researcher were confirmed by the formerly homeless parent who is now a mental-health professional in training.

> A lot of the concerns that I'm hearing now are trying to have child care and finding a job or having a job but trying to get back in enough time to pick the child up. I had one parent who said, 'There's no programs. I'm trying to save my money. I have a job. I'm making ten dollars an hour. But I can't get back at exactly six o'clock to get my kid.' Because her kids have special needs and they were acting out and really needed a one-to-one, they were eventually dismissed from the program. And now being dismissed, she had nobody to watch them after three o'clock. So she's resigned from her place of employment. If you're not working, you don't have money. You don't have money, you can't move out of the shelter. You have to choose your kids or your job. And you need your job to take care of your kids.

As the researcher summarized, "Different pieces of it keep falling out of alignment and trying to keep it all together is hard."

The difficulties of balancing low-wage work and child care are ameliorated with higher paying jobs. However, obtaining the education or skills training necessary to secure jobs that offer livable wages, flexibility to care for children, and benefits adds a third dimension to balance and maintain. For families employed in low-wage work, "There is definitely a challenge to getting people who are currently in low-wage jobs to take training programs. It's very, very difficult for people to work full-time, and to go to training, and to raise their families," said a policymaker. A "Catch-22" between child care and education exists even for unemployed parents, as "you can't bring your kids to the GED program. You have to have child care in order to take the GED that's going to allow you to set up for work to be eligible for child care," added an advocate.

When employment is not available or feasible, parents could access local benefit programs. Gaining access, however, can pose an additional structural paradox. The federal Temporary Assistance for Needy Families (TANF) program offers supplemental cash assistance to working parents as well as opportunities for employment training in lieu of work. The design of the program, however, serves as an obstacle for homeless parents to access job-skill training. The "barrier [to employment training] is that the TANF system does not fit our population," said one advocate. "The majority of moms are not on TANF, so therefore they are not eligible for the employment training that is there. Second part is, if they are on TANF, they are not getting any skill-based training that would qualify them for a job. They are getting 'resume 101' training. That system has totally failed."

A provider offered clarity on the types of knowledge required for homeless parents to find employment. "A lot of these parents can read; they just can't decode what things mean out in the world. We need to sort of embrace an educational agenda for these parents and give them the proper literacy skills to function in society, and that doesn't just mean being able to read a headline off a newspaper. It means really being able to function, quantitatively, qualitatively, in the world."

A provider, an advocate, and a researcher pointed out the transportation issues parents face as they struggle to access and maintain child care and low-wage work while seeking to improve their employability. Most homeless families cannot afford cars and must rely on public transit instead. For families living in shelter, insufficient access to transportation can be challenging; families must travel to child care, then to work, and then back again. Transportation becomes easier when child care is available through the shelter on-site. Therefore, homeless families need either "transportation or more services on-site," according to the provider, who favored the latter: "Just in bringing more services on-site instead of having the families go, and I know that might be codependent, but I think in some ways if we really want to serve them, we've got to provide the services on-site as much as possible, especially because of transportation."

Part II: Federal Policies That Have Positive and Negative Impacts on Families

Key informants were asked to discuss the implications, whether positive or problematic, of past or present federal policies for families experiencing homelessness. Many stakeholders offered multiple responses for one or both. Discussion of adverse policies ranged from more structural, macroeconomic effects to microlevel, implementation-related barriers and converged upon three primary themes. Four out of twelve interviewees, including two researchers, a policymaker, and an advocate, cited the history of policies that have perpetuated income inequality and limited the supply of affordable housing. All three advocates, along with three service providers and one researcher—seven stakeholders in total—agreed that recent homelessness policies have not afforded families the same amount of attention as chronically homeless individuals and veterans. Current bureaucratic rules and regulations that act as barriers to effectively serving families were cited by three interviewees (researcher, service provider, and advocate).

Perhaps the strongest statement, however, was that two advocates and a policy-maker did not name a single federal policy that benefitted homeless parents and their children. Other responses addressed both broader and homelessness-specific policies. A researcher and policymaker together accounted for three positive, pre-ventative legislative achievements: the Earned Income Tax Credit, the Homelessness Prevention and Rapid Re-housing Program, and the Affordable Care Act. A researcher, a policymaker, and a service provider favored the US Department of Housing and Urban Development's (HUD) forthcoming requirement to improve the efficiency of the homelessness services system by establishing a single point of entry for families to access needed services. Lastly, three service providers and an advocate described the benefits of the comprehensive umbrella of care for school-aged homeless students under the US Department of Education. Offering a unifying source of hope for the future of family homelessness assistance, two of these same key informants warned of the social and fiscal costs of not improving services for homeless families; neglecting to invest in the education of homeless children today will result in higher future costs to serve them when they are homeless adults.

Negative Impacts: Policies That Perpetuate Income Inequality

Setting the nation on a course to end family homelessness will require correcting harmful federal policies from the past and present. Many more families today are unable to secure housing that is considered affordable, leaving them vulnerable to homelessness. While adverse federal policies have resulted in more families with extremely low incomes or those who earn less than 30 % of their area median income, construction of affordable housing has not kept pace with the demand. One advocate noted that some areas around the nation have even experienced a loss of affordable housing, or units for which families contribute less than 30 % of their income toward rent and utilities. According to a researcher, "When you have roughly nine million households with very low incomes who are paying more than 50 % of their income on housing costs, it places them all in a very precarious position, and a certain percentage of them are going to become homeless every year."

To compensate for declining incomes and a lack of affordable housing, the fed-eral government offers rental assistance to income-eligible families. One researcher viewed this as the best federal family homelessness policy but noted that it is limited in scope: "There's a lot of research out there showing that federal rental assistance is highly effective at reducing housing instability and homelessness amongst fami-lies, in particular families with kids. On the other hand, since federal rental assis-tance is not an entitlement and we're assisting only about one in four eligible families, the need for assistance far outstrips the available resources."

While discretionary spending will likely continue to be limited in the foreseeable future, threatening both the prospect of expanding rental assistance and maintaining current levels, one researcher saw potential reforms to the tax code as an opportunity to make tax policies more balanced toward low-income renters. Current federal housing policies disproportionally support and promote homeowner rather than renter households. Roughly one-third of households are renters, who as a group receive only approximately one-quarter of federal housing assistance. Federal policies also favor homeowners with higher incomes; about three-quarters of homeowner tax benefits are accrued by families with annual incomes greater than $100,000. As the researcher explained, "Most of what we get from the mortgage interest deduction for instance is enabling higher-income households to purchase slightly more expensive houses, rather than really turning [lower-income households] into homeowners from renters, which is what the goal ought to be." The researcher suggested channeling some of the $100 billion annually spent on property tax, mortgage, and interest deductions to new low-income renter tax credits as one option to make housing affordable for more low-income families.

Negative Impacts: Homeless Families Are Not Policy Priorities

Seven of twelve key informants perceive that federal homelessness policy and fiscal resources have focused on eliminating chronic homelessness (experienced by an adult, who, as defined by HUD, has "been continuously homeless for a year or more or has experienced at least four episodes of homelessness in the last 3 years and has a disability") and veteran homelessness. Consequently, homeless parents and their children have not received the same level of attention or fiscal support. One service provider remarked, "The problem with federal policy is that it's so focused on individuals. I hate as a family provider being pitted against my colleagues who work on the individual side. Singles have always gotten a lot of focus, as they should, but not at the expense of children and families."

The national strategy calls for the end of chronic and veteran homelessness by 2015, with family homelessness to be resolved 5 years later. According to an advocate, prioritizing chronic and veteran homelessness and delaying assistance to families for 5 years miss a critical point: that the child becomes the adult. "It's not like there are a set number of chronically homeless people and once you get them into permanent housing, poof, they're gone." A provider also noted,

> Not every child is condemned to this life of poverty and perpetuating these cycles that they were born into. But the probability that you'll have more kids growing up with this kind of poverty-driven chaos is much higher. I think that we're only cutting off our nose to spite our face. We're foregoing an expenditure and policy priority today in order to have to at some point in the future confront even a harder, more expensive reality.

Stakeholders say that further evidence of the lack of emphasis on families is apparent in how the federal government chooses to spend its money. Over the years, HUD has provided bonus dollars to communities that show that they are implementing innovative strategies to reduce the number of chronically homeless adults. Separate programs have been created specifically for homeless veterans.

Such monies have not been allocated for homeless parents and their children until recently, with grants to be administered in 2013 including families in the definition of chronically homeless. As one researcher commented,

> There's just never been a point where they've stepped down and said, 'We have this extra money for communities that are doing great things to help families.' And if you can't show that you're doing it, you're not going to get the extra money. At the end of the day, financial incentives, especially in tight financial times... give the clearest impression of what federal agencies want you to do. Follow the money, I think, is lesson number one. Even if the rhetoric is 'Hey, families are important,' but the story when the money is getting handed out is that it's more important to help chronically homeless, then that's what people do.

With dedicated federal resources absent and community attention turned toward individuals, providers struggle to find alternative sources of funding for families. In part because chronic and veteran singles are often visible on the streets, while families are less likely to be unsheltered, providers find it challenging to raise community awareness for families.

Due to the success of "rapid re-housing" in reducing chronic and veteran homelessness, the entire homelessness services system is being converted to this model to the detriment of some families. Rather than employing the old system of longer shelter stays to treat the multifaceted causes that led to an adult's homelessness, rapid re-housing quickly moves individuals into permanent housing. However, key informants caution against the wholesale prescription of this strategy for families without considering their differing needs. One provider remarked,

> To base your kind of federal approach by saying the singular best thing you can do for a family is to put them in their own house, regardless of circumstance, is benefitting some and harming others. Why? Because there's nothing really wrong with having your own place, but if you only get your own place to lose it again and to destabilize again, you're just perpetuating a bad cycle that these families are in. ... I think you need a system that triages [assigns degrees of service need to] families and a federal recognition that one size does not fit all. There are those families who can move into housing very, very quickly. Others stay out a year, maybe two, and then return for a long stay. Some of them just return and return and return.

Rapid re-housing is an example of policies that may be well intentioned but can hurt families in the long term.

Negative Impacts: Homelessness Regulations

In addition to the conspicuous absence of homeless families from aspects of macrolevel federal policy, interviewees also identified bureaucratic impediments to serving these vulnerable populations. Foremost among them is the lack of a single federal definition of homelessness. Four programs that assist homeless families and their children, governed by four separate pieces of legislation, include living doubled-up with family or friends and in hotels or motels in their definitions of homelessness. The Education for Homeless Children and Youth program (under the McKinney–Vento Homeless Assistance Act), the Runaway and Homeless Youth Act, the Individuals with Disabilities Education Act, and the Head Start Act all recognize that these housing situations also have devastating negative effects on child development that are akin to, or worse than, as previous testimony underscored, living in shelters. These cohesive definitions are at odds with those of HUD, the agency that operates the largest homelessness programs, which restricts the definition of homelessness, with some exceptions, to living in shelter or "in places not meant for human habitation, such as the streets, campgrounds, abandoned buildings, vehicles, or parks." Providers who work with clients served by both of these definitions note that absence of a single definition hinders collaboration across governmental systems, and they are left struggling to effectively coordinate care. "I think it's just a bureaucratic nightmare that we have our public schools trying to deal with a whole set of families who are homeless and helping their kids get into school and stay in school, but our nation's housing agency doesn't think seventy-five percent of those kids are homeless," added a researcher. Bills to unify these definitions of homelessness were introduced in the 111th and 112th Congressional sessions but failed to receive support.

Other HUD regulations are perceived as being insensitive to the needs of parents and their children and as inhibiting service delivery. For example, in order to receive some forms of housing assistance, families must prove that they are homeless. This requires obtaining documentation, such as proof of eviction or loss of a doubled-up housing situation, which one advocate said can be difficult and can therefore delay the delivery of needed services. In addition, local Public Housing Authorities (PHA) who distribute long-term rental assistance from HUD have discretion to set admission and termination policies. Although HUD's rules for lifetime bans from assistance are limited, many PHAs regulate admission of ex-offenders based on additional criteria. The advocate praised a 2011 letter from HUD's Secretary Shaun Donovan urging PHAs to work with ex-offenders. However, many PHAs have not implemented the recommendation, and the key informant argued that the content of the letter should be codified into law to ensure compliance.

Positive Impacts: Legislative Measures

Interviewees cited three legislative measures as successfully preventing families from losing their homes and experiencing the negative effects of homelessness. The Earned Income Tax Credit, according to one researcher, helps to keep low-income families with employment income stable through cash tax refunds. The credit incentivizes families to work and is not time limited. Another researcher agreed that the credit is an extremely important tool to reduce poverty but said it is less than ideally conceptualized. The credit is annually claimed and distributed as one lump sum, which can pose challenges to budgeting for monthly rental payments. The interviewee would like the credit to be converted into a form that alleviates this stress on families and extended to cover more families with extremely low incomes.

A policymaker offered two more recent legislative measures that prevent family homelessness. The Homelessness Prevention and Rapid Re-housing Program, part of the American Recovery and Reinvestment Act of 2009 stimulus package, may have contributed to preventing a surge in family homelessness from the recent economic recession. The $1.5 billion program, which ended in 2012, offered financial assistance to keep precariously housed families in their homes and rapidly re-housed those who became homeless. Prevention and rapid re-housing have since been added as eligible activities to the new Emergency Solutions Grants Program (formerly the Emergency Shelter Grants Program, the main source of funding for emergency shelters).

The same policymaker also saw enormous potential for the Affordable Care Act to assist those families in which a health condition contributes to financial insecurity. The act will provide low-income families with greater access to affordable health insurance, which will also improve the health of parents and their children through preventative care.

Positive Impacts: Coordinated Intake

In addition to positive prevention policies, one researcher applauded HUD for forthcoming regulations requiring communities who receive federal homelessness funding to create coordinated intake assessment systems. A policymaker and a provider agreed that the change could more effectively and efficiently meet families' needs. Rather than compelling families to contact multiple shelters to find placement, this new system would establish a central point of contact for families seeking assistance. As the policymaker argued,

> If you think about the stress that occurs within that family unit and the stress that's happening between the parent and the child, within the child, within the parent, and between the parent and the system, if we can reduce that to one phone call as opposed to some documented cases where people had made 28 phone calls, that's a step in the right direction.

Coordinated assessment and intake will also allow communities to better evaluate and track families to reduce periods of housing instability. The provider bemoaned, "We see a lot of families that go from one shelter when their time runs out, to another shelter, another shelter and another shelter," which impairs parent and child well-being.

Positive Impacts: Education of Homeless Children and Youth

The educational component of the McKinney–Vento Homeless Assistance Act (McKinney–Vento), the EHCY Program, was cited by most interviewees (three service providers and one advocate) as the most positive federal measure in assisting homeless families. The law guarantees that all homeless students have equal access to education as their housed peers. Through the mandatory designation of a homeless school liaison in every school district to work with every school nation-wide, the legislation reduces school enrollment barriers, enforces outreach, and provides a wide range of additional services to homeless students, from housing to school uniforms. The advocate observed, "I think that McKinney-Vento, through the designation of a liaison to work with community agencies, has truly ended and prevented more homelessness than any other federal policy or program." By placing a homeless liaison in every school district, McKinney–Vento establishes a universal social safety net for homeless students. Not every area of the country has a shelter, and even when shelters are available, the level of nurturing care for children varies widely, as discussed earlier. However, every community has a public school where homeless children can be connected to services.

Furthermore, McKinney–Vento is one of the four pieces of federal legislation that includes precariously housed families in the definition of homelessness. According to one provider, this has significant implications for children and their parents: "The fact that the Department of Education has always had a much more broad definition for who they consider homeless certainly catches children earlier than a policy that defines it simply as living in shelter, and so there's fewer educational setbacks and there's less stresses on that family the sooner they can get some help."

Guaranteeing the educational rights of homeless students also helps to reduce disruptions to their schooling. Homelessness often necessitates frequent moves, to and from a shelter or doubled-up situation, for example, which can take a family outside the child's school district. McKinney–Vento gives students the right to remain in their original schools, regardless of districts to which they move, and receive transportation. This provides students with a sense of stability and helps to avoid additional education setbacks.

Despite the numerous benefits of EHCY, this effort remains severely under-funded. Only roughly $65 million is appropriated annually for the program. Because of the lack of funding, not all school districts receive monies and those that do often cannot afford dedicated staff to oversee the needs of homeless students full time. The only other limitation identified by stakeholders is that children who are not yet school aged are not eligible for assistance.

Conclusions

Key informants have provided a range of viewpoints regarding the many detrimental aspects of homelessness for parent and child well-being, both leading up to and during their experiences in shelter. The less time families are homeless and the sooner they can return to stable housing, the less they will experience these negative outcomes. However, the majority of stakeholders criticized the federal government for implementing a rapid re-housing approach. They fear that without the proper supports, families will return to homelessness. Therein lies a critical paradox; while long shelter stays adversely impact family well-being, additional episodes of homelessness experienced by families ill-prepared for stable housing are also detrimental. As a policymaker explained, "One of the tensions that we sometimes get into is that we want these shelters to be short stays. Yet there is an understandable pull to have these shelters be full-service daycare and family support systems, and that those two good instincts can be in tension."

Part of what fuels this debate is that no one really knows what happens to families if they are quickly moved into permanent housing. The policymaker stated,

> We don't know what is happening with a broad set of outcomes for a family besides not returning to shelter, and what's happening in terms of housing stability versus continued mobility for families when a rapid re-housing intervention occurs. The whole question of how the whole family assessment is occurring and then how we are connecting the family as part of short-term assistance back into larger mainstream systems, which should be able to continue that support after the homelessness is abated. I think those are all big questions.

This lack of information about what happens to families serves to support the belief among the majority of stakeholders that families are absent from the national conversation on how to end homelessness. The gaps in knowledge may be filled as the federal government turns its attention to ending family homelessness by 2020. In thinking about families, the policymaker noted,

> There are still more questions than there are answers. The good news is, there are some emerging ideas about a different way to think about the problem. And thinking about the problem in a different way might get us to a different result ... We need to augment that conversation with better data and more research so that we can figure out how to direct the resources that we have in the way that we can help the most families.

Index

M.E. Haskett et al. (eds.), *Supporting Families Experiencing Homelessness:*
Current Practices and Future Directions, DOI 10.1007/978-1-4614-8718-0,
© Springer Science+Business Media New York 2014